Clinical Challenges in Orthopaedics

The Hip

By

Martin D. Northmore-Ball MA MB BChir FRCS CIMechE

Honorary Consultant Orthopaedic Surgeon
The Robert Jones and Agnes Hunt Orthopaedic Hospital,
Oswestry, Shropshire, and Senior Clinical Lecturer, University of Keele, Staffordshire, UK

Gordon C. Bannister MD MCh Orth FRCS FRCS(Ed) FRCS(EdOrth)

Consultant Orthopaedic Surgeon, Southmead Hospital,
Westbury-on-Trym, and Senior Lecturer, University of Bristol, Avon, UK

Dana C. Mears BM,BCh PhD MRCP(UK) FACS FRCS(C)

Research Fellow, Johns Hopkins Bayview Medical Center, Baltimore, MD, USA

and

Sridhar M. Durbhakula, MD

Research Fellow, Division of Orthopedic Surgery, The Albany Medical College, Albany, NY, USA

With contributions from

Brian Bradnock BSc FRCS(Ed) FRCS(Orth)

Consultant Orthopaedic Surgeon, St Albans City Hospital, St Albans, UK

and

Guy Slowik MD

Orthopedic Research Fellow, Division of Orthopedic Surgery, The Albany Medical College, Albany, NY, USA

Martin Dunitz

First published in the United Kingdom in 2002
by Martin Dunitz Ltd, The Livery House, 7–9 Pratt Street, London NW1 0AE

Tel.: +44 (0) 20 74822202
Fax. +44 (0) 20 72670159
E-mail: info@dunitz.co.uk
Website: http://www.dunitz.co.uk

A CIP record for this book is available from the British Library.

ISBN 1-899066-83-7

Distributed in the USA by
Fulfilment Center
Taylor & Francis
7625 Empire Drive
Florence, KY 41042, USA
Toll Free Tel.: +1 800 634 7064
E-mail: cserve@routledge_ny.com

Distributed in Canada by
Taylor & Francis
74 Rolark Drive
Scarborough, Ontario M1R 4G2, Canada
Toll Free Tel.: +1 877 226 2237
E-mail: tal_fran@istar.ca

Distributed in the rest of the world by
ITPS Limited
Cheriton House
North Way
Andover, Hampshire SP10 5BE, UK
Tel.: +44 (0)1264 332424
E-mail: reception@itps.co.uk

Typesetting and image reproduction by Color Gallery, Malaysia
Printed and bound in Singapore by Kyodo Printing Co (S'pore) Pte Ltd

Contents

Acknowledgements

Martin Northmore-Ball had intended to acknowledge a number of people who had helped him with details in his chapters, but realized later that he had such a debt to numerous colleagues who have taught him so much over many years, and who could not be individually acknowledged, that he has had to forego this. He hopes they will accept this apology. He would like, however, to acknowledge the assistance of Miss Marie Carter, Librarian, Francis Costello Library, Institute of Orthopaedics, at The Robert Jones & Agnes Hunt Orthopaedic Hospital, Oswestry, and to thank his hard-pressed secretaries, Mrs Erica Hughes and Mrs Margaret Peach.

Dana Mears is grateful to acknowledge the assistance of his recent orthopaedic Fellows, Drs Sridhar Durbkhakula and John Velyvis, along with that of his secretary, Mrs Karen DiVirgilio.

Introduction

When one of us was approached about the preparation of this book, the objective was to concentrate on specific topics in reconstructive surgery of the hip where currently no one view is definitely correct. Later, as we began to list all these various areas, it became apparent that we needed to cover the whole subject. It was like being asked to pick out and describe the higher peaks in a mountain area. Eventually, there seemed to be so many peaks that it seemed best to describe the valleys as well. Nevertheless, we have tried to concentrate on the more contentious points.

The book has been almost entirely written by the three of us, and we hoped that not being a true multi-author text, the coverage is uniform and less subject to contradications between one part of the book and another. Nevertheless, we appreciate that there are some inevitable differences between our individual points of view, and we hope that the readers will understand this.

Variability will be found in emphasis in the book between some parts that are heavily referenced and others that are much more related to our own clinical and surgical techniques. The book, however, was originally conceived to give practical advice in clinical and operative situations, rather than as a guide to passing examinations. It seemed best to leave this variability rather than to try to add references where the main themes were based on our practical experience.

For us as authors, writing the book has necessitated a critical review of our own surgical indications and methods, and we very much hope that our readers will find that they can obtain guidance on diverse afflictions of the hip where currently suitable advice may not be immediately at hand.

MARTIN NORTHMORE-BALL
GORDON BANNISTER
DANA MEARS

SECTION I
The young adult hip

CHAPTER 1

The young adult: factors underlying choice of treatment

M. D. Northmore-Ball

The term 'young adult', in the context of hip surgery, is by no means a hard-and-fast one. Clearly, a 35-year-old patient with secondary osteoarthritis from a slipped epiphysis is a 'young adult', but the upper and lower limits are less clear. In this chapter, the lower limit is assumed to be the age of complete skeletal growth and, therefore, lies in the late teens. Although hips that are older than this still have a capacity for remodelling, this remodelling is of a subtle nature and quite distinct from the major changes of shape allowed by growth. The latter are in the province of the paediatric orthopaedic surgeon. The upper limit is even more vague. In this chapter, it is simply taken as the age below which the reader feels uncomfortable about carrying out his or her standard form of total hip replacement – usually about 50.

The disabilities and underlying hip pathology in this disparate group vary – from patients with extremely slight, almost absent, symptoms and hips that have only the most subtle of structural abnormalities to extremely severely disabled patients with gross hip disorganization.

The types of treatment considered range from none or minimally invasive measures to total hip replacement (and, indeed, revision hip replacement). Many patients referred for consideration of surgery, particularly if referred by general practitioners, prove, after assessment, to be inappropriate for any form of surgical treatment, at least without a significant period of initial non-surgical management. When surgery does appear to be appropriate, in general the younger patients require less radical measures, and older patients are more likely to require a total replacement. This is, however, an extremely poor correlation and a patient of 45 might be a candidate only for an arthroscopy, whereas a patient of

19 or less might, in some circumstances, be treatable only by total replacement.

This chapter reviews these two spectra of disability/hip pathology and treatment, and makes some statements about relating the two. Clearly, any proposals made can only be tentative and hedged about with reservations. As in some other fields, the subject does not have a solid base. New, apparently promising forms of treatment have been recommended and used, sometimes on quite a large scale, and have then proved disastrous; these failures, viewed retrospectively, have sometimes proved predictable, but this has not always been the case. If possible, the repetition of such mistakes clearly needs to be avoided. Nevertheless, if only those forms of treatment (such as a cemented total hip replacement) are used that, although having finite limitations, are to a very large extent predictable in the long term (i.e. 10–20 years), not only would the subject advance slowly, but numerous people would unnecessarily be subjected to the internal amputation and significant surrounding damage of total hip replacement, with the attendant high risk of serious disability late in life.

It has been suggested that newer, and possibly better, methods of treatment, particularly in terms of replacement, should first be used on elderly people, using more tried methods for younger people. Although this has some merit, unfortunately problems tend to occur in younger people, whilst a perfectly good solution is available for elderly people. It is, therefore, morally difficult to justify not allowing the second group to have the well-tried treatment. There are also those who enlarge and widen the indications for total hip replacement enormously, almost to the exclusion of other possibilities, on the basis that new techniques in revision surgery have stopped replacement being a 'one-way street', thus allowing several revisions to be carried out over the years with an expectation of satisfactory function on each occasion. Again this is an understandable view, but the necessary long-term data are not yet available; nor does it seem likely that revision could ever be so straightforward as to justify this approach as a general policy.

There is no dispute, however, that bone-conserving operations are, in principle, highly desirable. However, it must constantly be borne in mind that failure of an apparently conservative procedure can lead to early conversion to a very much more destructive operation than would have been the case had a less conservative (but effective) procedure been selected initially.

The following types of treatment are ranked, for convenience, in an order from very conservative to least conservative:

1. Arthroscopy
2. Osteotomy:
   (a) pelvic/acetabular
   (b) femoral
3. Arthrodesis
4. Resurfacing
5. Bipolar replacement
6. Total replacement.

One way of selecting the most conservative form of treatment that is likely to produce adequate and sufficiently long-lasting symptomatic relief in a given patient is discussed below. When an arthritic hip in a young adult is presented at a clinical conference, numerous different possibilities are usually suggested. A logical sequence of thought is needed to decide what to do in a given situation.

Initial outpatient assessment

The patient is first assessed in the ordinary way according to age, sex, and nature, duration, and severity of symptoms. A clinical examination is then done and standard radiographs taken. Usually, there is a clear idea of what can best be achieved at this stage, although, in a number of circumstances, further special tests are required.

Pain is the most common complaint; as with any other patient who has pain believed to come from the hip, it is essential, especially if surgery is contemplated,

to be as certain as possible that the pain does indeed come from the hip. This may not be obvious. There may, for example, be coexistent dysplasia and spondylolysis, and some forms of epiphyseal dysplasia may affect both the hip and the spine. Pain radiating into the groin or down to the knee is likely to come from the hip, but referred pain from the lumbar spine is also likely, especially if there is some backache. A careful analysis is therefore necessary. In cases of doubt, the opinion of a specialist spinal surgeon and a diagnostic injection of bupivacaine (Marcain) into the hip at limited arthrography must be requested. Such diagnostic injections frequently give a clear-cut and correct answer, although they may be equivocal or, at times, frankly misleading, especially if the patient misunderstands the reason for the injection. Occasionally, for example, a patient may think that the injection was supposed to be curative and will say later that it did not give pain relief; on enquiry, he or she may, however, recall that there was a transient improvement in the symptoms. The test is, however, the best that can be done.

The assessment may also be complicated by emotional factors. A young woman patient's parents may, for example, be heavily involved; in addition, the manifest uncertainty about what can or should be done to the patient's hip, perhaps associated with earlier opinion(s), may well have been communicated. Young patients with hip symptoms must, however, be allowed some measure of anxiety and, possibly, a feeling of resentment that they are unable to do those things that their friends can usually do.

For the correct navigation through these difficulties, an algorithm is necessary – the following sequence, in which patients are placed in specific groups, can be used.

Group A

Patients in this group, which is quite a problematical one, have mobile hips that are radiologically completely normal.

Assuming that it is clear or has been demonstrated that the symptoms come from the hip (and that any possibility of a localized form ['monopoly'] of an inflammatory polyarthropathy has been excluded), the possible diagnoses are: (1) labral tears and areas of true chondromalacia – for example, of the femoral head, loose bodies and other miscellaneous intra-articular causes; (2) one of the group of extra-articular causes (the 'snapping hip'), of which the most well-known variety is snapping from the iliotibial band; and (3) stage I avascular necrosis (AVN).

Labral tears and areas of true chondromalacia

These patients are seldom objectively disabled, except to quite a minor degree and, as with anterior knee pain, the symptoms may be out of proportion to any pathology present. Unfortunately, there is no complete uniformity in the nature of pain that is correctly ascribed to a labral tear. This may simply reflect the different shapes of tear possible. Thus, in the knee, a flap tear of the posterior third of the medial meniscus may produce a well-localized catching sensation, but it could also simply produce aching; the correct association between these symptoms and the pathology is seen in the reliable results of arthroscopic partial meniscectomy. At present, there is insufficient evidence about the labrum. Flaps, radial tears, and longitudinal tears, occurring in the meniscus, have certainly been shown to exist. A catching or locking sensation, sometimes with a giving-way, clearly suggests some well-localized problem, such as a flap tear of the labrum or a chondral flap, or some object getting caught, such as a very small (radiolucent) loose body.

Aching after activity might be caused by a labral tear or some surface abnormality in the articular cartilage. Clinical examination may be completely normal; unfortunately, as with the symptoms, there is no complete uniformity of opinion about the physical signs truly associated with a labral tear. Once again, this results partly from the different types and localization of the tear, such that it is pressed on, or tugs against, the synovium, in different positions of the hip; there is, however, a second source of unavoidable confusion resulting from the fact that labral tears may result from localized superolateral or anterosuperolateral overload in the earlier stages of degenerative change secondary to acetabular dysplasia.

Thus, groin pain in flexion and internal rotation may be produced by a labral tear (a positive 'impingement' sign), although pain on external rotation in extension or attempted hyperextension may be produced because the hip is starting to sublux anteriorly, rather than from pressure on the secondarily degenerated labrum in this area. However, it is the localized labral tear in the prescence of the normal hip which would best be treated, if possible by arthroscopic surgery, whereas to treat the latter situation in this way, even with improvement in

the symptoms, might simply result in acceleration of degenerative change due to the underlying structural abnormality of the hip. An attempt to identify and define labral tears properly using special investigations is difficult and, even in very skilled hands, may not give a definite result. Magnetic resonance imaging (MRI) arthrography appears, currently, to be the most promising technique.

This group of patients has a clear indication for arthroscopy.

The 'snapping hip'

At least seven causes for this symptom have been described. The most readily recognizable cause is that produced by the iliotibial band snapping backwards and forwards over the greater trochanter. The patient, invariably a young woman, quite often wrongly reports that the hip 'keeps coming out of joint'.

The diagnosis is very simply made by getting the patient to reproduce the snap – and this should be easily visible and palpable. In the great majority of cases, nothing more than an explanation is required. In those rare instances where the snapping is extremely frequent and pain is a genuine problem (as opposed to the snap being a party trick) – when the pain presumably results from secondary trochanteric bursitis – surgical treatment is needed. Of the different methods available, there has been some success with Z-plasty of the iliotibial band, as described by Brignall and Stainsby [1]. The technique has to be followed exactly, the Z being very carefully marked out on the fascia lata at and above the greater trochanter.

The other varieties of snapping hip are very difficult to pin down. A clunk at about 30° of flexion, when the hip is being extended from the flexed position with the patient supine, is suggestive of the variety resulting from the psoas tendon jumping over the iliopectineal eminence, although usually the diagnosis is likely to be one of exclusion. It is, in any case, surprising how often a completely asymptomatic click is audible from the hip when a patient's knee is examined for another reason; most patients can be adequately reassured that the problem is not of any consequence.

Avascular necrosis

The history here is of pain of insidious onset with or without a potential cause for AVN, as alluded to above. Examination and plain radiographs are completely normal, and the diagnosis is made by an MRI scan. The question then arises of whether the patient should be treated by core decompression. The procedure is quite often suggested, and is relatively straightforward; it may, therefore, appear tempting. Nevertheless, although large numbers of papers have been written on the subject, its indications still appear uncertain, and there is the very real risk of irrecoverable damage to a femoral head that, if it had been left to itself, would have recovered fully. The object of core decompression is to prevent later femoral head collapse. The likelihood of collapse seems, however, to depend at least as much on the size of the avascular segment as on the method of treatment; with less than 30% head involvement, Koo and Kim [2] found that no heads collapsed, whereas with more than 40% head involvement all collapsed. Others have found a much lower threshold.

The best results for core decompression have, not surprisingly, been seen with involvement of small volumes; as his indication for this method, Steinberg [3] cites the younger patient with no poor medical prognostic features, minimal symptoms and physical findings, and head involvement of less than 15%. However, such heads are also probably those that have the best chance of spontaneous recovery. Improvement without treatment has been seen by Sakamoto *et al.* [4] in no less than 45%. Markell *et al.* [5] were successful with core decompression in only 35% of patients in their series; in general, therefore, it seems better to wait. If symptoms continue and changes start to go into stage II, the patient may become a possible candidate for an osteotomy, as discussed below.

Group B

In this group, a clear radiographic abnormality in the hip is present. Certain patients are possible candidates for an osteotomy of some kind. The following are the main subdivisions in this group.

Hip with acetabular dysplasia

The hip has obvious acetabular dysplasia (Fig. 1.1a). The patient is quite young, usually under 30. Occasionally, there is a history of 'clicking' as a neonate, but usually the past history is completely negative and the symptoms are of insidious onset. There is some aching after activity and no other symptoms – initially this aching is extremely slight, but it very slowly increases.

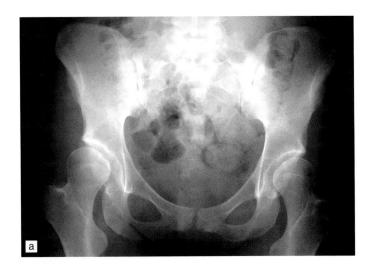

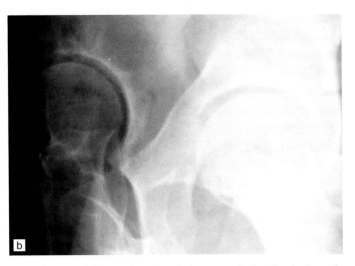

Figure 1.1 – *(a) Hip showing obvious acetabular dysplasia with sloping sourcil and low CE angle. (b) 'Faux profile' view, showing a very low VCE angle, with a cyst resulting from overload anteriorly. The femoral head is, in fact, round, the anterior appearance being a radiographic artefact.*

Examination shows a completely fit young (usually) woman with a hip of normal mobility or with some hypermobility. A pelvic radiograph shows a sloping acetabular roof with a normal or almost normal femur. A 'faux profile' view [6] (Fig. 1.1b) shows much reduced anterior coverage. Such a patient is potentially a candidate for a periacetabular osteotomy (PAO). This can produce good symptomatic relief in about 80% of patients for 10 years.

Unlike some osteotomies (e.g. an upper tibial osteotomy for the varus knee), a PAO attacks the root cause of the hip problem; in favourable circumstances, rather than simply postponing the need for a total hip replacement, it has the theoretical potential to abolish the need for such a replacement altogether. It is, therefore, appropriate to consider it even when symptoms are quite slight. In a child's hip, the concept of operating in the absence of symptoms, in order to produce a better future hip, is easy to accept, and this remains the case up until almost the end of growth. By extension, although, in the complete absence of symptoms, there would never be any question of a restorative osteotomy in the adult, such an osteotomy can be carried out when symptoms are mild. A PAO is, however, an operation of considerable magnitude. The earliest form of hip symptom occurs when the patient gradually realizes either that certain activities, which she (usually) was formerly able to do, become subtly restricted, or that she has simply stopped these activities, without being truly aware that this was the result of a hip problem. Although this may be an indication for surgery in a younger patient (e.g. in their early teens) in whom an obvious structural hip abnormality is present, in an adult it is necessary to consider a PAO only when a greater disability is present – one that is sufficient for the patient to feel that something needs to be done.

In the physical examination, a specific requirement is a sufficient degree of abduction to allow the equivalent degree of acetabular reorientation. The osteotomy will almost certainly imply flexion as well as abduction and, therefore, the patient's hip needs to be able to abduct to this degree in a position of some flexion. This is usually clinically obvious on outpatient examination, supplemented if necessary by a plain radiograph in abduction, although occasionally radiographic examination under an anaesthetic is needed. This procedure, which has other indications, is discussed further below. A PAO may still have a very good indication, even if the superolateral apparent joint space is reduced (Fig. 1.2). This appearance may simply be the result of early anterior subluxation of the head from under the anterosuperior acetabular lip. The subluxation is also clearly shown by the 'faux profile' view. In such cases, abduction on an awake patient in the outpatient department is sometimes limited and a film under anaesthetic, referred to above, may be needed. If the leg abducts and the hip reduces concentrically under anaesthetic, then a PAO will still be successful.

The narrowing of the anterolateral apparent joint space may also be caused by true thinning of the articular cartilage as a result of early osteoarthritis. In

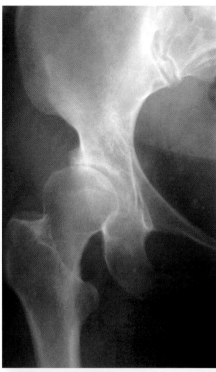

Figure 1.2 – *Marked reduction in superolateral 'joint space' resulting largely from anterior subluxation, and later completely reversed after periacetabular osteotomy.*

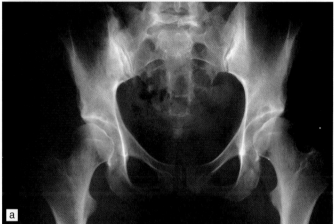

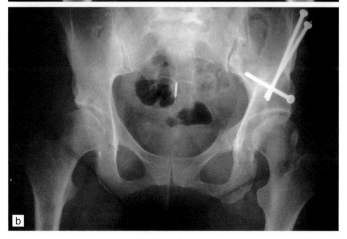

Figure 1.3 – *(a) Reversal of secondary overload changes (cyst) in left hip after periacetabular osteotomy (PAO). (b) Three-year film showing the appearance of an overload cyst on the right; the patient was listed for a right PAO.*

this case, there may be some sclerosis and small cysts in either the acetabulum or the femoral head. Provided that it is clear that the overload is the result of the inappropriately directed socket and that the hip abducts sufficiently, there is still a good indication for a PAO; but the patient must realize that the result is not as certain. Figure 1.3 demonstrates the disappearance of an overload cyst after a PAO.

A PAO is technically possible even with severe dysplasia that gives a marked slope to the acetabular roof and early subluxation. Lasting success is, however, unlikely if the cartilage responsible for load bearing after healing of the osteotomy is not the articular cartilage of the true acetabulum.

If, after the above considerations, a PAO appears to be a real possibility, it is best to arrange it without further delay, rather than procrastinate on the spurious basis of insufficient patient symptoms. Occasionally, a sequence is seen in a patient who, on initial presentation, is a definite candidate for a PAO, but for whom, after delays and various changes of surgeon, surgery is eventually decided on when the hip has deteriorated to such a degree that only a replacement is possible.

The valgus and/or anteverted femoral neck, which is commonly part of developmental dysplasia of the hip (DDH), appears to be less important than malorientation of the socket. Varus osteotomy is tempting because it is much easier to carry out than a PAO. The biomechanical explanation for its effectiveness is also quite straightforward. It has commonly been observed that protrusio-type osteoarthritis is associated with a varus deformity of the femoral neck (i.e. the centre of the femoral head is below the level of the tip of the greater trochanter); this appears to be a straightforward biomechanical effect resulting in too large a medially directed force component of the femoral head on the socket. Thus, a surgically produced varus neck can be expected to do the same thing, with the possibility, even in adults, of gradual secondary improvements in the acetabulum. An example is shown in Figure 1.4, which shows the reversal of established superolateral osteoarthritis.

In the treatment of symptomatic, but prearthritic, dysplasia, it is now recognized that varus osteotomy – which does not attack the most important abnormality – has much less of a place than it did. The procedure produces shortening and a prominence in the upper thigh in the region of the trochanter, which may be cosmetically unsatisfactory. Rarely, severe coxa valga with an almost horizontal sourcil, or acetabular roof presents a true indication for an isolated varus osteotomy; more frequently, the valgus deformity is such that a varus osteotomy is necessary as a planned sequel to a PAO. The PAO alone is, however, usually sufficient.

In contrast to varus osteotomy, a derotational intertrochanteric osteotomy may be necessary at the same time in a planned sequence after a PAO, and also occasionally as an isolated procedure. The rotational change means, of course, that, with the knee facing forwards, there is an apparent varus or reduction of valgus, even though the neck shaft angle has not been changed.

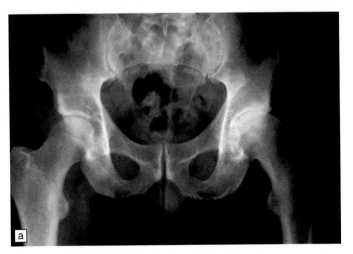
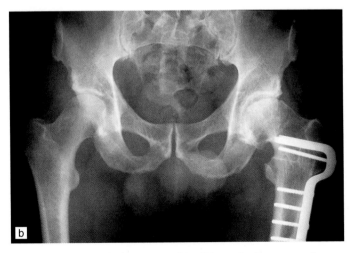

Figure 1.4 – *Reversal of established osteoarthritis by varus extension osteotomy. The wide 'joint space' in (b) gradually appeared postoperatively, showing it to be a true biological response to altered mechanics.*

DDH, with severe hip subluxation

In cases with obvious DDH, but severe subluxation of the hip (Fig. 1.5a), redirection of the acetabulum is no longer either possible or indicated for the reasons stated above; the patient is then a possible candidate for a Chiari osteotomy (Fig. 1.5b). Unlike a PAO, this is not a restorative operation and, in addition, as with virtually all osteotomies, successful relief of symptoms cannot be guaranteed. Therefore, a greater disability should be present for appropriate use of this procedure.

As the underlying condition is dysplasia, the patient is usually a woman; as the only other possible treatment is a total replacement, the patient is clearly far too young for this to be sensible (i.e. under 35). The patient walks with a definite limp and the leg is short with lack of abduction. The radiograph shows marked subluxation. The dividing line between a hip that is a potential candidate for a restorative PAO and one that can be treated only by the salvage procedure of a Chiari osteotomy is not hard and fast, and has been alluded to above. A hip that has no subluxation requires a PAO and one with severe subluxation requires a Chiari osteotomy. A bad or very short-lived result, after a PAO carried out with significant subluxation, would smack of being a technical exercise and therefore would be hard to justify; it is, however, the case that a well-performed Chiari osteotomy can give an excellent result in a poorly covered, but entirely concentric, hip. In these last circumstances, other forms of shelf surgery, numerous varieties of which have been described, may be appropriate. The Chiari osteotomy is, however, universally applicable in this situation, and has the merit that coverage of the femoral head is indubitably solid, can be adjusted by means of additional grafts, and is not, unlike other types of shelf surgery, subject to resorption.

Normal gross morphology but with stage II AVN

The gross morphology of the hip is completely normal, as is the 'joint space', although some part of the femoral head has an abnormal appearance, including increased density, as a result of stage II AVN (Fig. 1.6a). There may be an obvious cause for this, such as a patient on steroid treatment for a renal transplantation, or a possible cause in the past history, such as a brief period of high-dose steroids for asthma. The dosage and duration of steroids required to produce AVN are, however, not known. In many cases, the patient is otherwise well with no evident predisposing cause of any kind; this type of patient in particular is a potential candidate for an osteotomy. The diagnosis must be clarified by an MRI scan.

In such a case, osteotomy is a potentially restorative, rather than a salvage, procedure; it could be considered even when symptoms are not all that marked, in view of the strong possibility that, if not treated, the articular surface of the femoral head will collapse. On the basis that a flexion intertrochanteric osteotomy of the Willert type, as mentioned in Chapter 2, is the procedure under consideration, investigations are then needed to determine: (1) the size of the affected segment and (2) whether flexion of up to about 30–35° is enough to take a substantial amount of this segment out of the weight-

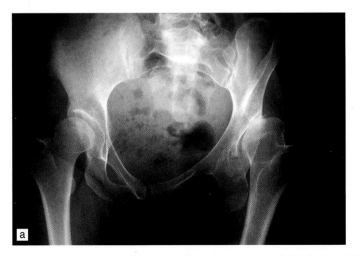
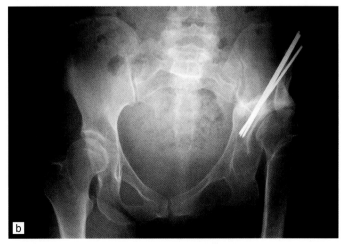

Figure 1.5 – *Severe subluxation from developmental dysplasia of the hip successfully treated by a Chiari osteotomy.*

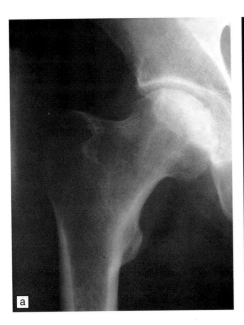
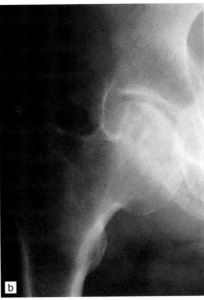

Figure 1.6 – *Avascular necrosis: (a) Ficat stage II and a possible candidate for osteotomy; (b) Schneider view.*

bearing area. The available techniques, in addition to normal anteroposterior (AP) and lateral radiographs, are:

■ Oblique plain radiographs (Schneider) (Fig. 1.6b) taken with the patient supine and in such a way that the X-ray beam penetrates the femoral head in a direction as though the hip were flexed at different angles (usually 30° and 60°)

■ Frontal and sagittal MRI scans.

The angle of the affected segment in the frontal plane is added to its angle in the lateral plane and this combined angle (Kerboul) is used as a measure of its size.

If the patient is very young (under 30, say), the combined angle is less than 200°, and the investigations, notably the Schneider and lateral plain films and sagittal MRI scan, strongly suggest that a flexion osteotomy (possibly with an associated varus or valgus element) will take much of the affected segment out of the weight-bearing area, then this operation should certainly be done. In a recent study by Mont *et al.* [7], 87% had a good or excellent clinical result. However, it is not sensible to carry out this procedure on a patient aged 45, in whom the precise demarcation of the affected segment in the head is not completely clear, and/or it is uncertain whether the angle is truly less than 200° in size or whether the segment can be adequately taken out of the weight-bearing area. The results of the procedure are much less certain and the patient is also reaching the age range in which some form of prosthesis seems entirely appropriate. At what point in the spectrum between these two clinical situations the cut-

off between osteotomy and a replacement (e.g. bipolar) is made depends on many factors, not least the surgeon and operating room team's familiarity with osteotomies around the hip; those who are confident about very good long-term results from replacement will set the cut-off point lower. Nevertheless, as the procedure is a potentially restorative one, which gives a good outlook for the natural hip, an over-prescription of replacement in this situation seems wrong. In cases of doubt, this group of patients is certainly one that should be referred, if appropriate, to another suitable colleague or centre.

Flattened femoral head

Patients in whom the femoral head is flattened or of 'mushroom' shape, with or without the presence of a degree of osteoarthritis (Fig. 1.7), are possible candidates for valgus extension osteotomy (VEO) as extensively advocated by Bombelli [8]. Using the indications described in this chapter and the surgical technique described in Chapter 2, this procedure has a survival rate (i.e. the patient's symptoms do not require total hip replacement) of about 70% at 10 years. The cause of the marked abnormality in the shape of the head is usually clear from the patient's history; it could be infection, such as tuberculosis, Perthe's disease, slipped upper femoral epiphysis (although, in this case, the term 'mushroom-shaped' is not a good one), or AVN, dating from either a childhood insult or adult disease, as referred to above. With the possible exception of Perthe's disease, however, the original cause of the ultimate abnormality of head shape has little relevance for the

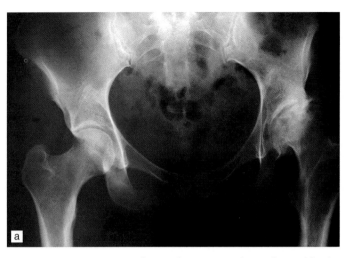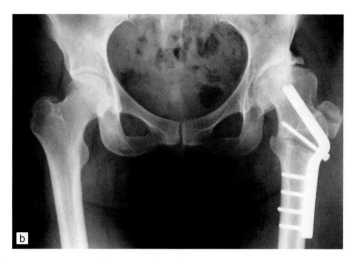

Figure 1.7 – *Treatment of secondary osteoarthritis from old tuberculosis in a 31-year-old patient by valgus extension osteotomy.*

treatment by VEO. The patient may be male or female, and of any age up to the age that is more appropriate for a total hip replacement.

When assessed in the initial outpatient appointment, the patient may walk with a definite limp and have a slightly short leg. The hip may lack abduction or have a fixed adduction deformity. A good range of flexion may be present, but marked loss of movement, especially in the presence of a normal opposite hip, does not necessarily rule out the procedure. It is not possible to tell at this stage whether the loss of movement is the result of contracture or of spasm secondary to pain. In the most favourable case, the plain AP radiograph shows a flattened femoral head, although relatively smooth in outline; there has to be definite evidence of excessive joint pressure anterosuperolaterally on both this film and a lateral one. Sclerosis should certainly be present, showing that the structure of the hip has the capacity to produce new bone, and there should be a floor osteophyte (of the type that has to be removed to get at the true floor in total hip replacement). A bonus is a 'capital drop' osteophyte medially on the femoral head, provided that this is not too large. A shoot-through lateral film should show poor anterior coverage of the femoral head and a very definite narrowing of the joint space as it runs from the back of the hip to the front, whether or not this amounts to frank osteoarthritis.

The biomechanical basis for VEO needs to be borne in mind constantly when using plain films for decision-making. By adducting the femoral head, the weight-bearing zone needs to move from the anterosuperolateral position to a fulcrum between the medial part of the head and the osteophytes deep in the acetabulum. A sufficient

degree of flattening or ovality of the femoral head is necessary for this to happen. In many cases, it is obvious from the plain film that the ovality is sufficient and that such a change in the weight-bearing area might occur with sufficient adduction (usually about 30°). Sometimes, however, one can say only that this might be a possibility.

A VEO in no way produces a normal hip. If a fixed deformity is present, this is alleviated (sometimes this by itself is beneficial), but only minor lengthening of a short leg in the absence of a fixed adduction deformity is possible; the total arc of movement is barely increased and, particularly if the hip is rather stiff, there is some loss of flexion. When considering a given patient as a possible candidate for this procedure, this end-result needs to be borne in mind. A male agricultural labourer in his mid-40s, in whom the hip shows a strong possibility of success after VEO, will receive good treatment from this procedure. He needs reduction in the pain, but may be perfectly happy to accept some residual discomfort. He may also not mind having a slightly short leg that is a little stiff, and in such a case replacement is clearly not a good proposition. On the other hand, a smartly turned-out woman of the same age may not be so happy with this and prefer to opt for replacement, in order to achieve complete pain relief, equality of leg lengths, and a very good range of hip movement; she will realize that she may have 'burnt her boats' as far as the distant future is concerned. A much younger woman may well, however, have learned from many sources that she is too young to have a total hip replacement and be ready to accept an osteotomy.

In the initial outpatient assessment, all that can be sensibly said is that the patient looks suitable and that it

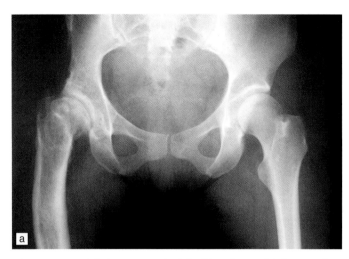

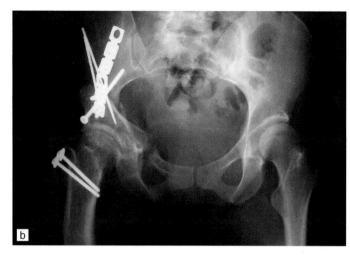

Figure 1.8 – (a) Symptomatic right hip after multiple procedures, including a Salter osteotomy for developmental dysplasia of the hip in a 27-year-old patient. (b) Appearances after periacetabular osteotomy (see text), combined with lateral and anterior displacement of the greater trochanter. The patient returned to competitive horse riding. In this film, union of the pubic osteotomy is still not fully complete.

is possible, after appropriate investigation, that a VEO will work. An investigation using a stress film under anaesthetic is necessary for the final answer.

Residua of treated DDH

Many of the hips in these patients are more properly in the province of the paediatric orthopaedic surgeon, although, not infrequently, young women are seen who have symptoms and markedly abnormal hip morphology that give rise to significant symptoms, but in whom any secondary changes are far too minor for replacement to be appropriate. Many will have had AVN of the femoral head from closed manipulation. This may result in a somewhat abnormal femoral head, which is oval in shape but with excellent articular cartilage; the striking finding is the height of the tip of the greater trochanter in relation to the centre of the head. The symptoms are aching and a limp after activity, believed to result from the fact that the abductors permanently function from a position of partial contraction. If it is clear that symptoms are sufficient for surgery to be warranted, such patients need advancement of the greater trochanter.

If the hip has been treated surgically, as is extremely common, often with several procedures, no general statements can be made. Some may well be candidates for a PAO. Figure 1.8 shows a patient, originally treated by a Salter procedure, as well as a femoral osteotomy, in whom a PAO (combined with trochanteric advancement) was very successful, and she returned to competitive horse riding. In other cases, a valgus osteotomy may be

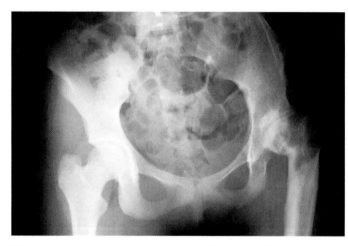

Figure 1.9 – A potential case for a valgus femoral osteotomy after childhood treatment for developmental dysplasia of the hip.

appropriate (Fig. 1.9). Such patients may, at some point in the past, have had a varus osteotomy, so that the effect of a valgus osteotomy largely neutralizes the previous surgery. Valgus osteotomy is particularly indicated if there is a fixed adduction deformity, as shown with this patient. In many such cases, an adequately definitive answer to whether an osteotomy should be done can only be achieved by screening the hip under anaesthesia, as described below.

The types in group B represent the major groups of patients in whom there is an obvious possibility for an osteotomy. It may be possible to make the decision quite definitively or, alternatively, stress films under anaesthesia are needed first.

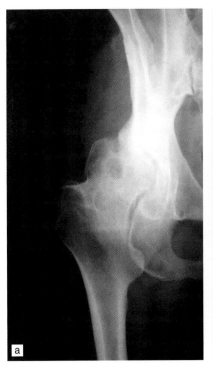
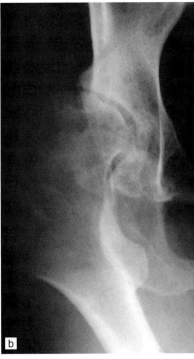

Figure 1.10 – *(a) Dysplasia with severe secondary osteoarthritis. (b) On the stress radiograph, the impingement between the capital drop and floor osteophytes, with separation superolaterally, can be seen easily. The patient was successfully treated by VEO.*

Examination under anaesthesia

The indications for this are chiefly hips in patients who are possible candidates for VEO and, much more rarely, hips that can hopefully be treated by PAO, but do not abduct properly. The hip is first re-examined under a general anaesthetic and on an appropriate table (often most conveniently in the radiology department). Usually, a very considerable increase in motion is seen. This increase in motion should be recorded.

In the hip with limited motion and a mushroom-shaped femoral head, there is often a substantial increase in flexion, and some increase in abduction and/or adduction, but not much change in rotation. The hip is then screened. In this case, the position of interest is marked adduction and some flexion. In this position, contact should be seen in the depth of the hip and physical separation, shown by a frank gap, should appear superolaterally. If this occurs in unequivocal fashion, then there is a good chance that a VEO (mimicking the angles produced at the stress examination, which should be noted) will produce effective symptomatic relief (Fig. 1.10).

It may be found that, even under anaesthesia, the hip adducts to only a very small degree. It has to be remembered that the only effect of the anaesthetic is to produce pain relief and to avoid muscular spasm. The procedure only partly mimics the possible position of the hip that can be achieved at open operation. Thus, a hip that does not adduct under general anaesthetic might, in theory, still be treatable by this procedure. Nevertheless, the outcome would be very much less certain and severely limited adduction is a contra-indication; in these circumstances, it should be

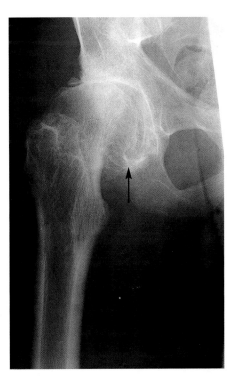

Figure 1.11 – *Old SUFE (SCFE) in a 28-year-old man who had a heavy manual job. Adduction of the hip was prevented by the large 'elephant's trunk' osteophyte (arrowed).*

concluded that VEO should not be carried out. A second reason for the inability to adduct may lie in the presence of an 'elephant's trunk' osteophyte (Fig. 1.11). An osteophyte of this type will certainly prevent the femoral head from rotating in the necessary fashion. Once again, in theory, an osteotomy at which this osteophyte is excised under direct vision may still be possible; this procedure has been described by Bombelli [8]. Nevertheless, the presence of such advanced changes, together with the fact that it is not possible to see the effect radiographically of moving the medial side of the head into the depth of the socket, means that there is bound to be greater uncertainty in the result. In most circumstances, therefore, VEO should probably be avoided in such hips.

Some hips adduct to a sufficient degree, but, instead of the head tipping on the medial osteophytes, a smooth sliding motion occurs, with the head moving laterally and with no change in the fit of the articulating surfaces (Fig. 1.12). The articulating surfaces of the normal head and acetabulum are spherical, with the centre of the sphere being in the centre of the femoral head. In the particular circumstance outlined here, the surfaces are still part of a sphere and move round the centre of that sphere, the only difference being that the diameter of the sphere is much greater than the diameter of the femoral head. In these circumstances, a VEO would be perfectly possible, but it would not produce the necessary change in the mechanics. Such hips are, therefore, not candidates for VEO.

Often, appearances are equivocal. With a marked adduction pressure, there is an impression from the image intensifier that some degree of superolateral opening is taking place, although the appearances are not at all striking (Fig. 1.13). In such hips, a VEO remains a possibility, although the chance of adequate symptomatic relief is clearly less than in more favourable circumstances. It then becomes a matter of weighing up the whole clinical situation and discussing the matter with the patient. Often, in such circumstances, if the only reasonable alternative is a form of replacement, it is best for the patient to persevere without surgery. This can be explained to patients in advance; often there is no problem for them to agree to have an osteotomy if the results of the stress examination are favourable, but to await worsening symptoms if only a replacement can be done.

The appearances seen during screening should be recorded by appropriate films. If and when the decision

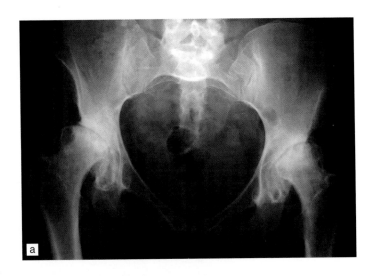

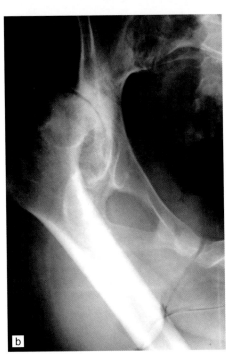

Figure 1.12 – *(a) Although this patient's right hip has a large capital drop and floor osteophytes, the concentric movement on (b) adduction stress is unfavourable for a VEO.*

to do an osteotomy is made, these films are useful at the later planning stage.

Arthrography is often recommended in these circumstances and useful information can be obtained. For example, in a case ideally suited to a VEO, initially there is pooling of the contrast medium medially, followed by the appearance of contrast medium laterally in adduction. The same appearances are, however, quite well seen in the absence of the medium. There is also the danger that arthrography is seen as a special test that has to be requested and it is carried out by someone else, such as a radiologist. Although it is perfectly possible that good and useful information will be obtained, it is

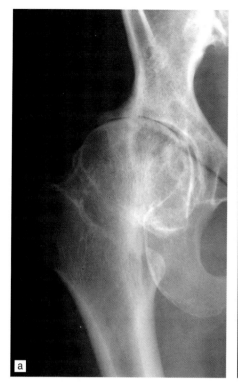
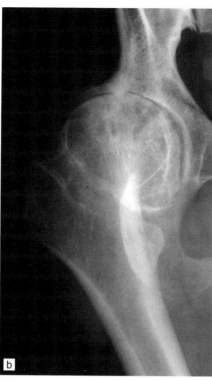

Figure 1.13 – *Stress films of a 47-year-old woman. The superolateral opening on adduction was felt to be insufficient to justify valgus extension osteotomy.*

much better if the examination is carried out personally by the surgeon doing the operation. As the hip is being screened, the whole situation can be thought about and a rational decision made then. In this context, arthrography seems less necessary.

If the examination is simply to determine whether a PAO (or, indeed, a varus osteotomy) is appropriate in the presence of limited abduction and, perhaps, diminution of superolateral articular cartilage, from either osteoarthritis or early subluxation, it becomes immediately clear whether the hip abducts and remains (or becomes) concentric. This can be documented by a radiograph. If the complete preliminary analysis of the case before screening has taken place, it is unlikely that effects such as 'hinge abduction' are seen. If there is any suggestion of this, then neither PAO nor a varus osteotomy should be considered (Fig. 1.14).

Finally, it is sometimes suggested (see below) that a valgus osteotomy should be carried out for early protrusio-type osteoarthritis, because this condition is always associated with a varus femoral neck. Such an indication is rare. However, if it is being considered seriously, it is necessary to screen the hip and make sure that it can adduct adequately. There is no question in this case of achieving any increased adduction (i.e. valgus) at surgery and, if a substantial degree of adduction cannot be achieved (so that, after a valgus osteotomy, the neck shaft angle would become normal or slightly valgus) at examination under anaesthesia, an osteotomy should not be done.

Group C

Patients in this group have radiologically abnormal hips with sufficient symptoms to merit treatment, but an osteotomy has been discounted either on initial presentation or after examination of a stress radiograph, and the patient's joint is not so irretrievably destroyed (for

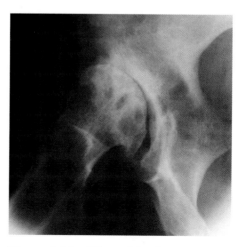

Figure 1.14 – *Hinge abduction.*

example, by complete loss of the femoral head from childhood sepsis) that only total hip replacement.

Among those patients with hips that are excluded as candidates for an osteotomy on the basis of their initial presentation, Figure 1.15 shows a patient's hip with a round head, but medial osteophytes, in which it is clear that a valgus (or a varus PAO) is inappropriate, and Figure 1.13 shows a patient with an old SUFE as an example of one excluded after taking stress radiographs. Previously, two now outmoded procedures might have been indicated for these patients, namely: the 'hanging hip' in which the hip was partially defunctioned by division of the psoas tendon, the adductors, and the greater part of the glutei; and the Maquet lateralization of the greater trochanter in the same fashion as the anterior translocation of the tibial tubercle in the knee. Isolated operations on the greater trochanter are, of course, still sometimes indicated, but only in cases where the lever arm is pathologically diminished rather than those in which the greater trochanter is in the normal position. The Maquet procedure clearly has a sound biomechanical basis, but it is not without possible complications, because it damages the femur significantly, at least when carried out following the described technique, with elevation of the lateral femoral cortex; it has, at best, unpredictable results. Nowadays, for these patients, arthroscopic débridement may be considered and, if this is not felt to be appropriate, or fails, then the patient is a candidate only for some form of replacement, with the exception of the possibility of arthrodesis – considered below.

Arthroscopic débridement

This procedure is still under evaluation. Its effect, even in the knee, is not universally accepted. As the hip is a ball-and-socket joint – its surfaces move in a much less complex way than in the knee – together with the fact that menisci are not present, it seems unlikely that this procedure will ever have more than a limited place in treatment of the hip. Nevertheless, medium-term improvement in patients aged under 50 has been reported, and results may improve with changes in instrumentation. It looks as though certain major limitations will inevitably remain (e.g. the inability to move the hip during arthroscopy), but improved arthroscopes with, for example, longer sheaths have already facilitated the procedure and further improvements can gradually be expected, particularly in relation to surgical instruments.

For effective débridement, however, it would certainly seem that some form of flexible-ended instrument, which can be manipulated within the hip (in the manner of a gastroscope), is essential. Figure 1.16 shows a patient in whom débridement, by including removal of loose bodies, certainly seems to be clearly indicated. It may be, however, that the principal role of hip arthroscopy in osteoarthritis will be in relation to cartilage grafting, if this becomes an effective treatment option.

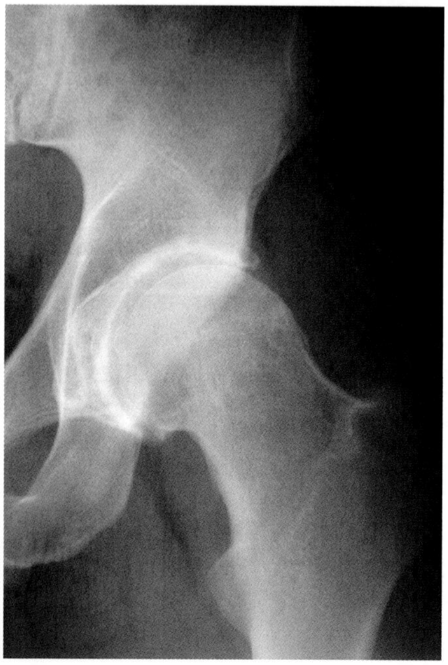

Figure 1.15 – *Hip with a large floor osteophyte, but a round head, which contraindicates a valgus extension osteotomy because there is no opposing fulcrum on the femoral head.*

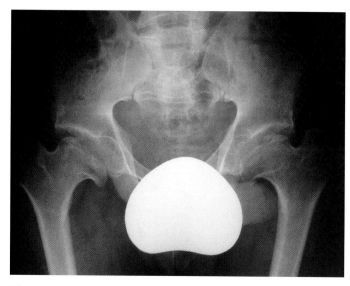

Figure 1.16 – *Patient with epiphyseal dysplasia and loose fragments in each femoral head – a potential case for arthroscopic surgery.*

Arthrodesis

Joint replacement techniques are certainly by no means advanced enough for this operation to be completely discounted. It is also striking how frequently patients are seen who, although needing conversion of an arthrodesis to a total hip replacement (usually for back pain), have had 20 or even up to 50 years of somewhat limited, but entirely acceptable, function with an arthrodesis. With the recent unfavourable publicity about certain types of joint replacement, young people may also be more inclined to agree to have a fusion. An appropriate candidate for this procedure is one in his early 20s, who is entirely normal musculoskeletally, apart from the affected hip (so that, with a pain-free hip, extremely vigorous activity would be expected), and particularly male with either a heavy manual job or wishing to participate in (with limitations) vigorous sports activities. On the initial proposal, patients are likely to be averse to it when they think of the apparently severe awkwardness of having a hip that does not move; if it is explained, however, that they will come to terms with these matters (such as sitting in a slightly awkward fashion), can drive a car, and can have a joint replacement much later, agreement is likely.

Among patients converted from arthrodesis to total hip replacement, women are quite often seen who appear to have had no particular difficulties. Nevertheless, it seems better to confine arthrodesis to young men.

Joint replacement

Although many will quite legitimately consider that joint replacement is, in this context, synonymous with total hip replacement, there is, in principle, more than one possibility. The theoretical places of these other procedures are quite simple to state. These are now given, followed later by a more detailed critique. The theoretical possibilities are:
- Bipolar replacement
- Resurfacing
- Total hip replacement, which is subdivided into (1) standard total hip replacement and (2) special or custom-made total hip replacement.

Bipolar replacement

The indication is a stage III AVN (Fig. 1.17); the hip has been ruled out as a possible candidate for osteotomy on the lines given above, and the acetabulum is still undamaged.

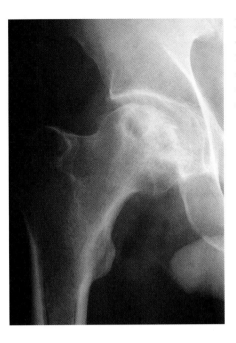

Figure 1.17 – *Stage III avascular necrosis beyond osteotomy, suitable only for some form of prosthesis.*

Resurfacing

The morphology of the hip is not grossly disturbed, so that, with replacement of the articulation only, the mechanics in terms of the centre of rotation, the position of the greater trochanter, and the abductor lever arm give adequate function. Clearly, it is not sensible to consider resurfacing a femoral head when the head itself is in a very unfavourable position (such as gross neck anteversion). The femoral head must itself be free from gross osteoporosis or large cysts.

Total hip replacement

This is indicated in the remainder. It is an unfortunate fact that, although idiopathic or primary osteoarthritis occurs in hips with relatively normal initial anatomy, secondary osteoarthritis occurring in the presence of anatomy that may be quite severely disturbed is often the type requiring total hip replacement in young people. In many patients, therefore, hip resurfacing, as part of a surgical armamentarium, is inevitably excluded, because the femoral head itself is either very small, extremely severely misshapen, in the wrong place, e.g. as a result of gross anteversion (Fig. 1.18), or, finally, absent; by the same token, the total replacement itself is likely to be less straightforward than in older people. Although in many cases, total hip replacement using off-the-shelf components, but often of special type, is possible, some may require 'custom-made' implants (Fig. 1.19).

This subject and the questions of textured surfaces, hydroxyapatite, and cement, and other related issues, are considered in greater detail in Chapters 3 and 6.

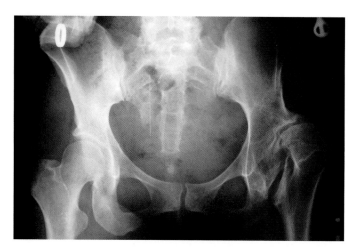

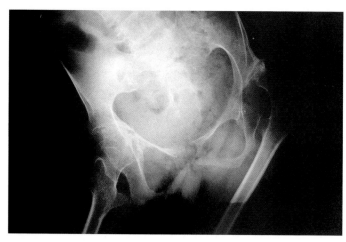

Figure 1.18 – *Hip with multiple childhood pelvic and femoral operations for developmental dysplasia of the hip, suitable only for total hip replacement.*

Figure 1.19 – *Patient with Still's disease in whom bilateral total hip replacement was decided on for pain relief; the femora were such that even the smallest proprietary prosthesis was much too large.*

References

1. Brignall CJ, Stainsby GD. The snapping hip. Treatment by Z-plasty. *J Bone Joint Surg* 1991; 73B: 253-4.
2. Koo K-H, Kim R. Quantifying the extent of osteonecrosis of the femoral head using MRI. *J Bone Joint Surg* 1995; 77B: 875–80.
3. Steinberg ME. Osteonecrosis of the femoral head (part 2). Care depression. *Hip International* 1998; 8: 145–53.
4. Sakamoto M, Shimizy K, Eida S *et al.* A prospective study with MRI. *J Bone Joint Surg* 1997; 79B: 213–19.
5. Markell DC, Miskovsky C, Sculco TP *et al.* Core decompression for osteonecrosis of the femoral head. *Clin Orthop* 1996; 323: 226–33
6. Lequesne M, De Sèze S. Periacetabular osteotomy. Le Faux profil du bassin. *Rev Rhumat* 1991; 58: 643–52.
7. Mont MA, Fairbank AC, Krackow KA, Hungerford DS. The results of a long-term follow-up study. *J Bone Joint Surg* 1996; 78A: 1032–8.
8. Bombelli R, Santore RF. Ten-year follow-up of 212 consecutive intertrochanteric osteotomies for osteoarthritis of the hip. Read at the Annual Meeting of the American Academy of Orthopaedic Surgeons, Anaheim, California, 14 March 1983. (Quoted by Poss R. *J Bone Joint Surg* 1984; 66A: 150.)
9. D'Souza S, Sadiq S, New AMR, Northmore-Ball MD. Femoral osteotomy as the primary surgical procedure for the young adult with arthrosis of the hip. *J Bone Joint Surg* 1998; 80A: 1428–1438.

Further reading

The labrum

Klaue K, Durnin CW, Ganz R. The labrum. The acetabular rim syndrome. A clinical presentation of dysplasia of the hip. *J Bone Joint Surg* 1991; 73B: 423–9.

Petersilge CA, Hague MA, Petersilge WJ *et al.* Acetabular labral tears: Evaluation with MR arthrography. *Radiology* 1996; 200: 231–5.

Tschauner Ch, Hofmann S, Graf R, Engel A. Labral lesions in acetabular dysplasia. Highlights of the First International Meeting, Vienna, 22 November 1997. *Hip Int* 1998; 8: 233–38.

The snapping hip

Brignall CJ, Stainsby GD. The snapping hip. Treatment by Z-plasty. *J Bone Joint Surg* 1991; 73B: 253–4.

Taylor GR, Clarke NMP. Surgical release of the snapping iliopsoas tendon. *J Bone Joint Surg* 1995; 77B: 881–3.

Avascular necrosis

Holman AJ, Gardner GC, Richardson MC, Simkin PA. Quantitative MRI predicts clinical outcome of core decompression for osteonecrosis of the femoral head. *J Rheumatol* 1995; 22: 1929–33.

Koo K-H, Kim R. Quantifying the extent of osteonecrosis of the femoral head using MRI. *J Bone Joint Surg* 1995; 77B: 875–80.

Willert HG, Buchhorn G, Zichner L. Results of flexion osteotomy on segmental femoral head necrosis in adults. In: Weil UH, ed. *Progress in Orthopaedic Surgery, Vol 5: Segmental Idiopathic Necrosis of the Femoral Head.* Berlin: Springer-Verlag, 1981; 63–80.

Osteonecrosis of the femoral head

Markell DC, Miskovsky C, Sculco TP *et al.* Core decompression for osteonecrosis of the femoral head. *Clin Orthop* 1996; 323: 226–33

Sakamoto M, Shimizy K, Eida S, Akita T, Moriya H, Nawata Y. A prospective study with MRI. *J Bone Joint Surg* 1997; 79B: 213–19.

Corrective osteotomy for osteonecrosis of the femoral head

EFORT Congress. Osteonecrosis of the Femoral Head: Mini-Symposium based on presentations at the European Hip Society Meeting at the 1997 EFORT Congress, Barcelona, 1997. Part I: *Hip Int* 1998; 8: 70–98. Part II: *Hip Int* 1998; 8(3): 145–66.

Lequesne M, De Sèze S. Periacetabular osteotomy. Le Faux profil du bassin. *Rev Rhumat* 1991; 58: 643–52.

Mont MA, Fairbank AC, Krackow KA, Hungerford DS. The results of a long-term follow-up study. *J Bone Joint Surg* 1996; 78A: 1032–8.

Triple osteotomy of the pelvis for acetabular dysplasia

de Kleuver M, Kooijman MAP, Pavlov PW, Vett RDH. Results at 8 to 15 years. *J Bone Joint Surg* 1997; 79B: 225–9.

Chiari

Graham S, Westin GW, Dawson E, Oppenheimer WL. The Chiari osteotomy. A review of 58 cases. *Clin Orthop* 1986; 208: 249–58.

Intertrochanteric osteotomy

Bombelli R, Santore RF. Ten-year follow-up of 212 consecutive intertrochanteric osteotomies for osteoarthritis of the hip. Read at the Annual Meeting of the American Academy of Orthopaedic Surgeons, Anaheim, California, 14 March 1983. (Quoted by Poss R. *J Bone Joint Surg* 1984; 66A: 150.)

Northmore-Ball MD. Experiences with a method of choosing between osteotomy, resurfacing and THR in the young adult. A long-term clinical survivorship study. Presented at the Second Domestic Meeting of the European Hip Society, Helsinki, 1996.

Sicre G, Favard L, JO Roy. Long-term outcome of upper femoral valgus osteotomy in the treatment of osteoarthritis of the hip: a retrospective study of 29 osteotomies. Presented at The Second Congress of the European Federation of National Associations of Orthopaedics and Traumatology (EFORT), Munich, July 4–7 1995.

Arthrodesis
Callaghan JJ, Brand RA, Pedersen DR. Hip arthrodesis. A long-term follow-up. *J Bone Joint Surg* 1985; 67A: 1328–35.

CHAPTER 2

Specific procedures in the young adult: preoperative planning and notes on technique in pelvic and upper femoral osteotomy

M. D. Northmore-Ball

Further details about procedures discussed in the previous chapter are given here. It is assumed, in each case, that a definite decision has been made to carry out a particular operation. In general, one technique is described, with commentary about other techniques, and references to places where further details may be obtained are given where appropriate.

Periacetabular osteotomy

General comments

As the adult skeleton does not have the flexibility of the child's, with the hip being deep seated and the acetabulum fused almost circumferentially with the rest of the pelvis, it is not surprising that free and unimpeded redirection in the adult is difficult, and that a number of techniques have been described. The operations vary, particularly in the position and number of the incisions and approaches used, the structures still attached to the osteotomized acetabulum, the radial distance from the centre of the acetabulum where the osteotomies are carried out, the shapes of the osteotomies themselves, and whether or not the pelvic ring is left intact. Some of the more established techniques also have very significant variations in the detailed way in which they can be carried out, as mentioned below.

Taking these matters in turn, one can say the following:

- One surgical incision and approach is clearly desirable, if possible, because otherwise it may be necessary to reposition the patient intraoperatively
- Residual attachments, such as the sacrospinous ligament, to the osteotomized acetabulum are likely to hinder free redirection
- The larger the radial distance from the centre of the acetabulum where the osteotomies are done, the greater the distortion of the overall shape of the hemipelvis and the greater the chance of some local adverse feature resulting
- Clearly, preservation of the pelvic ring must be desirable.

The most used redirectional acetabular osteotomies now are probably those of Wagner, Tönnis, and Ganz. The Wagner osteotomy is very different from the other two. It is the only one in which the osteotomy is truly acetabular rather than pelvic, being spherical and only just deep to the subchondral bone. It is done through one approach (Smith-Petersen), although radiological control throughout with an image intensifier is essential to control the precise direction of the special, spherically shaped osteotomes, to ensure that they remain concentric with the acetabulum. As the osteotomy is just lateral to the quadrilateral plate, rather than having any intrapelvic component, a slight degree of lateralization of the acetabulum, secondary to the dysplasia, facilitates the operation, which would not, in fact, be possible in the absence of dysplasia. This fact also produces one of the limitations of the procedure – that the acetabulum cannot be medialized and that, if anything, there may be a tendency for slight lateralization, which is clearly biomechanically undesirable in terms of transmitted load. The second disadvantage is that displacement may be somewhat limited, particularly in a flexion/extension sense, and may also be rather difficult to control.

Fixation is by a small plate fashioned distally into a fork shape, fitted on to the lateral wall of the ilium, with its prongs impacted into the cancellous, subchondral, acetabular surface. Such fixation is clearly somewhat limited and, were the acetabulum to be extensively mobilized to increase correction, it might not be adequate. The third potential disadvantage is usually given as avascular necrosis (AVN). AVN of the femoral head is, however, hardly likely to result simply from damage to the small branch of the obturator artery running in the ligamentum teres, and the blood supply of the acetabulum itself, which after osteotomy is simply supplied from the capsule, differs little from the supply in the Tönnis and Ganz procedures. In the last procedure, the quantity of bone to be supplied is also considerably greater. It seems rather doubtful, therefore, that the Wagner osteotomy is any more likely to suffer intrinsically from AVN than the others.

The Tönnis and Ganz osteotomies are rather similar, the main differences being that the latter, at least as originally described, is carried out through one approach; the former enters the greater sciatic notch, whereas the latter runs anterior to the notch and leaves the pelvic ring intact.

The next question relates to the nature and degree of the required acetabular displacement, and in particular the amount of abduction and extension and whether any ante- or retroversion should be incorporated. It seems almost certain that the results must to some substantial degree – at least in the absence of pre-existing degenerative change and a surgical complication – depend on the appropriateness of the various angular corrections. If the correction is too small, incomplete relief of symptoms results, with an impaired outlook; if correction in an abduction sense is too great, then late protrusio osteoarthritis might result; if too much extension is used, there will be significant limitation of hip flexion, and even a possibility of posterolateral instability. Precise correction must depend, in its turn, on appropriate preoperative planning. Although, from a normal anteroposterior radiograph, an estimate can be made of the required degree of abduction, the dysplasia

invariably affects the front of the hip and the deficiency in this area is critical. The degree of extension is much more difficult to estimate. An approximate assessment can be made from the 'faux profile' view, but, unfortunately, again as a result of variations in the side-to-side width of the articular surface from front to back, the two estimates are to some degree interdependent. Ante- or retroversion cannot be estimated in any way from plain radiographs.

To overcome these difficulties, an accurate picture of the coverage of the superior load-bearing section of the femoral head by the articular cartilage of the acetabulum has to be made from a very careful analysis of computed tomography (CT) scans. If the patient were standing and the femoral head, divided into anterolateral, anteromedial, posterolateral, and posteromedial quadrants, viewed in an imaginary sense from a position vertically above it, the percentage of each of these four quadrants hidden from view by the socket would be visible. In a normal hip, approximately 80% of the two medial quadrants and 50–55% of the two lateral quadrants are covered. From the CT scan, it is possible to measure the percentages of cover in the four quadrants in the dysplastic hip before periacetabular osteotomy (PAO). There is a computer program for producing these percentages directly from the CT information; this same program then indicates the most appropriate corrections, although an adequate, but less good and extremely time-consuming, calculation can be made using tracings on acetate (Figs 2.1–2.3).

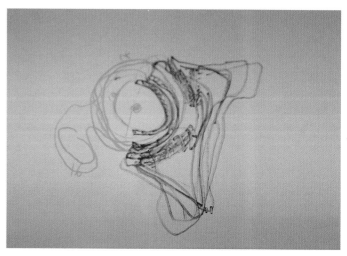

Figure 2.1 – *Tracings on acetate made from CT scans enlarged to actual size, before planning a periacetabular osteotomy. The CE angle of about 0° can easily be seen – the centre of the head is on a line with the edge of the socket.*

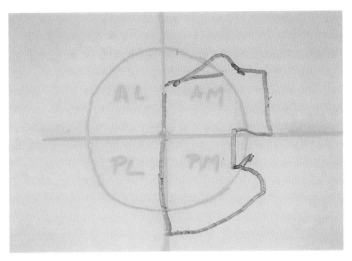

Figure 2.2 – *Outlines made from the same tracings showing the coverage in the anterolateral (AL), anteromedial (AM), posterolateral (PL), and posteromedial (PM) quadrants. There is zero cover in the AL and PL segments.*

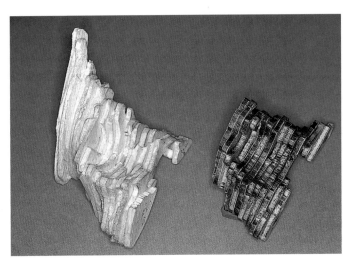

Figure 2.4 – *Examples of acetabular models made manually from tracings of enlarged CT scans.*

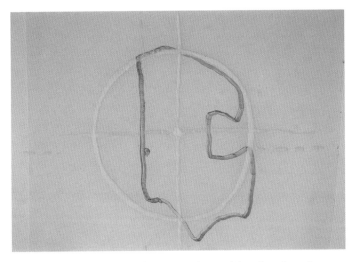

Figure 2.3 – *The selected compromise position showing almost normal anterolateral (AL) and posterolateral (PL) coverage, and an almost normal CE angle. The suggestion of lack of posteromedial (PM) coverage is illusory and is the one defect in this manual planning technique.*

The method requires the CT scans to be taken up to actual size; this can be done either directly from the CT computer disk, or photographically. By moving the traced outline of the acetabulum over that of the femoral head, a best compromise position can be arrived at. Displacements have to be converted to angles, knowing the diameter of the femoral head; ante- or retroversion can be measured directly. The method is, at best, an approximation and is in no way as effective as the computer-generated acetabular model; furthermore,

because the actual available articular surface of the acetabulum is likely to be less than normal, as well as being maldirected, even the ideal position can be only a compromise. The method does, however, give an estimate of the three axial corrections to be aimed at during surgery. A spin-off from the manual technique described above is that, if desired, an actual physical model of the acetabulum can be made (Fig. 2.4). Shapes, made from any convenient material of the same thickness as the CT scan slices, can be cut from tracings of the images and fixed together. The effect of the planned corrections on socket orientation can then be checked directly. The construction of physical models is, once again, something that is much more easily carried out using a computer-controlled process. Models made in this way have been available for a considerable time, but their availability is unfortunately restricted, largely for financial reasons.

Surgical technique for the Ganz PAO

The patient is placed supine in the centre of the operating table, and in such a way that an accurately centred, anteroposterior (AP), pelvic, plain radiograph can be taken. The precise positions of the X-ray machine and film need to be referenced so that an exactly equivalent repeat plain film can be done after the osteotomy. Only in this way can the accuracy of correction (i.e. in the abduction sense) be confirmed. Plain films take longer than image intensification, but the latter does not give adequate information in this situation.

In the method described below, a classic Smith-Petersen approach is used. Variations will be referred to subsequently. The interval between sartorius and tensor fascia lata (TFL) is identified just distal to the antero-superior iliac spine. The lateral cutaneous nerve of the thigh can seldom be preserved and it is best to ignore it. It is vitally important to identify the muscles in an ordered fashion in the deeper parts of the wound. The appearances may be initially confusing because there are several fascial webs, between rectus femoris and the underside of TFL, that need to be partially divided; underneath one of these lie the ascending and transverse branches of the lateral femoral circumflex vessels, the ascending branch of which needs to be identified and divided between ligatures. The origin of TFL is then marked with a stay suture and TFL and the glutei are taken off, leaving a small cuff of repairable fascia attached to the wing of the ilium. Glutei are then stripped from the lateral wing carefully from anteriorly all the way back to the greater sciatic notch, into which a finger may be placed for identification.

The straight and reflected heads of rectus are carefully identified. The tip of a pair of curved Mayo scissors can conveniently be put underneath the reflected head, and the tendon is then divided over them, giving a clearly recognizable stump for later repair. The straight head and the region between the anterosuperior and antero-inferior iliac spines is then carefully exposed; an anastomosis in this region means that there will be several small vessels to cauterize. A stay suture is put in the origin of sartorius and the muscles taken off medially in one sheet. Cutting diathermy can be used about half-way across the iliac crest, so that there is soft tissue for subsequent repair still on the top of the crest and lateral to it. An alternative technique is given later.

The soft tissues can now be taken medially down to the greater sciatic notch, and it should be possible to put a curved instrument, such as a Moynihan, through from one side and to feel it with the fingertip from the other (see also 'Chiari osteotomy' below). The extracapsular fat anteriorly needs to be dissected off and the lateral edge of iliacus clearly seen. Once the plane underneath this has been defined, the straight head of rectus can be transfixed with a final marker suture and taken off the AIIS. Using a combination of sharp and blunt dissection, the iliopectineal eminence and the pubis medial to this can next be progressively exposed. Iliacus is taken off the capsule anteriorly and inferomedially. The hip has to be

progressively flexed on to some form of covered support, allowing it to go progressively up to an angle of about 60 or 70°. This slackens off the anteromedial structures.

With a retractor impacted into the pubis, a good enough view can then be obtained of the latter to place a curved instrument safely through the top of the obturator foramen and feel its tip with a fingertip from the opposite side. The final part of the soft tissue dissection requires palpation of the ischium with an instrument from anteriorly. This is not particularly difficult once the feel of it has been recognized. Rehearsal of this complete exposure in an anatomy department (or, preferably, on a fresh postmortem specimen) is mandatory. A long, curved pair of Mayo scissors, held in one hand with the blades kept firmly closed and passed inferomedial to the capsule, is convenient. This can be put medial and then lateral to the posterior part of the teardrop. Finally, it is necessary to confirm that adequate access can be obtained to the medial surface of the quadrilateral plate, and once again it should be possible to palpate the tip of a Moynihan placed to run medially from the posterior end of the teardrop, with a fingertip placed on the inner surface of the quadrilateral plate. The inner surface of the quadrilateral plate is difficult to see directly, although it should be possible to glimpse it at this stage. The surgeon needs to be very familiar with the bony landmarks in this region; a pelvic model, made as described above and giving the dimensions of the actual patient being operated on, is very helpful. The quadrilateral plate becomes somewhat more visible before completion of the osteotomy.

The osteotomies are then carried out. First, the superior pubic ramus is divided, protecting the obturator nerve immediately behind it with curved Homan levers (Fig. 2.5). The hip is kept flexed throughout this. Next, a Cobb periosteal elevator is placed on the ischium and the junction of the teardrop region and the ischium is scraped with its tip, defining the position of the ischial osteotomy, which cuts part way into the ischium. A special angled osteotome is then placed between the capsule and the Cobb elevator to make this osteotomy (Fig. 2.6). The leg is then once again extended and the ilium marked with an osteotome, and an osteotomy is made with a saw starting anteriorly, just distal to the ASIS and running in a coronal plane to about the region of the pelvic brim. From the lateral side, this osteotomy is continued a short way in the direction of the ischial

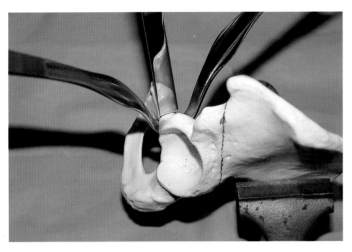

Figure 2.5 – *Periacetabular osteotomy: the pubic osteotomy.*

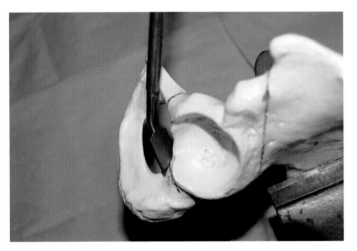

Figure 2.6 – *The pubic osteotomy has been made. The incomplete ischial osteotomy is now being made from anteriorly with one of the special chisels. The position for the first limb of the iliac osteotomy is seen.*

spine, running parallel to the distal edge of the greater sciatic notch (Fig. 2.7). The leg is then again flexed and, partly under direct vision and partly by feel, the osteotomy is continued from medially in exactly the same direction.

Care is needed to make sure that the osteotomy does not enter the greater sciatic notch, producing a pelvic disruption. At this stage, a Shanz screw can be inserted into the AIIS, with a T-handle to manipulate the acetabulum, and appropriate Kirschner wires inserted, so that when brought parallel the planned degree of correction is made. The osteotomy is then completed between the limit of the osteotomy just made and the previous ischial osteotomy from the inner surface of the quadrilateral plate (Fig. 2.8). Although there is concern about entering the hip, inspection of a model shows that this is very unlikely. Some special instruments, such as the angled osteotome mentioned previously, are required. As the osteotomy is made, a laminar spreader can be put in the iliac osteotomy and the acetabulum gradually displaces, giving a better view of the quadrilateral plate.

When the osteotomy is completed, there may well be initial difficulty in moving it to any great degree. This must be overcome. There may be residual attachments posteriorly and distally. When the acetabulum is properly mobilized (and assuming that the hip itself has sufficient mobility), it is possible to rotate the acetabulum to bring the Kirschner wires parallel, while at the same time noting its position mediolaterally. It should be

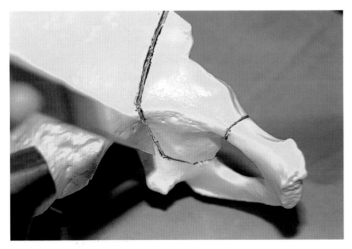

Figure 2.7 – *The iliac osteotomy has been made down to just above the pelvic brim with a saw. The second limb of the iliac osteotomy is now being made about parallel to the distal edge of the greater sciatic notch and about a finger's breadth from it.*

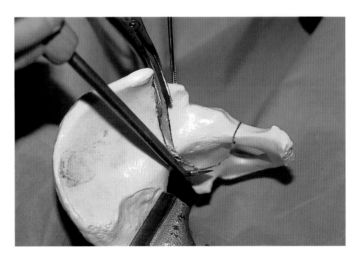

Figure 2.8 – *The iliac and previous ischial osteotomies are now being joined up from within, along the inner surface of the quadrilateral plate. A Shanz screw has been inserted in the AIIS and a laminar spreader has been inserted into the iliac osteotomy.*

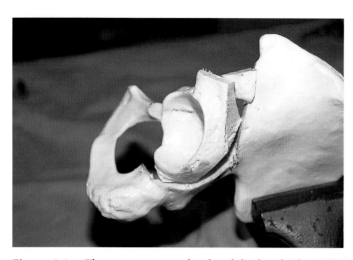

Figure 2.9 – *The osteotomy completed and displaced. The AIIS has been sawn off and put inside the anterior limb of the iliac osteotomy.*

possible to put the acetabulum into almost any position at this stage. Once the displacement has been made (Fig. 2.9), it can be held with threaded pins inserted into the iliac crest, entering the displaced acetabulum under direct vision. A radiograph is then taken. If all appears well, the osteotomy has to be fixed. The Shanz screw is taken out, and the AIIS, which will now be prominent anteriorly, is trimmed with a saw, producing a triangular piece of graft, and a long untapped 4.5-mm cortical screw is inserted into the strong bar of bone running down towards the sacroiliac joint. The threaded pins are then progressively removed and two further long cortical screws are inserted (see Fig. 1.3). This is not particularly easy although, provided that the iliac osteotomy has been started just below the AIIS, there will be sufficient bone to insert two screws alongside the one already inserted. The graft from the AIIS can now be put in the opened-out anterior part of the iliac osteotomy, and the straight head of rectus, easily identified by the stay suture, is sutured back through a drill hole. The reflected head can then be repaired. With the hip in flexion, the glutei can be brought up quite readily to the iliac crest, and the abdominal muscles are sutured through the cuff of tissue on the crest to the fascia over the glutei. Drill holes may be needed in the iliac crest to get a sound repair, and the previously marked origins of sartorius and TFL can be sutured back through drill holes in their correct position.

Postoperatively, the leg can be suspended in slings attached to long springs, so that it floats gently above the bed and can be actively moved easily by the patient. The

time when the patient is remobilized depends somewhat on the solidity of the fixation, but a period of 10 days of bedrest is usually tolerated very well. This is succeeded by a period of 6 weeks of non-weight-bearing, followed by progressive removal of walking aids – this is determined by the apparent rate of clinical and radiological union.

Variations on the above technique are given below:
- In an attempt to preserve the lateral cutaneous nerve of the thigh, the distal part of the approach may be carried out within the sheath of TFL; the muscle is taken off its sheath from within.
- TFL and glutei can be taken from the iliac crest by means of an osteotomy, as can the origin of sartorius; these osteotomies are then fixed with screws. This is reported to give improved function, but the suture technique described above seems perfectly satisfactory.
- The blood supply to the acetabulum may possibly be improved by preservation of some of the origin of gluteus minimus near to the reflected head of rectus. This, however, makes the osteotomy itself slightly more difficult.
- Variations in the fixation system are sometimes also needed. In, for example, the case shown in Figure 1.8, the patient had as a child had a Salter osteotomy, with removal of a large graft from the iliac wing. The resulting wing was very thin and it was necessary to fix the osteotomy with a reconstruction plate.

The same osteotomy can also be carried out using a somewhat different surgical approach, such as an ilio-inguinal approach, almost entirely from within. The theoretical advantage of this is that there is a lesser disturbance of the abductors. Other, less well-established variations include carrying out the pubic and ischial osteotomies through separate incisions, in some cases using radiographic control with an image intensifier. The latter is not required in the method described above.

Chiari osteotomy

This procedure works by producing a solid load-bearing buttress immediately above the subluxing femoral head. As a result of the side-to-side movement of the osteotomy, there is probably some rotational change of the hip in an effectively valgus sense, but this is unlikely to be significant. The best height above the hip at which a Chiari osteotomy should be carried out has occasionally been disputed in the past, on the basis of its function, although there seems little doubt that it should be as close to the capsule of the hip as possible. The capsule is now in a position to take load directly and capsular metaplasia can, at least in theory, result; if the osteotomy is too high then there is no way in which this can occur. The direction should be medially and slightly upwards. Planning is very limited, but a line can be drawn along the proposed site of the osteotomy across the ilium just above the hip, and if the hip is spherical and only moderately subluxed this does not present any problems.

In more severe subluxation, however, the same inclined line may seem hardly to enter the greater sciatic notch, running more up towards the sacroiliac joint and, although this does not mean necessarily that the Chiari osteotomy cannot be done, it makes it clear that care may be required in the posterior part of the cut. Clearly, also, the more subluxed the hip, the less easy it is to incline an osteotomy upwards and medially for a similar reason. Finally, the shape of the subluxed part of the femoral head itself may make a lesser or greater degree of upward inclination seem appropriate, bearing in mind the concept that the displaced piece of ilium is intended to be in a load-bearing position above the subluxed head. It has to be borne in mind, however, that an attempt is made intraoperatively (see under 'Surgical technique' below) to reduce the subluxation of the head, and grafting is also used.

In addition to the possible variations in height and angle, the osteotomy itself can be carried out in different ways. Different approaches can be used, different shapes for the osteotomy achieved, and different tools used to make it, and the osteotomy may or may not be supplemented by grafts and may be fixed in different ways. Many of these variations are interrelated. One technique is described and commentary made on the variations.

Surgical technique

The following method is based on one used in Berne. The patient is placed supine on a radiolucent table, so that an AP view of the hip can be obtained using an image intensifier. As it is necessary only to check the height of the osteotomy and its direction, and the magnitude of subsequent displacement, image intensification, giving a relatively restricted view of one hip only, is sufficient; this is unlike a PAO.

A Smith-Petersen approach is then used, and the surgical approach follows exactly the parts of the PAO description given earlier. It may not be necessary, however, to divide the lateral femoral circumflex vessels running across the gap between rectus femoris and TFL, although their position must be very carefully established. The metaphyseal region of the femur, somewhere at or just above the lesser trochanter, must be palpated anteriorly. In the proximal part of the wound, the TFL and glutei are taken off laterally, as far back as the greater sciatic notch, into which a fingertip may be placed, and then one medial sheet is fashioned by detaching sartorius and iliacus as far back as the notch; this part of the dissection is usually easy. The tip of a curved instrument, such as a Moynihan, placed through the notch from one side or the other, can then be palpated with a fingertip from the other side. Sometimes the fingertips themselves can be palpated directly across the notch. As far as the proximity of the sciatic nerve is concerned, the obvious space is reassuring.

A curved pair of Mayo scissors can be put underneath the reflected head of rectus, hard by its junction with the straight head; the reflected head is then neatly divided over them and dissected off the ilium in the region of the superolateral acetabular margin. In theory, the tendon can be preserved for later repair, but this is not

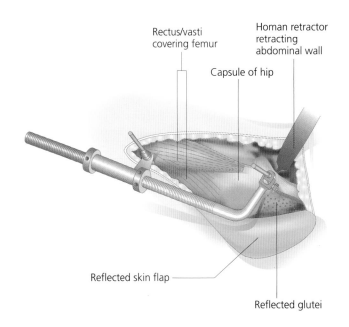

Figure 2.10 – *Chiari osteotomy: drawing showing the position of the ASIF fracture distractor, with one Shanz screw in the anterior cortex of the femur near the lesser trochanter and the second screw in the iliac crest.*

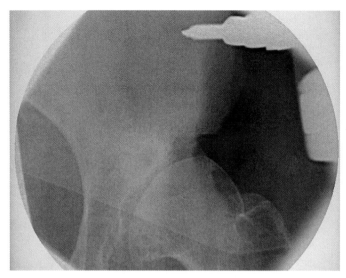 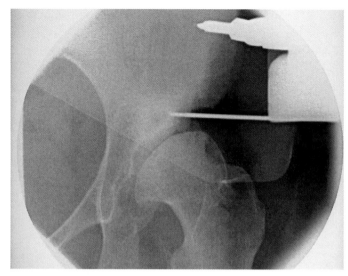

Figure 2.11 – *Intraoperative image intensifier views: (a) before distraction, the correct entry point is obscured by the subluxed femoral head; (b) after distraction, the ideal point has been selected. The rather horizontal direction in this case was chosen to match the shape of the head.*

always practicable. The superior capsule is then cleaned. An ASIF femoral distractor (Fig. 2.10) is placed with its distal fixation rod inserted through a unicortical hole in the femoral metaphysis, in the region previously identified. A Shanz screw is an alternative. The proximal rod or Shanz screw is then placed in the iliac crest. The bar in between is positioned so as to allow an AP view of the hip using the image intensifier. A moderate distraction force is then applied, and the precise position of the joint found with a needle or Kirschner wire. Soft tissues need to be scraped from the ilium immediately above the hip; with the femoral head suitably distalized, the optimal entry point for an osteotome laterally, immediately above the capsular attachment, can be chosen, and its site marked by a thin threaded AO pin inserted with a drill (Fig. 2.11). Using this technique, an extremely fine and certain adjustment of the level and direction of the osteotomy is possible. Once the line is determined, another threaded pin can be inserted just above it to give the direction, and the previous pin is removed, taking care that the entry position is still easily visible.

Alternatively, the pin can be left in place and the osteotomy begun using thin, flat osteotomes immediately above and below it. The position for these osteotomes is very close to the acetabular margin, and it is sometimes better to make drill hole perforations in the cortex in this area to avoid any possibility of fragmentation. The anterior part of the osteotomy is then carefully marked. It runs anteriorly and distally underneath the straight head of rectus femoris, emerging at the level of the anteror inferior iliac spine. The way in which this anterior and distal extension of the osteotomy can be fashioned when a Chiari osteotomy is carried out in this way is clearly of great importance, because the acetabulum is deficient anteriorly in all cases in which a Chiari osteotomy is done. The line of the osteotomy in this region can be marked from laterally and medially using needlepoint cutting diathermy. The posterior part of the osteotomy runs directly backwards in a straight line into the greater sciatic notch. Having marked the osteotomy, it is progressively fashioned with osteotomes (Fig. 2.12); there is a significant curvature anteriorly, so relatively narrow ones are required in this area. Some fragmentation of the internal iliac cortex may occur, but this is not of any consequence. When the osteotomy is continued posteriorly, curved Homan levers should be placed for protection through the sciatic notch.

Once the osteotomy is completed, it is displaced by direct pressure and it will probably be necessary to abduct the hip, having removed the femoral distractor. If the osteotomy does not displace initially, this is probably the result of a posterior spike of bone on the medial side. Further careful work with an osteotome is needed. Occasionally, this can be supplemented with a Gigli saw, simply to make sure that the osteotomy is posteriorly completed, although this is not usually required.

The osteotomy has to be displaced to achieve the desired femoral head coverage. A very substantial

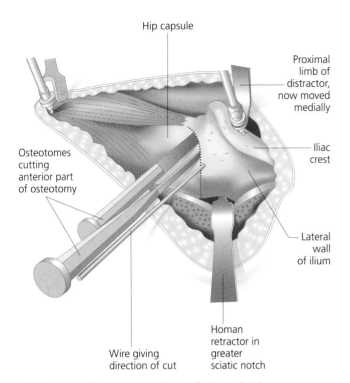

Osteotomes cutting anterior part of osteotomy

Hip capsule

Proximal limb of distractor, now moved medially

Iliac crest

Lateral wall of ilium

Wire giving direction of cut

Homan retractor in greater sciatic notch

Figure 2.12 – *The osteotomy being fashioned. The narrow osteotomes used to curve the anterior part of the cut distally can be seen.*

displacement is usually needed (see Fig. 1.5). Much has been written about the degree of displacement theoretically needed, although it is, in fact, obvious from the radiographic appearances whether the displacement is sufficient, bearing in mind the function of the iliac buttress. Quite frequently, the initial displacement is seen to be inadequate because the requirement is for the maximum that can be achieved. The osteotomy is fixed with AO threaded pins, which are passed through the iliac crest and enter the distal fragment under direct vision. The proximal ends are cut off short, leaving just enough for their later identification and removal.

Finally, a graft that is about 2–3 cm square is taken with a saw and a curved osteotome from the lateral wall of the ilium. If the removal site is chosen carefully, then, after minor trimming, it should fit neatly underneath the displaced anterior part of the osteotomy between the osteotomy and the capsule, further increasing the anterior coverage significantly. It is important, however, to check that the graft is not displaced with maximal hip flexion. Wound closure is then as for a PAO.

Postoperatively, suspension of the limb in slings attached to long springs works very well. Loss of position of the osteotomy is unlikely and the patient can

in theory be mobilized after 2–3 days in bed, although nothing is lost by a slightly longer period of bedrest, provided that the leg is kept actively moving, and the appropriate anti-deep vein thrombosis prophylaxis is used; the author's practice is to use a very similar postoperative regimen to that described above for PAO.

Variations
A fracture distractor was not used in Chiari's originally described technique, but its use confers very considerable advantages. Instead of osteotomes, a Gigli saw can be used, although, as with so many easier techniques, the result is likely to be much less satisfactory, with a higher cut at a poorly controlled level and an inability to curve the cut round towards the front to provide the vital anterior cover; some of these deficiencies can, however, probably be made up with supplementary grafting. Advocates of the technique have stated that avascular necrosis of the acetabular margin can take place if the osteotomy is too near, although whether this has been truly established is doubtful. Another version is to carry out a trochanteric osteotomy and fashion the iliac osteotomy in a curved fashion, using a narrow-bladed saw from laterally. The relatively poor definition of the critical area around the anteroinferior iliac spine, and the inability to view the pelvis from within, seem to be distinct disadvantages of this technique.

Chiari osteotomy and later total hip replacement
A Chiari osteotomy is sometimes stated to be little more than a preparation for subsequent replacement. This not only seriously under-estimates the effect of a well-executed Chiari osteotomy, but is quite incorrect as far as simplification of total hip replacement is concerned. Unless the Chiari osteotomy is being used for a hip that has minimal subluxation (in which almost certainly a PAO would be better), the iliac buttress will be much too proximal to be of any value at replacement, when the prosthetic socket needs to be put distally and medially into the true acetabulum to give proper function. Furthermore, although the increased anterior coverage might possibly be useful for support of the socket, the persisting, almost complete, posterolateral deficiency is very unhelpful. The Chiari osteotomy has to be considered as a definitive operation by itself, with a good chance of producing long-lasting symptomatic relief, but accepting that the total hip replacement – almost certainly eventually required – will be made

slightly more difficult (although not to a great degree), rather than facilitated.

Labral tears

After remodelling of a successful Chiari osteotomy, the effective acetabular roof consists of the original articular cartilage medially and metaplastic capsule laterally. Between the two is the acetabular labrum, and this structure therefore occupies a completely different position in relation to the weight-bearing part of the acetabulum from the one that it occupies normally. Any loading on therefore is certain to change. If the labrum has some functionally significant abnormality, it is unfortunately possible for symptoms to persist, and perhaps increase, after an otherwise technically successful Chiari osteotomy, causing symptomatic failure. In theory, to avoid this problem symptomatic labral tears need to be treated either simultaneously or as part of a planned sequence with the Chiari osteotomy, and by this means the clinical success rate of the surgery should increase. Nevertheless, as noted elsewhere, both the diagnosis and the treatment of labral tears are by no means well established. In principle, the diagnosis should be made, or at least strongly suggested, by clinical signs and appropriate imaging studies (such as magnetic resonance imaging [MRI] arthrography) and the lesion treated arthroscopically. The labral tear can be treated directly by opening the capsule at the same time as the Chiari osteotomy; the integrity of the capsule beneath the newly weight-bearing buttress is, however, important and, if the capsular disruption were too significant, then this in itself could be a cause of the procedure's failure.

Similar comments apply to labral tears and PAO. This subject is touched on elsewhere (see Chapter 1). Although it has been suggested that they should also be treated either in a planned sequence or concurrently with a PAO, in a PAO the labrum moves with the acetabulum so that it remains on the less highly stressed acetabular lip. It would, therefore, seem in principle that it is less likely to be a cause of persisting symptoms than in a Chiari osteotomy.

Other forms of shelf

These procedures are much easier to perform than a Chiari osteotomy, although they rely on rather unpredictable graft consolidation and remodelling before they function. Their place is probably best considered as supplementary to a more major form of osteotomy

carried out at the same time. Of the many varieties, the slotted acetabular augmentation technique described by Staheli *et al.* [7] is recommended. The paper also has a commentary on earlier forms of shelf augmentation [7].

Intertrochanteric femoral osteotomy

Valgus extension osteotomy

The following description is based on that of Bombelli [8]. As well as producing a major alteration in the mechanics of the joint itself, with medialization of the fulcrum, a Voss effect is produced by temporary weakening of the abductors and psoas tenotomy. The amount of valgus required is estimated from the stress radiographs. This can, however, be measured only very approximately and 30° of valgus is usually appropriate. The amount of extension is decided intraoperatively and is usually between 10° and 40°. The extension is the mechanical equivalent of the extension produced at PAO and the anterior coverage achieved at Chiari osteotomy. In some circumstances, only a very small amount of extension is needed. This applies particularly to secondary osteoarthritis after slipped upper femoral epiphysis, where the articular surface of the head is already in a pathologically posterior position.

The osteotomy is customarily fixed with a 130° angled ASIF blade plate, and the operative planning consists of working out and then drawing the precise position for insertion of this blade plate before and after fashioning the osteotomy. Unless this is carried out in good time before surgery, the chance of a successful operation is very much diminished. The author has seen numerous failures with removal of inaccurately planned wedges, perhaps at an incorrect level and often in association with badly positioned blade plates. Complete failure of symptomatic relief or non-union may result. This can occur even in experienced hands as a direct result of lack of detailed planning.

These same strictures apply to all varieties of modern precision osteotomy, and not just to the valgus extension osteotomy (VEO) considered in this section. A tracing needs to be made and the osteotomy marked at 90° to the femoral shaft at the upper end of the lesser trochanter (which immediately shows the position for the

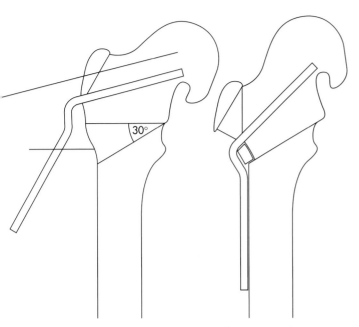

Figure 2.13 – *Typical planning drawings for a 30° valgus extension osteotomy.*

lateral end of the first transverse cut; this is usually considerably higher than initially expected). Assuming that a 30° valgus is intended and a 130° angled blade plate is to be used, the blade of the blade plate needs to be inserted at an angle of 80° to the axis of the femur (Fig. 2.13). The entry point needs to be about 1.5 cm proximal to the lateral end of the intertrochanteric osteotomy (ITO) to give an adequate bone bridge. A second tracing is made of the femoral shaft distal to the ITO, and on this a 30° wedge is marked. A small, rather lateral, trochanteric osteotomy can also be drawn in. The second tracing is then put on top of the first, with the osteotomy reduced, and a decision can be made about lateralization of the distal fragment. It is possible to see the amount by which the blade plate needs to protrude from the proximal fragment to allow for this lateralization. The length of the blade of the blade plate can then be measured. The more lateral the distal fragment, the greater the eventual length of the leg, although, if the displacement is too great (bearing in mind that there will also be extension and alterations of rotation, resulting in an apparent fit of the osteotomy surfaces on the tracing that is artificially high), the solidity of fixation may be compromised.

Surgical technique

Image intensification is desirable. A long lateral incision is made, the capsule cleared anteriorly, and vastus lateralis split far enough down the femur to allow for the

insertion of a compression device at the bottom of the blade plate.

Vastus is elevated at the upper end anteriorly and the femur is cleared at the back at the level of the osteotomy and the wedge. The lesser trochanter is palpated with a fingertip from behind the femur and the position of its upper end marked. A drill can be inserted at 90° to the shaft and its position checked. An extracapsular and quite lateral trochanteric osteotomy is then made, leaving a soft tissue attachment at the front and back, which creates a pouch. Through the distal end of this osteotomy, a guidewire is inserted at 80° to the lateral cortex of the shaft. The capsule is opened and, if planning has shown that the blade needs to be quite inferior in the head, the head/neck junction inferiorly is defined. Synovium must be removed with rongeurs. A guidewire is inserted anterior to the neck, to show the amount of neck anteversion, and a definitive guidewire is inserted parallel to the first wire looked at from the front and to the second wire in the anteversion sense. It is convenient to put this guidewire through the upper part of the trochanteric bed. The previous wires are removed and the entry position for the seating chisel suitably prepared.

As the trochanter is a posterior structure, the entry point is at the anterior edge of the trochanteric bed. The drill is inserted parallel to the definitive wire and its position checked. The length of the blade of the blade plate can also be confirmed at this stage. The hip is now flexed and the knee put on some form of soft support while the anterior coverage of the head is inspected directly. To make sure that this degree of extension is produced by the osteotomy, it is necessary to put the guide of the seating chisel at 130° and to insert the seating chisel (Fig. 2.14a) with the plate part of the guide in a horizontal plane. If the seating chisel is simply inserted in a vertical plane, the planned degree of correction does not necessarily happen when the blade of the blade plate is put up against the lateral femoral cortex.

As with any intertrochanteric osteotomy, it may be necessary to drill some way into the femur before inserting the seating chisel. It is also important to withdraw the chisel repeatedly during insertion to avoid it jamming. It is vital to make absolutely sure that the lateral portion of the seating chisel track is so well defined that the blade of the blade plate cannot possibly go into a 'false passage'; omission of this point can easily

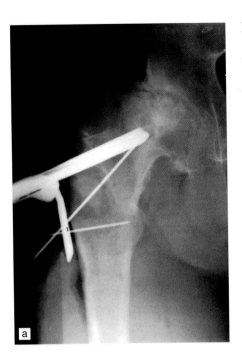

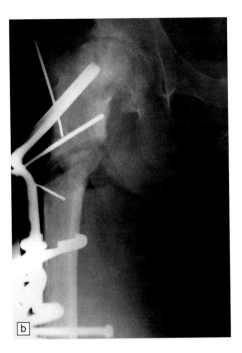

Figure 2.14 –
(a) Intraoperative radiograph of valgus extension osteotomy in a 27-year-old man with avascular necrosis and collapse secondary to steroid therapy for a head injury. Guidewires to indicate the level of the lesser trochanter and the angle of neck anteversion are seen and the seating chisel is in situ.

(b) The osteotomy has been made and displaced. The opening of the hip superiorly can be seen. The two wires were to mark rotation. This particular patient still has satisfactory function 14 years later.

cause complete failure. If it is inconvenient or impossible to insert the blade plate before completing the ITO, failure to ensure that the blade plate can enter the defined seating chisel track easily can entirely vitiate the operation. As a precaution, it is best to leave the definitive guidewire in place until the last possible moment. Fortunately, in most cases the blade plate can be partially inserted before making the osteotomy, while the femur is still in one piece. Assuming that this has been done, a wedge is marked distally with a 30° angle anteroposteriorly and an angle equivalent to the degree of extension laterally. The osteotomy is then made, producing what is a very large wedge, in most cases. If correctly made, the residue of the lesser trochanter (some will have been removed with the wedge) is still present on the distal fragment, increasing the osteotomy contact area. The distal fragment is then withdrawn from the wound and the psoas tendon taken off the lesser trochanter. The blade plate is impacted until it protrudes the planned amount. The excised wedge is cut in two and part of it is inserted under the knuckle of the blade plate. A long untapped cortical screw is inserted through the upper hole of the plate, and the hole in the piece of graft needs to be overdrilled. The leg is extended and brought to neutral rotation, some traction is applied and the osteotomy reduced (Fig. 2.14b).

It is necessary to make sure that there are no projections from the lateral surface of the femur underneath the necessary position for the plate or it will

not sit correctly. It is usually necessary to put in a spike or lever into the front of the osteotomy to prevent the distal fragment slipping backwards. After a little work, the osteotomy can usually be made to fit extremely well. The compression device is then applied and the blade screwed to the shaft. As a result of the oblique direction of the osteotomy surfaces, care is required to avoid displacement when the compression is applied. Very solid fixation should be achievable. The remainder of the wedge is then placed in the trochanteric pouch (see Fig. 2.13). This piece of graft can, if necessary, be held temporarily in position with a wire, while the trochanteric fragment is sutured to vastus lateralis over the knuckle of the plate. The wedge tends to maintain the abductor lever arm, which would otherwise, at least in theory, be somewhat reduced. The transfixion wire, if used, is removed.

Postoperatively, the patient can be got up quite early and assisted active exercises are started. The patient should be instructed in a planned sequence of exercises, including flexion, abduction, and, particularly, adduction. After 30° of valgus, the leg may tend to be held in a slightly abducted position, and it is important to ask the patient to overcome this, so that the planned alteration in hip mechanics can take place. Although shadow walking with controlled, but very slight, weight-bearing is certainly theoretically desirable, this is often difficult to achieve and it is probably safest to have the patient non-weight-bearing for the first 6 weeks. Originally,

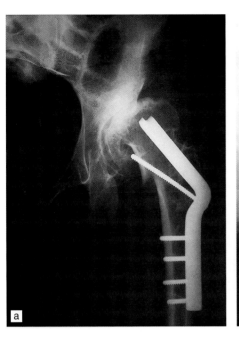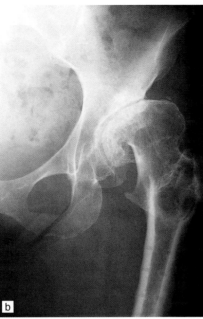

Figure 2.15 – *Showing the slow biological response to valgus extension osteotomy that is sometimes seen. (a) The initial postoperative appearance in this 39-year old woman was disappointing, but (b) cartilage gradually appeared together with symptomatic relief, as seen in this radiograph at 3 years. An additional shelf procedure might have been appropriate in this case, but the patient's symptoms were too slight to justify it.*

very long periods of restricted weight-bearing were recommended and, in theory, this should increase the chance of cartilage regeneration; such long periods are not, however, practicable and it does not seem sensible to advise patients deliberately to restrict weight-bearing beyond 3 months. The prolonged rehabilitation period, compared with replacement, is one of the drawbacks of most hip osteotomies.

In the days of uncontrolled intertrochanteric osteotomies of the McMurray type, it used to be said that it was possible to tell immediately whether the operation had been successful in terms of pain relief. This is certainly not the case for VEO. The operation is fairly complex; the hip is put in a completely different position, and is usually initially held rather stiffly. Whether the operation has achieved the desired pain relief gradually becomes apparent only over a number of weeks, and sometimes months (Fig. 2.15).

Variants
The description above relates to how the operation may be carried out using quite limited hip screening and with fixation by fixed angle-blade plates. If more extensive image intensification is used, it may not be necessary to open the hip; however, it is possible that the capsulotomy necessary in the described method has some biological effect, for example, in terms of the avoidance of raised postoperative intracapsular pressure. The seating chisel and fixed angle-blade plate technique, formerly widely

used in fracture fixation, has now been to some degree supplanted. Nevertheless, the system has considerable advantages. The blade in the head is, unlike a screw, rotationally stable as far as the extension angle is concerned. This does mean that, provided the seating chisel is correctly inserted, the correction at the osteotomy is bound to be correct. It is not possible to quantify the effects of psoas tenotomy and the elevation of the abductors. The long-term results of the procedure, quoted briefly earlier, include these two elements and, without the trochanteric elevation, the insertion of the abductors would be unfavourable in many cases after a substantial valgus osteotomy. The description given here also includes the use of a separate compression device. This is necessary even in the presence of a DCP plate, because the shaft has to move a significant distance along the blade of the blade plate to achieve proper compression with a large oblique wedge osteotomy, and the excursion allowed by the ovality of the DCP holes would be insufficient for this. The DCP holes are, therefore, simply used as a supplementary compression device.

VEO and later total hip replacement
Although VEO does make subsequent total hip replacement, when required, more difficult, the fact that the corrections at the osteotomy are of an angular nature means, in fact, that a standard type of femoral component can be inserted with no particular difficulty. The

33

difficulties of total hip replacement after earlier osteotomy are more commonly associated with the older types of McMurray osteotomy, in which there was medial displacement of the distal fragment, often to an extreme degree. In such cases, an excessively valgus position is necessary for the stem, or a stem with very little offset, or in extreme cases it may even be necessary to carry the resection level down to the actual level of the osteotomy itself – something that is clearly very undesirable. This is not the case with a VEO. Although the angular changes may be quite considerable, the upper femur is still in line, making femoral preparation relatively straightforward.

Varus and/or derotation osteotomy

Careful planning is still needed, but this is much easier than in VEO. Fixation is by an offset 90° blade plate. The osteotomy is at the same level as the upper cut of the VEO wedge (see Fig 1.4). A trochanteric osteotomy is not usually required. The order of insertion of guidewires is as for a VEO. A wedge does not need to be excised; after insertion of the blade plate, strong compression ensures a degree of impaction, which will be sufficient for sound fixation, union, and subsequent full remodelling. If the osteotomy has been done for derotation, then Kirschner wires should be inserted above and below the osteotomy before completing it at the planned angle. If this step is omitted, it is all too easy to produce inadequate correction.

Trochanteric osteotomy for AVN

General comments

The principle of osteotomy for early AVN, as already described, is simply to rotate the affected segment out of the weight-bearing zone. This can be done by rotating the femoral head and neck either around the axis of the femoral neck, as in the osteotomy of Sugioka, or around the normal transverse flexion/extension axis of the hips (Willert), as already referred to. The former procedure is a logical one and has the merit of allowing, at least in principle, an extremely large correction – greater than that achieved by an intertrochanteric osteotomy. Nevertheless, the procedure is particularly difficult and, although in the hands of the originator the results have been very good, others have not always been able to reproduce these results. Flexion intertrochanteric osteotomy is, therefore, recommended as the procedure when needed for AVN.

Flexion osteotomy

This is as for varus osteotomy with certain special additional points. The main problem to overcome is that the hip does not necessarily go easily into the necessary hyperextended position. To overcome this, it is necessary to carry out as extensive a capsulotomy as possible, and the leg itself should be flexed upwards off the table to give the planned flexion before, or immediately after, making the ITO. With the leg still up in this position, and with the planned flexion correction, the hip itself is then in neutral position, so that the osteotomy lies relatively comfortably while the blade plate is inserted and compression applied. When the leg is brought down on to the table, the hip rotates backwards, extending to the planned degree. If attempts are made to extend the hip before fixing the osteotomy, there will be considerable difficulties. Postoperatively, exercises are required to discourage a flexion deformity, and it may be necessary for the patient to be on his or her side or to spend periods in a prone position.

Variants

The above technique only allows flexion of up to 30°. If attempts are made to produce a greater angle, then a flexion deformity in the hip subsequently results. By carrying out a laterally placed trochanteric osteotomy as described above for VEO, an increase of up to about 40° in the correction can be achieved if necessary. This is important for two reasons. First, a circumferential capsulotomy is possible; second, after the leg is brought down to neutral and the hip hyperextends, the abductors are still in their normal neutral position. It is also possible, as Willert has done for many years, to curette out and graft the necrotic segment by making a small fenestration in the anterior aspect of the femoral neck. This is best done after the blade of the blade plate has been inserted; if done earlier, it may be difficult to achieve adequate seating. Alternatively, a vascularized graft can be added simultaneously. Both these techniques have theoretical attractions, but, unfortunately, there is no clear evidence about whether they are strictly necessary. An intertrochanteric osteotomy alone, with appropriate indications can certainly be effective.

Further reading

Henry AK. *Extensile Exposure*, 2nd edn. Edinburgh: Churchill Livingstone, 1973.

Klaue K, Wallin A, Ganz R. CT evaluation of coverage and congruency of the hip prior to osteotomy. *Clin Orthop Rel Res* 1988; 232: 15–25.

Ganz R, Klaue K, Vinh TS, Mast JW. A new periacetabular osteotomy for the treatment of hip dysplasias. Technique and preliminary results. *Clin Orthop Rel Res* 1988; 232: 23–36.

Tönnis D, Behrens K, Tscharani F. A modified technique of the triple pelvic osteotomy: early results. *J Pediatr Orthop* 1981; 1: 241–9.

Fernandez DL, Isler B, Müller ME. Chiari's osteotomy. A note on technique. *Clin Orthop Rel Res* 1984; 185: 53–8.

Nishina T, Saito S, Ohzono K *et al.* Chiari pelvic osteotomy for osteoarthritis. The influence of the torn and detached acetabular labrum. *J Bone Joint Surg* 1990; 72: 765–9.

Staheli T, Chew DE. Slotted acetabular augmentation in childhood and adolescence. *J Pediatr Orthop* 1992; 12: 569–80.

Bombelli R. Structure and function in normal and abnormal hips. In: *How to Rescue Jeopardized Hips*. Berlin: Springer-Verlag, 1993.

CHAPTER 3

The young adult: replacement arthroplasty, with notes on arthroscopy and arthrodesis

M. D. Northmore-Ball

As in the previous chapter, it is assumed that it has been decided to carry out a particular procedure; where appropriate, further discussions of indications and limitations are given.

Resurfacing

The theoretical attraction of resurfacing is very clear and has been for a long time. In most cases of degenerative hip disease, at least in the presence of anatomy that is not grossly disturbed, all that is required in principle is to replace the damaged bearing surfaces. To do more than this destroys normal material which, particularly in the femoral head and upper femur, becomes no longer available for later surgery. The two fundamental difficulties in resurfacing are also very apparent, namely: the small space available for the implants and fixative material, and the higher frictional resistance caused by the large radius in comparison with total hip replacement. Charnley dismissed resurfacing as impracticable very early on for the latter reason and it could very well be argued that subsequent events have proved him right. When the difficulties sometimes associated with revisions of total hip replacements became obvious, the advantages of resurfacing (often called 'double cups') was seized upon and, in the later 1970s and early 1980s, a considerable number of designs were formulated and used. The early results at that time were very good and it seemed that resurfacing might supplant total replacement as the standard treatment for osteoarthritis.

Failure of the procedure began, however, to be seen and it soon became obvious that the results were very poor. The rates of early loosening and other problems, such as subcapital fractures, were quite unacceptably high. In addition, it was found that revision to total replacement was often quite difficult as a result of loss of acetabular bone stock, both at the time of the initial operation and resulting from the loosening process. As a result of these problems, resurfacing was abandoned as rapidly, and almost as universally, as it had been taken up in the first place. For some years, only two implants were left: those of Wagner (Fig. 3.1) and those of

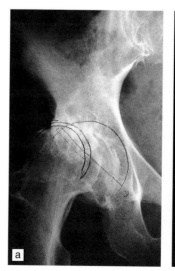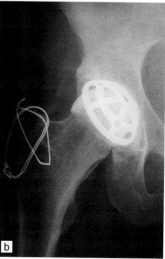

Figure 3.1 – *Wagner resurfacing using a cemented high-density polyethylene (HDP) socket with perforated metal back and cemented ceramic femoral component.*

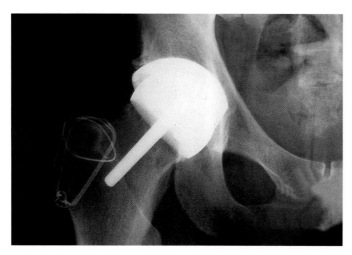

Figure 3.2 – *Beuchel-Pappas, cementless, nitrided, titanium/HDP resurfacing.*

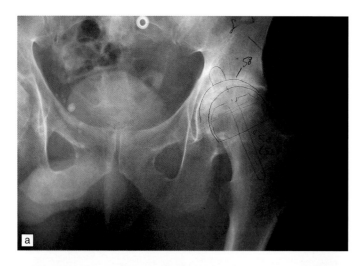

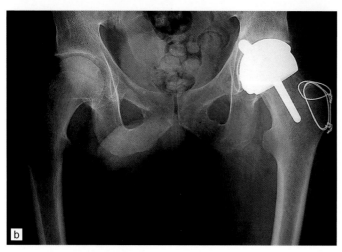

Figure 3.3 – *Planning drawing, and McMinn metal/metal resurfacing with a cementless hydroxyapatite-covered socket and cemented femoral component.*

Amstutz. A few other designs, such as the Beuchel-Pappas (Fig. 3.2) and, most recently, the metal-to-metal McMinn (Fig. 3.3), and its Cormet 2000 and Birmingham Hip Resurfacing (BHR) (Fig. 3.4) variants, have become available, but at the time of writing the most widely held view about resurfacing is that it is something that has been tried in the past and found not to work; although possibly better than before, it still remains very experimental.

Difficulties, solutions, and unresolved problems

Femoral neck fracture
A high incidence of this was seen, particularly in the early Imperial College London Hospital (ICLH) implant. The possible causes have been:

- The use of a trochanteric osteotomy in the surgical approach. It seems, however, that, provided that a laterally placed, extracapsular, trochanteric osteotomy is used (see 'Surgical technique', below) rather than the much deeper osteotomy used in the classic Charnley approach, this possible cause of subcapital femoral neck fracture is eliminated.

- Notching of the upper surface of the femoral neck when the femoral head is reamed and the femoral cup implanted. This potential cause is quite easily eliminated as soon as its possibility is realized.

- Avascular necrosis (AVN) of the femoral head. It is still not entirely clear whether this commonly comes about as a primary event. In the Wagner procedure, care is taken to preserve the posterior part of the head/neck junction in an attempt to retain the blood supply coming up on the outside of the femoral neck in this region. The Wagner technique also uses a Smith-Petersen approach, preserving all the muscular attachments to the upper femur, with their associated blood supply. However, when other approaches are used and no vessels around the outside of the femoral neck are in continuity, the prepared surface of the femoral head still bleeds, as originally pointed out by Freeman.

- Lysis from whatever cause (but probably in considerable measure associated with wear products) can gradually cause obvious thinning of the femoral neck on the radiograph. Meanwhile the patient may continue to have good function. Eventually, however, the residual neck becomes too thin and suddenly

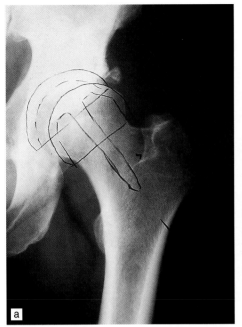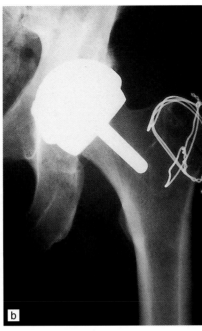

Figure 3.4 – *(a) Pre- and (b) postoperative appearances with the most recent BHR resurfacing in a 40-year-old farmer.*

breaks. It is in an attempt to prevent this problem that some resurfacing designs have incorporated a short stem to cross and splint the head/neck junction. Such a stem, however, can only delay a failure through this cause and its presence is not necessarily desirable.

It can be seen that two of the four causes of subcapital fracture can be readily eliminated and only one (AVN), which may or may not occur to any significant degree, is intrinsic.

Loosening

Impingement
Early designs of resurfacing (Fig. 3.5) had a fully hemispherical acetabular component, the shape being derived from a standard type of hemispherical acetabular component for total hip replacement with the bearing surface taken out to an appropriate diameter. Unfortunately, this is likely to cause impingement between the retained femoral neck and the edge of the socket. The human acetabulum is, in fact, considerably less than a hemisphere and it is necessary to mimic this in the acetabular component in resurfacing. This feature was realized some time ago, notably by Freeman, and incorporated into a number of designs (Fig. 3.6). Surprisingly, however, simply testing of explanted specimens of some quite recent designs shows that impingement between the femoral neck and the edge of the

prosthetic socket has not been fully eliminated. It seems very likely that such impingement (analogous to impingement seen in captive sockets in total hip replacement) is one cause of loosening through repeated shock loading of the rim of the socket.

Poor initial fixation
Most early resurfacing designs used cement fixation as with total hip replacement. In the latter, there has been a cycle that has now almost come round full circle from cemented, through cementless, to a situation in which cemented fixation using better techniques is considered an entirely legitimate procedure. This cycle has not yet been completed with resurfacing, and the advances in 'cementology' that have been developed in total hip replacement have not yet been significantly applied. The addition of cement to an implant designed primarily to be fixed with an interference fit without cement, is not a good principle and is extremely unlikely to take the best advantage of the cement; the carefully prepared surfaces have to be altered in an ad hoc way to give room for the cement, and late insertion of the implant on to a bed of pressurized cement may well be impracticable. In the acetabulum also, the relatively large external diameter of the component may make proper cementation less easy.

Although it is not proposed that cement should necessarily be used for both components, it is clear that resurfacing has not in general had the advantages of modern thinking about the use of cement.

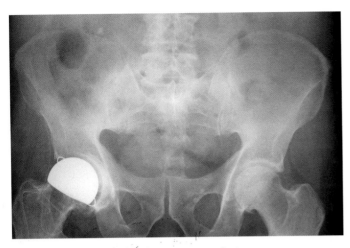

Figure 3.5 – *Early type of Wagner resurfacing.*

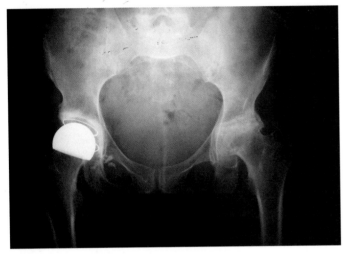

Figure 3.6 – *ICLH/Freeman resurfacing before the same procedure was done on the opposite hip. Inserted in 1984, this replacement is still functioning satisfactorily.*

Wear products

Early designs of resurfacing had high-density polyethylene (HDP) and metal as the bearing surfaces. The subsequent developments in bearing surfaces to reduce or eliminate HDP wear products has parri-passu (in parallel with) with bearing surface development in total hip replacement. Ceramic (see Fig. 3.1) and nitrided titanium against HDP (see Fig. 3.2) and metal-to-metal (see Figs. 3.3, 3.4) have been, or are, in use. All produce less debris, but none is without potential problems. A ceramic femoral shell can break (Fig. 3.7a), with the potential for large sharp dangerous fragments within the hip; a nitrided titanium surface can sometimes fragment, producing rapid wear and, although metal-to-metal has been used very successfully in total hip replacement, it has the potential disadvantage that, in order to retain the

carefully controlled equatorial tolerances, no distortion can be allowed and so the walls have to be comparatively thick. There is also the possibility of systemic toxicity and a lingering concern about late carcinogenesis, particularly because these implants may be inserted in young people and, if successful, be *in situ* for a very long period.

Component sizing and subsequent revision

Early designs of resurfacing reamed the acetabulum to as large a size as possible. As already indicated, this gave significant problems at conversion to total hip replacement. When this problem was appreciated, the tendency was to reduce the size of the femoral head instead. Conversion to total hip replacement of such a resurfacing should not be greatly different from primary total hip replacement (Fig. 3.7).

It will be seen that there is no theoretical reason why a very considerable improvement should not be made in all the causes of loosening.

Current situation

The above analysis shows that many of the problems associated with early failures in resurfacing, unsolved at the time that the procedure was largely abandoned, either have been solved or appear potentially capable of solution. Certainly, with suitable attention to design features, not only of the implant, but also of its insertion and fixation system, and using materials now under development, major improvements should be achievable. A design study for this is under way in the Unit for Joint Reconstruction, Oswestry, in association with the IRC in Biomedical Materials at Queen Mary and Westfield College, London. In a comparatively small personal series, carried out over a large number of years and using several different types of resurfacing implants, virtually all now obsolete, the author found a survival rate in terms of non-conversion to total hip replacement of 70% at 10 years (Fig. 3.8). Although this figure is extremely poor in relation to the survival rate in established types of total hip replacement, it seems certain that it can be very substantially improved with newer implants. In view of the fact that, with a proper design, revision would not be much different from primary total hip replacement, a tenable view is that not all that great an improvement in survival statistics would be required for resurfacing to become something of much wider applicability.

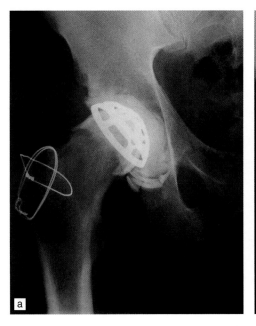

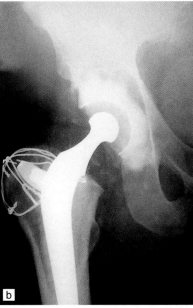

Figure 3.7 – *(a) Fracture of the ceramic femoral component of Wagner resurfacing. Large fragments are seen in the hip inferiorly. (b) In this late type of resurfacing in which the socket has not been enlarged, the radiograph after total hip replacement is virtually indistinguishable from a primary case.*

Surgical technique

As the technique is largely determined by the implant to be used, only very brief general comments are appropriate here. Adequate access is essential and this is considerably more difficult than in a total hip replacement, because the retained head tends to obscure the view of the acetabulum. The author uses a lateral transtrochanteric approach with the patient in the supine position, but a carefully developed posterior approach is

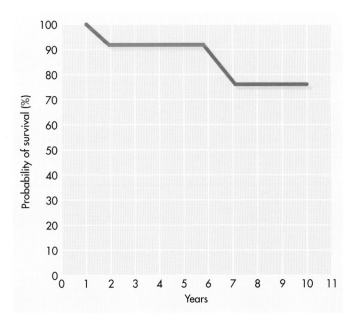

Figure 3.8 – *The author's personal survival curve for resurfacing in patients under the age of 50 years at the time of the operation.*

also suitable. If this approach is used, the gluteus maximus insertion on to the linea aspera has to be tagged and divided, a complete capsulotomy done, and sufficient soft tissue elevation carried out to allow the femoral head to be displaced anterosuperiorly during acetabular preparation.

If a transtrochanteric approach is used, it is important to avoid allowing the osteotomy to run deeply at the upper end. This is best done by beginning the osteotomy a few millimetres distal to the vastus ridge. A chevron osteotomy made with a power saw can be carried out almost parallel to the lateral cortex of the greater trochanter. This avoids any possibility of damage to the upper surface of the femoral neck. If, however, it is too lateral, it will be very thin posteriorly, none of the external rotators will be removed with it, and there will be some concern about fragmentation. An instrument, such as a Moynihan clamp, can be put down intracapsularly, and a very good view is obtained if the superior capsule is elevated with the trochanter. The exposure also has to be somewhat more developed anteriorly and the inferomedial capsule divided before dislocation. After dislocation, the femoral head then needs to be mobilized to bring it right out of the wound laterally, in order to enable acetabular access in the presence of the retained head. With a little work, a good view of both sides of the joint simultaneously can be achieved. *Sizing* will have been done from the planning, but may or not prove correct, owing to variability in radiographic magnification. It may well be necessary to ream the acetabulum up to what appears to be the right size, and then to see whether the femoral head can be taken down to the appropriate size. If not, a decision has to be made about whether to enlarge the acetabulum or to reduce the head further. Further reduction of the head will, however, be possible only if great care has been taken in centring the femoral head reaming in relation to the femoral neck. If this has been rather medial, it may be difficult to avoid notching of the femoral neck laterally when the diameter is decreased. Over-reaming on the medial side (see Fig. 3.1) does not appear to be so important.

Similarly, it is important to note that the normal femoral head overhangs the neck posteriorly to a considerable extent. The *orientation* of the femoral component will be largely (though not completely, especially if a non-stemmed component system is used) determined by the geometry of the upper femur, and in particular the degree of anteversion. It is necessary to be able to carry out a trial reduction to determine the optimum orientation for the acetabular component. If (as has been practised in the past) the acetabulum is put in in relation to fixed landmarks, as in a standard total hip replacement, impingement and/or instability may result. During *component* implantation, if an interference-fit, cementless, acetabular component is used, the external diameters of the reamers need be carefully checked and probably measured intraoperatively (Fig. 3.9). Reamers by no means necessarily ream to their given dimension and, unless this is checked, it may be found difficult or impossible to impact the acetabular component.

If the femoral component is based on a design originally intended for cementless fixation, there is likely to be very little room for the cement and low-viscosity cement, poured into the implant and used at a very early stage, is essential, or it is impossible to impact the component. This system has the theoretical disadvantage of producing very uneven pressurization of the cement with low pressure around the skirt. A better system is probably first to wash and dry the prepared head, and then to pressurize cement directly into it (if necessary, simply by covering it in glove rubber and a swab, which is then squeezed – some more sophisticated system is preferable); in this technique, it must first be clearly established that the component goes fully home easily before cementation, with an adequate gap for cement egress. Finally, if wires are used for trochanteric re-attachment, these should be inserted before putting on

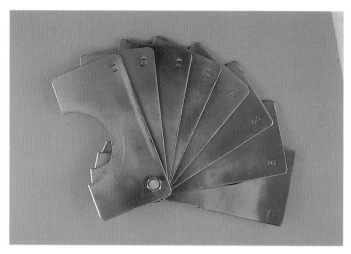

Figure 3.9 – *Set of gauges for accurate measurement of the dimensions of acetabular reamers.*

the femoral component. If a vertical wire is used, emerging from somewhere near the digital fossa, there could be a danger of scratching the femoral component. Post-operatively, the patient should certainly be kept in bed for a week, possibly 2 weeks, and then be allowed up strictly non-weight-bearing until 6 weeks from operation, to give the maximum possible chance of osseointegration.

Total replacement

This subject is thoroughly discussed in Section II and only restricted comments are appropriate here.

If the hip has not been operated on before and the morphology is not particularly abnormal, no special remarks apply, except that more than the customary care should be devoted to it. It should be carried out by the surgeon with the greatest experience available. Total hip replacement by a surgeon who is comparatively new to it, or under supervision, should be restricted to elderly patients because a hip replacement in a young person is likely to have more than the usual demands made on it, and there is also no question of 'the implant outliving the patient'. The procedure should not, therefore, be hurried and should be carried out with every possible attention to detail. Furthermore, total replacement in the younger age group, especially if felt to be indicated only after the exclusion of other possible measures of treatment, is likely to be carried out in the presence of very significant developmental structural abnormalities and/or scarring from previous surgery. As this type of problem frequently occurs in patients of a more conventional age for total hip replacement, the reader is referred to Chapter 7 for a full discussion of the subject; only selected information is given here.

Planning

As in revision surgery, careful thought at this stage can avoid numerous later problems. The socket should be drawn in at as near to a true anatomical position as possible. A good estimate can be made of whether the socket will be adequately covered or whether grafting, probably from the femoral head, will be needed. If the condition is bilateral and the femoral heads are spherical, quite a good estimate of the anteroposterior (AP) dimension of the acetabulum, and therefore of the socket size, can be obtained by measuring the diameter of the opposite femoral head, allowing for articular cartilage thickness with a magnification-adjusted ruler. It is surprising how whose diameters are very obviously such that the antero-posterior diameter of the socket of the acetabulum could in no way accommodate them. If the acetabulum is displaced extremely superolaterally, the coverage of the floor by osteophytes and its probable initial appearance on exposure should be assessed to avoid surprises. This avoids any possibility of the socket being placed on the osteophytes rather than down deep on the true floor.

In cases of previous fracture dislocation, a computed tomography (CT) scan is useful to determine any wall defects, particularly posterosuperiorly. If such defects are present, it may be appropriate to have reinforcement rings available. A line should then be drawn across the pelvis at the level of a convenient landmark, e.g. the tear-drops, upper or lower limits of the obturator foramina, or the bottom of the ischial tuberosities, and the position of the lesser trochanters measured (allowing for their possible different appearance on the two sides as a result of alterations of femoral rotation), to give an estimate of the true shortening; this should confirm the distance previously measured clinically. The height necessary for the centre of the femoral component to compensate for this shortening can be marked, the position of the centre of the acetabulum having already been decided on, at least provisionally.

Usually, the complete leg length difference can be made up. In cases of high CDH, however, it is unlikely to be either possible or safe to bring the femur down by more than about 4 cm. This is mentioned again later.

Frequently, a narrower or straighter stem, such as a reduced offset (for example, 35 mm) or CDH stem, is indicated. To get the component down to the right level, it may look as if femoral cortex should be reamed using powered instruments. If so, the operating room staff can be forewarned. If planning shows that the femoral component may have to be sunk a long way into the femur, it may be better to decide to place the socket a few millimetres higher. It must, however, always be very close to the true acetabulum. Generally speaking, plates and other metal fixation devices should always be removed at a first operation some weeks before total hip replacement (Fig. 3.10), so that they are no longer present at this planning stage. However, occasionally, paediatric femoral plates used for femoral osteotomy can be so deeply embedded in the femur that they can be left alone, provided that they are sufficiently distal (Fig. 3.11).

In terms of the surgical approach, many factors apart from the radiographic appearances influence this; these are discussed at several points in this book. If a cement-less stem is to be used, the greater trochanter must be retained, but otherwise, if in doubt and particularly if the anatomy is very distorted, the use of a transtrochanteric approach (see Fig. 3.10) is hardly ever regretted. In addition, it may very well be the case that, because of the dysplasia or dislocation itself, or of a previous upper femoral osteotomy, the greater trochanter may be medially displaced (as the result of an old varus osteotomy, for example) or markedly posterior; in extreme cases it is barely apparent on the AP radiographs. In these circumstances, it is seen on the lateral view or very obviously on a CT scan, if taken. In these cases, part of the replacement should be to correct the mechanics by putting the greater trochanter in an appropriate position to restore the abductor lever arm (Fig. 3.12). In addition, if an abnormally medial trochanter is left in this position from a varus osteotomy, it is very seriously eroded in the femoral reaming process (Fig. 3.13).

Type of total hip replacement

This subject is discussed in Chapter 6, so only brief comments are appropriate here. In older age groups, the main distinctions from total hip replacement are not only that the hip must have a high likelihood of long-lasting survival, despite the large loads that will be put on it, but also that the necessity for eventual revision is a

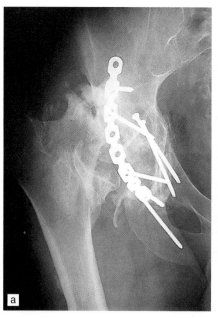

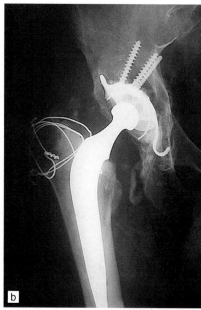

Figure 3.10 – *Radiographs of the right hip of a 24-year-old man with multiple injuries, including fracture dislocation of the right hip. (a) Radiograph of right hip at the time of referral. There was a partial sciatic nerve palsy. This and the other injuries contra-indicated treatment by arthrodesis, which would otherwise have been correct. (b) The plate and all the screws were first removed and the hip replacement, using autografting of the socket, was carried out as a second procedure.*

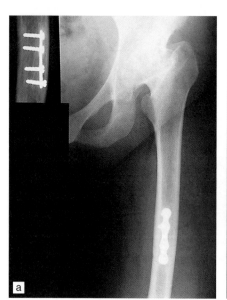

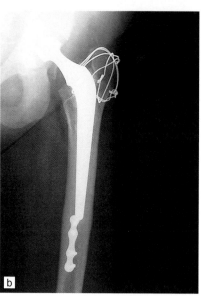

Figure 3.11 – *(a, and inset) Small plate used for childhood derotation osteotomy, which had become intramedullary; removal would have meant fenestrating the femur. (b) A specially shortened stem was prepared, although, in fact, this was not required.*

certainty, so a later revision must be planned from the outset. However, to put too great an emphasis on the second of these is clearly wrong; this was the situation in the not-too-distant past, with advocacy for easily revisable, smooth-surfaced, cementless implants in this age group; the effect of this was often that revision was necessary far too early. On the other hand, certain types of hip used, although producing satisfactory longevity, have been almost unrevisable; among these are those with very rough surfaces, such as the original Madréporique.

Returning to longevity, the best type of hip is one that has the smallest production of particulate debris (notably from the articulating surfaces, but also from intracomponent movement in modular systems), with the best possible bone-implant junctions, particularly at the exposed edges (making the interface more resistant to particle invasion); at the same time it must be subsequently revisable. The best combinations of bearing material and the best fixation design for achieving these objectives are still controversial, with wide differences of well-informed opinion. Although there are sound arguments for newer bearing combinations, such as HDP on ceramic, and for fixation by hydroxyapatite, both of these have also produced new problems (such as ceramic head fracture and increased wear through release of hydroxyapatite particles). Although the earlier

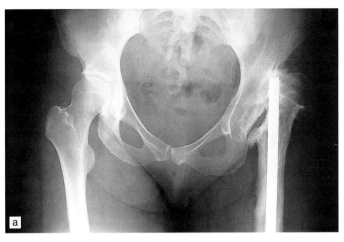
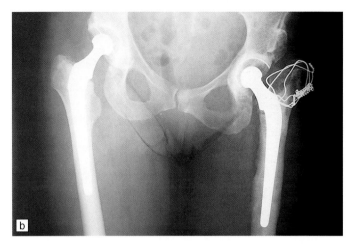

Figure 3.12 – *A 39-year-old woman with old, unreduced congenital displacement of the hip (CDH) and a nailed femoral shaft fracture after a riding accident. (a) Radiograph at referral; (b) 9-year film. The eccentricity of the femoral head within the wire marker is caused by the extra thickness of plastic in the weight-bearing zone in this special CDH ('offset bore') component. The trochanter was moved laterally from a posterior position, giving a substantial lever arm.*

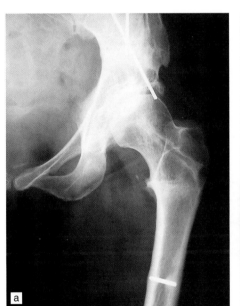
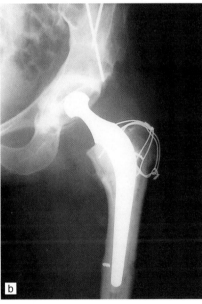

Figure 3.13 – *(a) A patient with an old varus osteotomy, giving a very medial position for the trochanter. (b) At the total hip replacement, the trochanter was lateralized to a more functional position.*

(and too often quoted) papers on the results of cemented total hip replacement in young people gave very bad results, more recent studies, often using traditional metal against HDP-bearing surfaces and cemented fixation, have given remarkably good long-term results. Considerable caution needs to be exercised and little regret should be felt if it proves necessary to use these combinations in a young person, even today, provided that the procedure is done extremely carefully.

The author's preference is to use a Freeman cementless total hip replacement (Fig. 3.14) when the anatomy is not too disorganized. The stem in this implant has proximal hydroxyapatite coating, and torsional loads are transmitted by retention of the femoral neck and by longitudinal ridges. The distal part is quite steeply tapered and polished. A Zirconia ceramic modular with a 28-mm diameter head is available. Migration studies and statistics for survival [1] of this implant appear to be very favourable and the stem is certainly revision-friendly, as a result of retention of the femoral neck and the largely virgin condition of the femoral shaft. The stem can be used with a superolateral flanged socket. This socket has a central spigot, which ensures a certain orientation; unlike some other spherical press-fit sockets, it has two anti-rotational, radially directed fins or flanges,

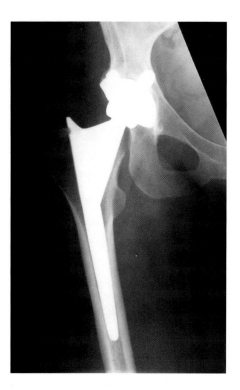

Figure 3.14 – *The Freeman cementless total hip replacement (see the text).*

and is coated in hydroxyapatite around the periphery, although not centrally.

Insertion technique for Freeman cementless total hip replacement

Any approach can be used that preserves the greater trochanter and allows a straight instrument to be passed down the femur from the neighbourhood of the piriform fossa. If the supine position is used (e.g. with a transgluteal approach), then a sandbag is necessary to tilt the patient slightly and make the femur somewhat more horizontal after hip dislocation, in view of the length and relative complexity of the instrumentation used in the femur. A straight rod is passed first down the femur from the pyriformis fossa and the canal is reamed by hand with a straight fluted reamer. Tapered reamers are then used, which need power and are of exactly the same shape as the stem. The apex, front, and back of the head are then cut off and a slot is cut through the residuum of the head and into the femoral neck; its depth is measured by an outrigger registering with the medial, outside surface of the neck. A trial femoral stem is then inserted and the acetabulum reamed spherically to fit one of four sizes (diameters from 46 mm up to 58 mm) of a special acetabular trial, which can subsequently be articulated with the femoral trial and its modular head neck. The best position for the acetabular component is then established, a particular feature being

that the angle of anteversion can be defined accurately by reference to a groove on the trial head, and the acetabular trial, which is itself modular, can be locked in position. The hip is then dislocated and the central hole for the spigot on the acetabular component can be drilled, because it is certain that the real socket goes exactly into this planned position. The external diameter of the socket is the same as the nominal size of the last reamer, an interference fit not being a feature. The modular socket is then impacted and the HDP insert put in, followed by insertion of the stem. As a result of the preservation of the femoral neck, some care has to be taken to ensure that osteophytes are fully removed so that impingement does not occur, particularly with the hip flexed to 90° and internally rotated.

As an example of a more anatomically distorted case, the surgical technique for total hip replacement in old CDH is discussed. As stated, a transtrochanteric approach, although not mandatory, is strongly recommended. A very carefully executed posterior approach and various forms of lateral approach that preserve the vastogluteal sling can be used; the commonly performed, purely soft tissue, transgluteal approaches are, however, very unlikely to be adequate if the case is of any severity.

Previous incisions dating from childhood surgery can usually be ignored. The incision through the skin and later the fascia runs along the front of the shaft of the femur to about four fingers' breadth above the estimated top of the trochanter, then curving quite steeply backwards to a level well posterior to the greater trochanter. A marker stitch in this greatly facilitates later closure. After opening the fascia lata, it is frequently found that strong adhesions lateral to vastus lateralis have to be divided by sharp dissection before the posterior flap can be properly mobilized. At the upper end, the fascia may need to be taken off gluteus medius by sharp dissection while the medius/maximus interval is carefully defined. Although, in normal cases, the leading edge of medius can be stripped by blunt dissection, it is often best to define it in a more formal fashion in these cases. The small size, peculiar shape, and posterior position of the trochanter, together with an abnormal, virtually coronal direction of the leading edge of medius, are then noticed. Careful extracapsular clearance has to be done and, running from laterally to medially, it should be possible to elevate the psoas tendon and iliacus from the capsule, and 'climb' quite steeply upwards (assuming that the patient is in a supine position) on to the anterior column of the acetabulum; a Homan lever can then be placed there. The hip can be flexed to some degree during this dissection. The trochanteric osteotomy is best done with a saw.

If it looks as if the trochanter is going to need simply to go back in the same place or be moved distally and laterally, then a chevron made with a saw is satisfactory. If, however, it looks as if the trochanter will need to be moved somewhat anteriorly, a flat osteotomy may be easier, because a new bed can be created (in theory, a cylindrical osteotomy would be best, if it could be accurately fashioned). After trochanteric mobilization and dislocation, the femoral head can be prepared as a bone graft if necessary. Its surface is scarified and a suitably shaped piece cut from its superomedial section with a saw. The remainder of the head is then removed and the region of the true acetabulum properly identified. It is deep and distal and may at first appear almost non-existent. The anterior wall is very rudimentary and, if some true floor is visible after the teardrop has been identified and a retractor put in, it is largely covered, either by osteophytes or by the lateral cortex of the ischium, which protrudes a long way anteriorly.

Preparation needs to start with gouges or osteotomes before an appropriate centring position for a small reamer (e.g. 36 mm) can be established. This reamer needs to be cautiously taken down to the quadrilateral plate, with bone impacted using a punch ahead of the reamer superomedially where it is often extremely porotic,

to avoid too much loss. There will be virtually nothing to ream anteriorly and it is necessary deliberately to make the reamer cut posteriorly. It will usually be possible to ream to 40 mm, in which case a socket designed for CDH use should be implantable (in the current Charnley system, this would consist of a CDH offset-bore socket, the external diameter of which, without the flange, is 36 mm). Once an appropriate position is found, it should be possible to see whether the acetabulum has to be grafted. If the socket is fully covered (see Fig. 3.12b), then clearly this is not necessary. However, grafting should be employed, even if the lack of cover is very slight (Fig. 3.15), in view of the near certainty that a revision will eventually be needed.

The easiest way to fix the graft is to put the matching, previously articular surfaces together after scarification, and this is certainly a perfectly acceptable technique. However, more certain bony union of the graft is likely to result if the head is turned around so that the cancellous surface is medial. Work is needed to produce an adequate fit and bone mush must be put in any residual gaps. Insertion of the screws is, however, considerably easier because there is a cortical surface underneath the head. With the cortical surfaces together, there is some danger that the screws will hold the surfaces slightly apart because it may not be possible to 'lag' them. After the graft has been solidly fixed (Fig. 3.16), the acetabulum should be re-reamed so that the distal surface of the graft matches that of the reamed socket. The socket is then inserted in at about 10° of

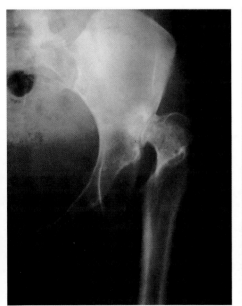
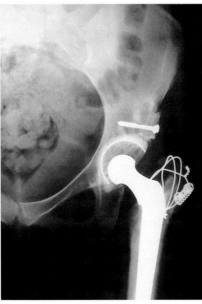

Figure 3.15 – *Total hip replacement for old, unreduced CDH (same socket as in Figs 3.12b and 3.16). Autografting of the socket is mainly to retain bone stock for subsequent revision in this 25-year-old woman.*

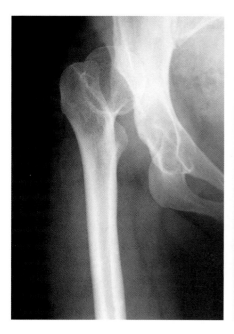 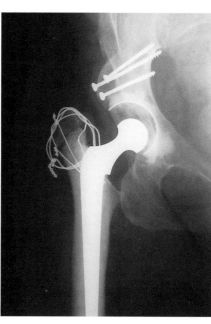

Figure 3.16 – *In this case of CDH, the acetabular roof is seriously deficient and a solidly fixed head autograft, capable of bearing load, is essential.*

anteversion. Assuming that cement is used, the pressurizers available to date are seldom sufficiently small to be used in this situation. A largely cancellous surface, however, favours cementation. Pulsed lavage should be used, but care is needed to avoid washing any mush out from between the graft and the acetabulum superiorly.

The femur is then reamed using rotary reamers. It is very unlikely that the standard proprietary rasps are sufficient. The femur has to be shortened gradually, about 2 mm at a time, until the hip can be reduced. It is often necessary to repeat the use of the powered reamers, to allow the trial prosthesis to sink further with each cut. Moderate traction is entirely acceptable. The lengthening achieved is governed by the overall elasticity of the soft tissue and fascial structures in the hip and thigh. A sciatic palsy is always a concern and the patient should have been warned about this possibility preoperatively, although this is unlikely, on the assumption however that a very careful soft tissue dissection has been done at the outset, and provided that the lengthening is limited by the soft tissues as described, and that major other measures, such as extensive soft tissue releases around the upper end of the femur, and levers or skids to reduce the hip, are not used, this is unlikely. Preoperatively, the patient may also have had a degree of flexion deformity, and the relief achieved by the replacement tends to slacken the sciatic nerve. It is sometimes felt that only an extremely small amount of true lengthening is allowable, but this would commonly produce an

unsatisfactory clinical result which could itself be a cause of dissatisfaction. Furthermore, sciatic nerve palsy can occur even in total hip replacement carried out for straightforward osteoarthritis without any apparent intraoperative complication. The possibility would not, therefore, be entirely removed by a deliberate policy of minimal lengthening.

After definitive trial reduction and choice of stem, and again assuming that cement is to be used, it is necessary to be particularly sure that there is sufficient space around the stem for the cement. It is most important that the stem should not be a tight fit within the femur. The inner surface of the tube is almost entirely cortical and if, in addition to this potential weakness, there is metal/bone contact with an imperfect mantle, fixation may be inadequate. A cruciate wiring system is then inserted. It may be necessary to make indentations in the upper femur with a burr to accommodate these if the space is extremely small. The femur is plugged with either a small plug or, alternatively, vanes removed from one of the proprietary plugs (if of the vaned type) before insertion. If attempts are made to knock one of these vanes down a very narrow canal, the central part of the plug could be completely detached from the vanes. Before cementation, it may be desirable to create some indentations or longitudinal slots in the upper femur with a burr, to improve the fixation in a torsional sense, the femur being in many cases virtually circular. After reduction, the leg should be fully abducted. Adductor

48

tenotomy is sometimes needed, but more often, after an initial tight feeling, the leg will come out some considerable way as a result of stretching (and probably a degree of rupture) of the adductors. The trochanter is then reattached. In many cases, this is found to be surprisingly free from problems because the abductors have, in fact, been stretched by the displaced femoral head. If this is not the case, the trochanter must be mobilized by elevation of muscle from the lateral wall of the ilium.

It is best if the trochanter can be advanced to a slight degree so that its distal cortical rim can fit over the distal end of the trochanteric bed. Provided that a soundly executed wiring system (see Chapter 11 for a fuller description) is used, moderate tension on the reattachment is acceptable. The patient should, in any case, be kept in bed for at least 10 days postoperatively, to help osseointegration of the main components; the leg can be kept in some abduction during this time. If, however, it is necessary to abduct the leg markedly and the tension is very high, trochanteric separation will result.

Postoperatively, the patient should be kept in bed, as already stated, with appropriate anti-deep vein thrombosis measures, and then should be mobilized strictly non-weight-bearing until 6 weeks after surgery. For patients who are young and otherwise fit, this is seldom a problem and patients are perfectly happy to comply with this once the reasons are explained.

Variants

Rather than building up the roof of a deficient socket by superolateral grafting, it is possible deliberately to break the floor of the acetabulum (cotyloplasty), to autograft this area, and to cement in a socket in a rather medial position. The potential difficulty with this procedure is that the medialization of the socket is rather difficult to control and gross immediate failure of fixation with medial migration of the socket could occur in theory. In skilled hands, however, the procedure can certainly work effectively, and the medialization of the socket is favourable as far as hip loading is concerned.

If, in the conventional grafting technique described above, a graft is needed that occupies a major part of the weight-bearing zone, and particularly if it proves difficult to insert screws in a direction other than largely transverse, the reconstruction should be supplemented with either a roof reinforcement ring or a hooked ring. This is described more fully in Section III; in CDH, the procedure is simply a miniature version of that tech-

nique. A disadvantage of rings, however, is that, for any given outside diameter of cup, it is necessary to ream the acetabulum 4 mm larger. An example of the use of one of these rings in the case of a revision of a failed total hip replacement for CDH is shown in Figures 3.17 and 3.18.

If the trochanter is not osteotomized (e.g. in a posterior approach), shortening of the limb can be done by a femoral osteotomy. The osteotomy is fully displaced and the hip reduced with the stem in the upper, but outside the distal, section. The necessary degree of shortening in the femur can then be estimated and produced. The procedure has the merit that a rotational change can be made in the upper femur as well as shortening it. The osteotomy will, however, need to be fixed and an endosteal grafting technique used to prevent cement causing non-union of the osteotomy.

Cementless total hip replacement for CDH

Cementless total hip replacement, if desired, can readily be done in minor or moderate degrees of dysplasia when a proprietary implant can be used. In more severe degrees of dysplasia or frank CDH, the smallest available cementless implant is almost certainly too large. The choices are between using cemented fixation (as described above) and having a 'custom'-made cementless replacement. The latter has been done quite extensively using hydroxyapatite-coated components made by CAD-CAM.

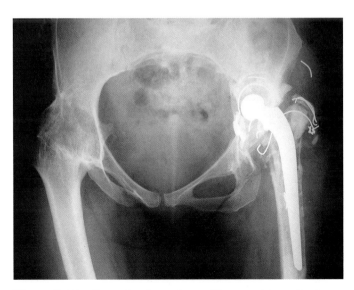

Figure 3.17 – *Example of massive grafting requiring a hook ring: radiograph at referral. The total hip replacement had originally been carried out for an unreduced congenital dislocation of the hip.*

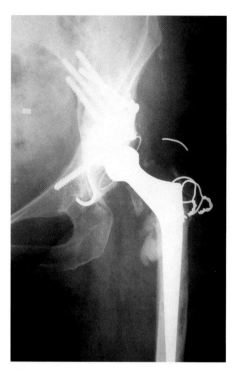

Figure 3.18 – *The same patient as in Fig. 3.17 after massive acetabular grafting supplemented by a Ganz hooked ring and endosteal grafting of the femur. Some cement leakage has occurred through the femur medially. The stem is the smallest one commercially available in the AO system for CDH. Revision in this case was done in two stages, with a long gap to allow for solid graft fixation before component reimplantation.*

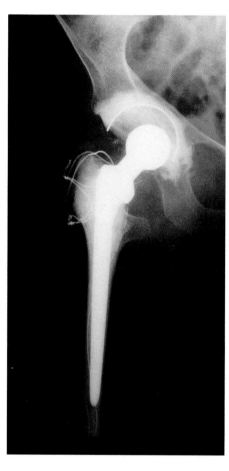

Figure 3.19 – *Total hip replacement in Still's disease (same case as in Fig. 1.19). The size of the specially made stem can be gauged from the fact that the head has a diameter of 22.25 mm.*

Although technologically of great interest, it is, however, doubtful whether this has any real advantage.

Total hip replacement in severe Still's disease

In some of these patients, and others with pathologically small skeletons, even the smallest, commercially available, cemented implants are too large. If it is elected to use cement fixation, very small implants can be manufactured quite adequately from plain radiographs because an exact fit is not important. Figure 3.19 shows an example of such a case. The stem used in this very low-demand patient was about the thickness of an ordinary lead pencil.

Bipolar replacement

If the acetabulum is completely normal, then it is logical to replace the femoral head only; this is the situation in stage III avascular necrosis (AVN) – resurfacing may occasionally be possible if the avascular segment is not

too large, as advocated by Amstutz, using the Conserve system (Wright Medical Technology Inc.), and by some others, but this is strictly a research technique at present. The operation then becomes analogous to the treatment of a subcapital fracture, where improved results in terms of acetabular wear and migration of the head have been seen using a bipolar stem, although the actual movement that takes place in bipolar heads in the long term is not entirely beyond dispute. A number of systems are available with stems of different types, some for use with cement, such as the Hastings, which were originally thought of largely as a treatment for subcapital fractures in elderly people, and some without, such as the Bateman. In general, however, the cementless stems, as with so many other cementless stem designs, have not done well.

Unfortunately, the apparently straightforward issue of the use of a bipolar component in AVN has been clouded by two matters. The first of these [2] is that probably the most widely known early implant (Monk) had a cementless stem, and the advocates of bipolarity have also tended to be advocates of cementless stem fixation. As enthusiasm for the latter has somewhat waned, the implants associated with them, even though they incorporate a completely different principle at the upper end, have failed to gain further popularity. Secondly, bipolar implants have also been used in the treatment of osteoarthritis. This can work, but the results are not sufficiently reliable for the technique to be recommended (except, perhaps, in very old people, in whom replacement of any kind is, however, probably contraindicated); once again, this has limited the use of bipolar implants.

Figure 3.20 shows a bipolar implant with a cement-less stem used for osteoarthritis in a young person who would now present quite a difficult case for revision. In this case, the socket is easy to replace, but the necessary modular head/neck unit, with a sufficiently long neck, is unlikely to be available, and the stem therefore needs to be changed; however, the stem in this case (unlike many) looks very soundly fixed – it was tight enough at the original operation to produce an intraoperative fracture. One of the potential advantages of the use of a bipolar replacement for stage III AVN is that, should acetabular wear become a problem necessitating

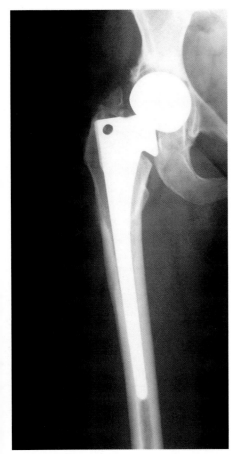

Figure 3.20 – *Bipolar Bateman prosthesis originally used for osteoarthritis in a young woman, before revision (see text).*

acetabular replacement, the head/neck unit can, in theory, be replaced with one suitable for total hip replacement. This is a sound concept in principle, but it has its drawbacks. The conversion operation is equivalent to changing the socket only in a failed total hip replacement. Provided that the orientation of the stem is correct, stability should be achievable if a head/neck unit of suitable length is available. If this is not the case, or the stem is to some degree malorientated, it is necessary to change the stem as well or instability will result.

The production life of implants tends to be limited, so that, at the time of conversion, a suitable head/neck unit may no longer be available. Although it might be possible to have manufactured one of suitable dimensions, an exact fit of the Morse taper or trunnion is essential to avoid production of wear debris. The advantages of the bipolar system in this type of case may be more theoretical than actual; figures do not appear to be available for the number of times that bipolar replacements have been converted to total hip replacement or for the success of this procedure. Although bipolar replacement with a well-tried stem and an adequate range of head sizes, resulting in a good match, should certainly be recommended in AVN, acetabular replacement in this type of case is straightforward and there should be little regret about carrying out a total hip replacement.

Arthroscopy

Arthroscopy of the hip is considerably more time-consuming and complicated than arthroscopy of the knee. This is principally because traction is required, together with radiological control using an image intensifier. The two main available techniques are to have the patient (1) in the supine position on an ordinary fracture table, and (2) in the lateral position using a special hip distractor. The latter is almost certainly the better system, and it may well transpire that arthroscopy of the hip should not be carried out unless such an apparatus is available. Certainly quite a good view of the hip can be obtained and some limited arthroscopic surgery can be done using a fracture table. In this technique, the patient is set up in a similar fashion to that for the fixation of a trochanteric fracture, so that AP and lateral radiographs of the hip can readily be obtained. A special plastic drape, of the type used for trochanteric fracture treatment, is very convenient. Care needs to be taken with the position of the X-ray screen and the arthroscopic television monitor, so that both can easily be seen at the same time.

The leg on the operated side is in the extended position with some internal rotation. A moderate degree of tension is applied to the limb (the inability to control this is one of the major defects of this technique) and a spinal epidural needle inserted under image intensifier control from just above the greater trochanter into the hip. Appropriate skin markings should be made with the hip screened in the AP and lateral positions at the outset; if desired, the exact position of the femoral head can be drawn on the skin anteriorly. Once the needle has entered the hip, the slight distraction that has already (in a favourable case) taken place becomes very much greater and the fluid is sucked from the syringe. Distraction has to be sufficient for it to be obvious that there is enough space for the arthroscope and its sheath to enter the hip. If the space is insufficient, then significant damage can result to the articular surfaces. Through appropriate entry portals near the front and back of the upper end of the trochanter, cardiac needles can then be inserted, usually without particular difficulty, into the hip and it can be verified that fluid can pass from one to the other. Crowding of the tips can be avoided by checking the position on the lateral film.

A stab wound is then made around one of the entry points, the line of the needle very carefully memorized, the needle withdrawn and the arthroscope sheath with trochar inserted along the same line. Several different types of tip are available to help perforate the capsule. Minor resistance needs to be overcome, but force should not be used. Both 70° and 30° arthroscopes should be available and, although special long arthroscopes are not strictly necessary, it is essential to have a sheath of adequate length. Some varieties of sheath have a bridge, which limits the depth to which the arthroscope can be inserted. An appropriate instrument (usually an endoscopic shaver) can then be inserted in a similar fashion along the track of the other needle. One of the merits of the shaver is that no separate outflow is required. At the end of the procedure, the traction should be gradually released with a needle in the hip, bupivacaine (Marcaine) may be instilled, although this is probably not necessary, and the postoperative regimen is as for arthroscopy of the knee.

The great advantages of the use of a special distractor with the patient in the lateral position are that a lateral distraction force can be applied by means of pubic or groin support, and that the distraction force (about 20–25 kg) can be accurately measured. It is possible for the patient to be, to some degree, suspended by the groin or pubic support, making the patient's own body weight responsible for the lateral distraction force. Such a procedure also tensions the capsule in a more controlled fashion and may facilitate entry of instruments. Regrettably, no suitable traction device is commercially available at the time of writing.

Certain types of hip undergo arthroscopy more easily than others, and in some this may be impossible without risk of significant damage. The more mobile the hip, the more likely it is to distract. This is, however, less likely to be a problem in the types of hip that are appropriate for arthroscopy; there will probably never be a place for arthroscopy in the stiff hips that may be found with full-blown osteoarthritis. Arthroscopy is also more difficult in hips with certain types of morphology than in others. This applies particularly to hips that have a slightly protrusio configuration and those in which the greater trochanter is rather high. Unless the hip is easily distractable, it may not be possible to advance a straight instrument across into the middle of the joint above the femoral head from the ordinary (and safest) supratrochanteric route.

Arthrodesis

Arthrodesis of the hip has a long and extremely interesting history. The difficulties have always been, first, to achieve union and, second, to achieve union in an adequate position. As well as intra-articular scarification of the surfaces, extra-articular struts, particularly iliofemoral and ischiofemoral ones, were used, often combined with an upper femoral osteotomy. The methods also required long periods of plaster fixation.

With the development, notably in Switzerland, of internal fixation of fractures, but before the widespread use of hip replacement, it was possible to be much more certain about obtaining the desired position for the fusion; at the same time, the scientific approach to primary fracture healing, in association with rigid fixation and compression, enabled much more rapid mobilization of the patient without the use of a hip spica. This was the situation in the early 1960s.

Later, with the advent of hip replacement, a secondary disadvantage of these methods (and, in fact, one not always found in earlier techniques, such as the central dislocation method of Charnley) became apparent in that they produced, however carefully carried out, a significant degree of abductor damage. Atrophy of the abductors clearly always results from arthrodesis, but with conversion to total hip replacement they have the potential for a very good (albeit slow) recovery (see Chapter 8). This recovery will, however, be vitiated if serious damage to either the muscles or the greater trochanter occurs at the arthrodesis, as tends to occur in techniques using a lateral Cobra plate. This problem can, in principle, be overcome in two different ways, namely by using an anterior rather than a lateral plate or, in marked contrast, by using external fixation. These three techniques are the main choices available at present, although it is unclear which is best.

Unfortunately, there are no comparative studies of complications or outcome, nor do such studies seem likely to be available in the future, in view of the small numbers of patients treated in this way. External fixation has the merit of operative simplicity, but is associated with all the known problems of external fixators and the use of fixation pins, a potential source for infection, in a femur in which later joint replacement is very likely is not attractive. The method is also less applicable to the strong otherwise fit young men, not all of whom will necessarily be in a position to cooperate perfectly with outpatient management, in whom hip arthrodesis is likely to be appropriate. Internal fixation with an anterior plate is very attractive in principle, but the method currently is still under evaluation.

Position for fusion
This should be flexion of 15–20°, just sufficient abduction (maximum 5°) to ensure that there is no adduction, and 5–10° of external rotation. In the days before joint replacement, hips were often placed in abduction to attempt to gain some length. This may, however, bring on both an earlier onset of back pain and an earlier conversion of the arthrodesis to total hip replacement – something that the fusion should delay; it is not, therefore, recommended any longer.

Brief summaries of the techniques used in arthrodesis are given below – that of Schneider [5] using a laterally placed Cobra plate, that of Matta *et al.* [6] using an

anterior plate, and that of Agostini and Lavini [7] using an external fixator.

Arthrodesis with a laterally placed Cobra plate
In summary, the patient is positioned supine with both legs prepared and draped free so that leg lengths can be verified by inspection of the medial malleoli. A rather laterally placed trochanteric osteotomy is carried out through a long straight lateral incision, and the abductors carefully mobilized upwards to above the level of the joint. A transverse pelvic osteotomy is then carried out through the extreme upper limit of the femoral head, similar to a pathologically low Chiari osteotomy, and this is then displaced slightly. Bone is removed from the trochanteric bed until a Cobra plate can be made to fit from the lateral wall of the ilium across the trochanteric bed and on to the lateral cortex of the femur. The upper end of the plate is fixed to the ilium with one screw and the compression device applied.

At this stage, the hip has to be in a slightly adducted position to allow for the slight change in alignment as a result of the subsequent compression. Compression is then applied and the position of the leg very carefully checked (in Schneider's description a special form of sterilizable goniometer was used in relation to pins placed in the anterosuperior iliac spines) and the remaining screws inserted. The trimmed part of the trochanteric bed and any other excised bone are then used as a graft. Finally, one of the screws can be removed from the region of the trochanteric bed and the greater trochanter fixed, using this screw hole, on to the outer side of the plate. When the Cobra plate is later removed, the greater trochanter can be put back in its previous position (albeit more medially).

Variants
It may not always be necessary to carry out a pelvic osteotomy. This depends very much on the local conditions present and the shape of the hip. In the Schneider technique, the hip is not dislocated, but this can obviously be done if this is likely to bring better surfaces into contact after scarification.

Arthrodesis using an anterior plate
The surgical approach in this technique is similar to the earlier parts of the technique for periacetabular osteotomy. The inner wall of the ilium is exposed down to the pelvic brim. Access to the upper part of the anterior and anteromedial parts of the shaft of the femur

is created after ligating the lateral femoral circumflex vessels and elevating the vasti, reflecting them medially. The hip is then distracted in exactly the same fashion as described above for Chiari osteotomy, using an ASIF femoral fracture distractor and the joint surfaces scarified and made to fit, so that an adequate area comes into contact. The distraction force is then released, the surfaces apposed, the position checked using a radiograph, and a long 6.5-mm cancellous lag screw is placed from the lateral aspect of the greater trochanter, across proximal to the femoral head and into the ilium. The arthrodesis is then fixed by a 12- to 18-holed plate, preferably of low-contact DCP type, which, in addition to its other advantages, allows much easier accurate contouring. The plate is initially fixed proximally and compressed with a compression device, as in the Cobra plate technique.

Arthrodesis using an external fixator

A standard fixator with a T-clamp proximally on the ilium is used. The description referred to relies largely on radiological control and the hip itself is not opened; fusion is aimed at via prolonged compression only. Easier and more reliable placement of the screws is, however, achieved if the procedure is carried out as an open one and, certainly, it does not seem possible to lose anything by opening the hip for scarification. The fixation can also be supplemented by a long screw passed up the femoral neck into the ilium, rather like that described in the anterior plate technique. The external fixator will need to be kept *in situ* for 3–5 months.

References

1. Donnelli WJ, Kobiashi A, Freeman MAR *et al*. Radiological and survival comparison of four methods of fixation of a proximal femoral stem. *J Bone Joint Surg* 1997; 79B: 351–60.
2. Takaoka K, Nishina T, Ohzono K *et al*. Bipolar prosthetic replacement for the treatment of avascular necrosis of the femoral head. *Clin Orthop Rel Res* 1992; 277: 121–7.
3. Villar R. *Hip Arthroscopy*. Oxford: Butterworth-Heinemann, 1992.
4. Leichti R. *Hip Arthrodesis and Associated Problems*. Berlin: Springer-Verlag, 1978.
5. Schneider R. Hip arthrodesis using a Cobra-plate. In: *Manual of Internal Fixation. Techniques recommended by the AO Group*, 2nd edn. Berlin: Springer-Verlag, 1979; 388–9.
6. Matta JM, Siebenrock KA, Gautier E *et al*. Hip fusion through an anterior approach with the use of a ventral plate. *Clin Orthop Rel Res* 1997; 337: 129–39.
7. Agostini S, Lavini F. Arthrodesis using the orthofix external fixator. In: *Orthofix Modulsystem Manual on Arthrodesis*. Orthofix Srl, 8–14.
8. Northmore-Ball MD, D'Souza S, Varughese J *et al*. Experience and indication of osteotomy resurfacing and total arthroplasty in the young adult. Long-term clinical and survivorship study. Proceedings of the European Hip Society. *J Bone Joint Surg* 1997; 79B: 295.

SECTION II
Total hip replacement

CHAPTER 4

History and basic science

G. C. Bannister

Treatment of osteoarthritis before hip replacement

Before the advent of hip replacement, the treatment of osteoarthritis of the hip comprised manipulation, cheilectomy (excision of osteophytes), arthrodesis, osteotomy and excision, interposition, and replacement arthroplasty. Results were highly variable and surgical intervention confined to the severest cases. Over the 11 years between 1946 and 1957, surgeons at the Middlesex Hospital performed a total of 260 interventions for hip arthritis [1]. Cheilectomy afforded only temporary relief [2]. Arthrodesis abolished pain and gave a stable hip but it was a protracted operation. At one time, it was staged because of high perioperative mortality [3], and failed to unite in 50% of cases, when spica immobilization alone was used. It either produced or aggravated low back pain in the older population and, although non-union was reduced by internal fixation, the results remained uncertain.

Intertrochanteric osteotomy was popularized by McMurray in Liverpool, who performed the procedure regularly from 1929 [4]. Hey Groves [2] performed the operation principally to correct adduction deformity, but recognized that more benefit accrued from it than just this. McMurray's procedure was defined precisely as a 40° oblique osteotomy performed under direct vision to ensure that the femur was divided just proximal to the lesser trochanter. The distal fragment was displaced proximally and medially to appose the inferior margin of the acetabulum and the procedure was sufficiently successful to enjoy wide popularity. Osborne and Fahrni [5], reviewing McMurray's patients 10 years after surgery, recorded that 81% had relief of pain, flexion exceeded 60° in 23%, and mean shortening was 2.5 cm (1 inch). A variety of osteotomies was widely performed before

the advent of hip replacement. Overall, osteotomy offered relative relief of pain, with retention of some movement. Nicol and Holden [6] recorded abolition of pain in 52% and relief in 36%, with ankylosis in 34%.

Excision arthroplasty was initially employed in the management of septic arthritis, but was subsequently adopted for osteoarthritis. Girdlestone resected the head and neck in line with the trochanters and excised the outer lip of the acetabulum [7]. There was good pain relief in just under 90% of cases and average shortening was 3.8 cm (1.5 inches), but instability was the main problem. Hey Groves [2] noted that patients were dependent on crutches after the procedure. Shepherd [8] recorded good or excellent function in only 27%, although functional results improved after 5 years. Early arthroplasty involved surgical procedures that lasted for between 4 and 6 hours, bedrest for weeks, and exercises and protected weight-bearing for months, followed by years of rehabilitation [9], before there was relative freedom from pain, residual limp, and dependence on orthoses. Hey Groves summarized the three requirements of a good arthroplasty as 'freedom from pain, mobility and stability'.

During the first half century of hip arthroplasty, interposition with zinc, tin, rubber, celluloid, metal plate, or gold leaf was used. Biological interpositions included muscle transplantation, fascia and fat [10a], xenograft [10b], and interventions ivory femoral head replacement [11]. In 1923, Smith-Petersen [12] began to experiment with inorganic interposition arthroplasty. Smith-Petersen's cup arthroplasty was one of the most intellectually appealing procedures in the history of hip replacement. The concept was that smooth, inert, inorganic material was placed between two decorticated joint surfaces, sufficiently loosely to allow space for soft tissue ingrowth, which could then undergo metaplasia to fibrocartilage. Glass and then Pyrex were used; both

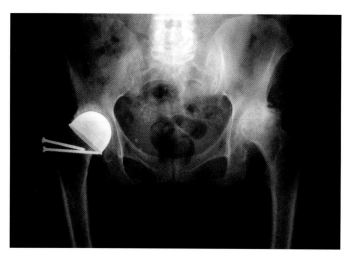

Figure 4.1 – *Smith-Petersen cup arthroplasty.*

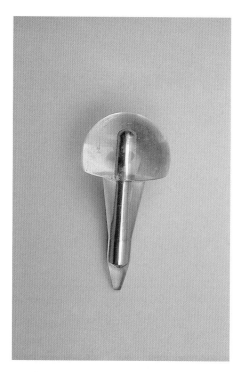

Figure 4.2 – *Judet arthroplasty. Note the metal reinforcement because the original acrylic prostheses fractured.*

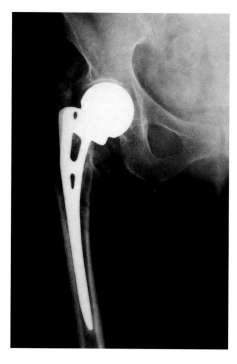

Figure 4.3 – *Austin Moore hemiarthroplasty.*

broke. Celluloid caused a foreign body reaction and, in 1938, cobalt–chrome was employed (Fig. 4.1), rendering the procedure sufficiently reliable for its widespread adoption. The surgical procedure was followed by a protracted period of rehabilitation. Up to a third of patients required further surgery, principally to correct stiffness. Results improved over a 5-year period [9] and walking support was required for 1-5 years for short distances and indefinitely for longer [13]. In the UK, cup arthroplasty was unsatisfactory in 30% of cases after between 1 and 3 years [14].

In the hands of the originators, cup arthroplasty maintained pain relief in patients with rheumatoid arthritis for 20 years in 80% of cases, but only 7% could walk without a stick and only 14% achieved more than 50% of normal mobility. In the general population treated by cup arthroplasty, 22% of patients were pain free, 31% experienced discomfort on weight-bearing, 50% could walk a mile, but 66% required a stick. Of the patients treated, 22% required further surgery, and 30% of those from a number of British centres [14] were worse than before surgery. Results peaked at 3–4 years and deteriorated thereafter.

In 1948, an acrylic prosthetic femoral head was introduced by the Judet brothers, with a significantly quicker recovery than that seen after vitallium mould arthroplasty (Fig. 4.2). After 18 months, 80% of cases were satisfactory, although 66% needed to use a stick. The acrylic fractured, caused a foreign body granuloma, and was eventually abandoned.

In 1950, Austin Moore collaborated with R.M. Sumwalt, Professor of Engineering at the University of South Carolina, to produce a modification of an earlier vitallium resection prosthesis (Fig. 4.3). The shorter fenestrated stem was used predominantly for displaced intracapsular femoral neck fractures, but 55% of patients treated for degenerative arthritis of the hip had satisfactory results after 5 years [15]. These results were not confined to Moore's unit, because they were reproduced at the Royal National Hospital, Stanmore, England [16]. Thompson [17] had noted the unpredictable resorption

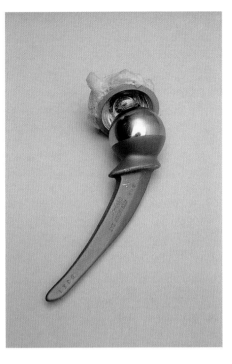

Figure 4.4 – *McKee–Farrar metal on metal total hip replacement.*

survey of the American Academy of Orthopedic Surgeons. Of these, only 61% could walk at all after surgery and 71% required a stick. Five per cent of surgeons had given up the operation and almost 70% had changed prosthesis after failure with the Judet one. Shepherd [8] reviewed the pioneer procedures for osteoarthritis. Of cup arthroplasties, 30% were good or excellent and 42% were either worse than before surgery or had undergone revision. Of Judet prostheses, 28% were good or excellent and 80% showed radiological signs of failure. Of osteotomies, 48% were good or excellent after 10 years and 90% of excision arthroplasties had pain relief, accompanied by poor function. McKee [21] (1966) summarized the situation:

> Operation was never a satisfactory procedure. In fact, many of the older orthopaedic surgeons would be only too willing to admit that whenever they tried to carry out an arthroplasty, i.e. form a new joint, they obtained an arthrodesis and vice versa.

The development of total hip replacement

Philip Wiles of the Middlesex Hospital experimented first on animals, using a pre-formed acetabulum and femoral head. The acetabulum was held by two screws

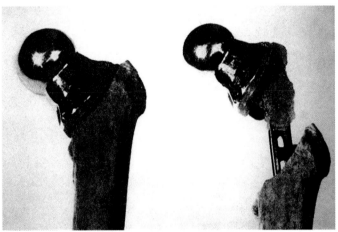

Figure 4.5 – *Bone cement used by Haboush.*

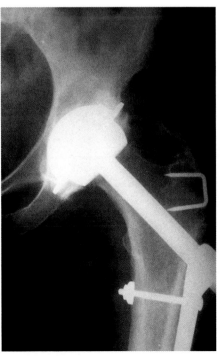

Figure 4.6 – *Wiles' total hip arthroplasty.*

of the femoral neck after displaced intracapsular fractures, and produced a vitallium prosthesis with a collar, bearing weight on both the trochanters. This prosthesis would become the femoral component of the McKee–Farrar vitallium total hip replacement (Fig. 4.4). The mistrust of the proximal femur as a source of fixation was most graphically demonstrated by McBride [18], who produced a threaded prosthesis designed to be screwed into cortical bone of the femoral shaft. The first surgeon to attempt metaphyseal fixation was Haboush [19], who used acrylic bone cement (Fig. 4.5).

The results of prosthetic hemiarthroplasty for osteoarthritis were erratic. King *et al.* [20] reported the results of 10 274 patients with hemiarthroplasties culled from a and the femoral head by a bolt and a plate (Fig. 4.6). In 1938, he operated on a small number of patients, predominantly with juvenile chronic arthritis, who had been bedridden or were just able to walk. Results were only tolerable in 25% of cases. In 1940, McKee adopted the same approach. His first prosthesis used an uncemented Thompson's stem and a screw-in acetabular component; 50% of cases were successful. Although a metallic sludge was produced by the metal-on-metal joint, McKee felt that the main problem in hip replacement was fixation of prostheses to bone. In 1960, he supplemented fixation with acrylic bone cement, with satisfactory results in 90% of cases after 5 years [22], the results lasting for about 13 years [23]. In the 1950s, Charnley observed a squeaking noise coming from the early arthroplasties and attributed this to friction of the joint. He then concentrated on lower friction arthroplasties, starting initially with a cup-and-socket arthroplasty made of Teflon [24a]. The femoral neck underwent aseptic necrosis, after which Teflon was retained for a socket with partial sacrifice of the neck, and a Moore or Thompson prosthesis was cemented into the femoral medullary cavity with dental acrylic. The head was reduced in size as a further concession to friction, but the socket wore and a foreign body reaction resulted in his having to revise over 200 cases. In 1962, Charnley pioneered the use of high-density polyethylene as a socket, and the metal-on-polyethylene joint remains the standard bearing in the overwhelming majority of total hips implanted today.

Charnley undoubtedly produced a lower friction joint than other pioneers, but the higher friction of the metal-on-metal articulation employed by McKee, and subsequently in the uncemented form by Peter Ring [24b] (Fig. 4.7), produced results that were only slightly inferior and certainly did not reflect the difference in friction alone. Other factors contribute to the outcome of total hip replacement and these are the quality of the bone, bone cement, metallic properties of the stem, and polyethylene.

Bone

The bone into which prostheses are fixed is characterized by wide variation. Bone is a composite structure, strongest in the direction of the strains imposed on it *in vivo*. The direction of such strains cannot be computed by simple mechanics on cadaveric material. Bone varies in its strength by a factor of 10 according to the strain rate of testing. Its properties after death and preservation alter. The postmortem changes of compliance, recognized in soft tissues as rigor mortis, occur in bone within 5 hours of death [25]. Fresh bone is over half as strong again as that fixed in formalin [26]. In the femur, the cancellous bone at the isthmus and distal to the trochanters is coarse, whereas, in the metaphysis, the structure condenses centrifugally until it coalesces into cortical bone. The shear strength of human cancellous bone in the central 4 mm of the metaphysis is of the order of 1.5 MPa, whereas it is nearer 4 MPa at the corticocancellous junction[27].

Bone cement

Acrylic bone cement was originally used in dentistry, principally in prosthetics. Chemically, it is polymethylmethacrylate (PMMA). Compressed PMMA is Perspex which was the material employed by the Judet brothers [28] for the first widely used hip prosthesis. PMMA was first employed in prosthetic fixation by Haboush [19] in New York, although the major development was carried forward by Charnley. Although PMMA is heated and compressed to manufacture Perspex and dental plates, it is used in self-curing form in orthopaedic surgery. Methylmethacrylate monomer is in a liquid state and boils at 100°C. It is activated by 2% benzoyl peroxide and is prevented from polymerizing in its glass container by the addition of 0.01% hydroquinone. The monomer is added to powered PMMA and polymerization is initiated by 2% *p*-toluidine. The different properties of commercial bone cements depend on the molecular weight of the polymer, the texture of the

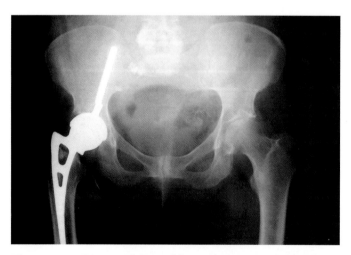

Figure 4.7 – *Ring mark II total hip replacement, implanted originally rather too medially, hence the fracture and readjustment of the acetabular component.*

powder, and the proportions of activator and initiator and liquid and powder. Ambient temperature and humidity also affect the rate of curing. In the process of setting, a mix of 40 g expands by 4 cm^3 and contracts by 0.5 cm^3 [29]. Of the widely used cements, there is variation in dough time by 1.25 minutes and solidification by 3.75 minutes under standardized conditions [30]. The strength of bone cement depends on the strain rate at which it is tested, the temperature at which it sets, and the degree of constraint when it is tested. Traditional mixing techniques in a bowl allow air contamination. The quicker the mixing, the greater the air contamination. The strength of bone cement prepared in operating room conditions varies by a factor as high as 3 [30–33].

Methylmethacrylate in its original form was radiolucent and the addition of radio-opaque markers slightly weakens the material. Antibiotic addition, particularly in the operating room, is often uneven and can reduce the strength of the composite by almost a fifth [34]. Having been mixed, air and blood laminations further reduce cement strength. Blood lamination in cement prepared in operating rooms reduces the strength by some 12% on average, but can do so by up to 30% [33]. Lee et al. [35] demonstrated that delayed insertion and air lamination reduced the strength of cement by 30%, and that blood lamination rendered some specimens so weak that they fractured merely on handling. Cement is strongest in compression and weakest in tension and shear. Gruen et al. [36] recorded a reduction of shear strength of up to 61% in blood-laminated cement. By contrast, Lee et al. [37] were unable to break cement that was constrained in aluminium tubing, although the material was subjected to over four times the compressive force required for fracture. Vacuum mixing and centrifugation both increase cement strength but, apart from constraint, in clinical practice the capacity to weaken bone cement exceeds that of strengthening it.

The effect of the biological environment on bone cement appears to be less noxious. Lee et al. [35] noted some weakening of cement stored in saline, but storage in bovine serum at 37°C either had no effect [38] or improved fatigue strength [39]. Sharkey and Bargar [40] were unable to demonstrate any difference in strengths of specimens of bone cement taken from revision hip replacement after a mean of 5.5 years. Bannister and Miles [33] found that the shear strength of bone cement, similarly retrieved at revision hip arthroplasty, was

significantly stronger than blood-contaminated cement prepared in operating rooms, and equivalent to that of pure cement.

Cement–bone interface

Cement fracture [36, 41] and failure at the cement–bone interface [42] are both associated with aseptic loosening. Charnley [43] encouraged patients with hips that had been successful for at least 3 years to donate their arthroplasties after death. Charnley found no cracks in the cement and no fibrous tissue between the cement and the bone load-bearing areas. By contrast, the cemented socket universally had a layer of fibrous tissue of between 0.5 and 1.5 mm between cement and bone. Malcolm [44] and Muller [45] also failed to demonstrate cracks in cement in well-functioning prostheses, although Jasty et al. [46] (1991) recorded cracks radiating from stress raisers in a number of salvaged successful hip replacements.

The cement–bone interface is undoubtedly the weakest link in total hip arthroplasty. The shear strength of the cement bone interface achieved by most investigators varies between 5 and 15 MPa, whereas the shear strength of cement is 40 MPa. The strength of the cement–bone interface depends on the quality of the component materials, cleaning, pressure, and reduced cement viscosity. Halawa et al. [27] recorded an increase in the shear strength of the cement–bone interface of 200% when bone was cleaned under high pressure. These results were reproduced by Krause et al. [47], Askew et al. [48], and Majkowski et al. [49]. The degree of pressure required to achieve cement penetration appears to be finite, and Bean et al. [50] (1988) found that 0.37 MPa (60 lb/in^2) was as effective as 0.53 MPa (80 lb/in^2). The least important variable identified by Halawa et al. was reduced cement viscosity. Krause combined low-viscosity cement with increased pressure and demonstrated a two- to fourfold improvement in the tensile strength of the cement–bone interface. Bean et al. [50] found that low-viscosity cement penetrated bone further, but gave an interface that was no stronger than cement of normal dough thickness.

As pressure appeared to be the most consistent variable that could be influenced by the surgeon, pressures induced by varying surgical techniques were measured by Markolf and Amstutz [51]. Distal restriction increased distal pressures, particularly if prostheses were inserted early. There was, however, little difference on late

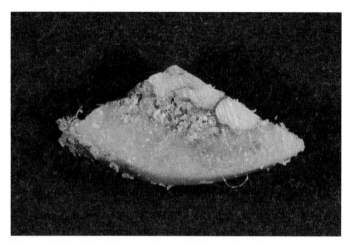

Figure 4.8 – *Blood laminations with low-viscosity cement.*

prosthetic insertion. Charnley [52] proposed that cement pressurization occurred on insertion of a wedge-shaped prosthesis, and this concept was extended by the Exeter group who designed a tapered stem to enhance this effect. Turner *et al.* [53] confirmed this, noting that prostheses of broad proximal geometric configuration enhanced interface pressures. Bannister *et al.* [54] compared cement–bone interfaces of the press-fit straight stem Muller type with other devices and found the former to be superior. In surgical practice, blood frequently contaminates the cement–bone interface. Bannister and Miles [33] examined first-, second-, and third-generation cementing techniques, using low-viscosity cement in the last of these. In clean bone, the strength of the cement–bone interface increased fivefold but, when blood was smeared on the cement–bone interface, the beneficial effects of the second- and third-generation cementing techniques were lost. Low-viscosity cement, in particular, became heavily contaminated with blood (Fig. 4.8) and Scandinavian studies have shown that it is inferior clinically to cement of greater viscosity.

Metallic implants
Metallic implants are composed of three groups of alloys. Cobalt–chrome (cobalt 70%, chromium 30%) was the original material used in Smith-Petersen's cup arthroplasty and subsequently the McKee–Farrar total hip replacement. The original Charnley stem was composed of 316-L stainless steel (classically 18% chromium, 10% nickel, and 3% molybdenum, with the remaining 66% ferrous iron); 316-L stainless steel fractured in the Charnley and other stems, and the

response was to change to the high-nitrogen stainless steel Rex 734, which has been employed for most stainless steel stem manufacture since 1979. The fatigue strength of Rex 734 is double that of 316-L. Titanium was employed in an attempt to achieve greater biocompatibility, because it is three times as elastic as stainless steel. Titanium may be pure, or in the alloy Ti 6Al 4V (90% titanium, 6% aluminium, 4% vanadium).

Of the three types of alloy, cobalt–chrome is the hardest and titanium the softest. This means that cobalt–chrome is the only material from which it is practical to manufacture a metal-on-metal prosthetic joint. Soft titanium prosthetic heads scratch easily and are associated with excessive polyethylene wear in metal-on-ultra-high-density polyethylene joints.

The practical problems that beset the orthopaedic surgeon in the choice of metal in prostheses are fracture, production of wear particles and corrosion.

Fracture
The original Charnley stem made of 316-L stainless steel fractured at the junction of the distal third and proximal two-thirds. The response to such fractures was to use high-nitrogen stainless steel, and increase the cross-sectional diameter of the implant, employing both new material and a different structure to overcome the problem. The rigidity of a structure is proportional to the fourth power of its radius. Thus, second-generation Charnley stems are very much more rigid than the first-generation ones, and, by virtue of being broader, allow less room for bone cement. Bone cement is elastic and acts to reduce movement between metal and bone. The effect of this rigidity has been that, instead of the fracture taking place in the stem itself, it now occurs either within the cement or at the cemen–bone interface. Attempts to modify the rigidity of the construct saw the introduction of titanium alloy. Tripling the elasticity of the material is, however, vastly overwhelmed by the effects of increasing the radius of the structure, and titanium, particularly with a matt surface, brings its own problems.

Wear particles
There is continuing debate about whether the initiating factor in loosening is breakdown of the cement–stem or the cement–bone interface [42]. If it is the former, a rough surface on the stem increases the surface area for bonding with cement and ought to reduce loosening. If,

however, dissociation of the stem and the cement takes place in such designs, the loose prosthesis acts as a rasp and is correspondingly more destructive. If the metal from which the prosthesis is manufactured is soft, loose particles are released in greater profusion than if it is hard, and in practice a number of matt titanium-cemented stem designs have had unacceptably high loosening rates, being associated with metallosis and bone lysis.

Corrosion

Corrosion releases metal ions, which can be found as far from the site of implantation as the frontal cortex, lung, liver and spleen [55]. There is an association with tumours of the lymphopoietic system [56]. The surface of a metal implant oxidizes, and it is the stability of the oxide layer that determines how resistant that implant will be to corrosion. The most stable oxide layer is that overlying titanium, and the least stable stainless steel. The addition of chromium, nickel and molybdenum to steel renders the surface oxide very much more stable than that of ferrous material alone. Corrosion is not merely a function of the material, but also of the movement imposed on it in the human body. Movement between components of the same metal causes corrosion, such as in the McKee–Farrar hip or, in modern practice, the junction between the Morse taper in the modular stem and the head [57]. The combination of a hard cobalt–chrome head with a soft titanium stem increases the risk of corrosion, as does instability of a prosthesis, causing fretting of its surface.

Overall, titanium is a safe metal to use, provided that it is stable. It is, therefore, a very much better surface for acetabular, than femoral, components, the length of which increases potential fretting against relatively elastic bone. Cobalt–chrome has the potential to produce an all-metal joint if the surfaces are prepared to sufficiently high tolerances. Stainless steel is highly likely to corrode, particularly in contact with other metals, such as wires or screws used for bone fixation.

Ultra-high-molecular-weight polyethylene

The weakest link in the construct of a total joint replacement is polyethylene, because of wear. Wear properties of ultra-high-molecular-weight polyethylene are very much greater than high-density polyethylene. The strength of the former depends on bonding of long chains of polyethylene, and this can be disturbed either by poorly adherent particles or by oxidation reducing the long to short chains. Gamma irradiation is the most widely used method of sterilization, but, in the presence of oxygen, oxidizes ultra-high-molecular-weight to high-density polyethylene.

Oxidation takes place in the human body and there is little evidence that oxidation by irradiation is responsible for excessive polyethylene wear in hip arthroplasty. By contrast, the structure in which polyethylene is placed is of paramount importance. A thin mantle of polyethylene subjected to the shear forces of a 32-mm head, scratches on the femoral head, friction against uncemented acetabular components, and loose metal particles from fretting uncemented femoral components all contribute to polyethylene wear. The optimum structural environment to minimize polyethylene wear is the use of a cemented, all-polyethylene, acetabular component and a monoblock cemented stem with a 22.25-mm head. A ceramic head would appear to have slight advantages over those of cobalt–chrome or stainless steel.

References

1. Wiles P. The surgery of the osteoarthritic hip. *Br J Surg* 1957–8; 45: 488–97.

2. Hey Groves EW. Surgical treatment of osteoarthritis of the hip. *Br Med J* 1933; i: 3–5.

3. Watson-Jones R. Arthrodesis of the osteoarthritic hip. *JAMA* 1938; 110: 278–86.

4. McMurray TP. Osteoarthritis of the hip joint. *J Bone Joint Surg* 1939; 21: 1–11.

5. Osborne GC, Fahrni WH. Oblique displacement osteotomy for osteoarthritis of the hip joint. *J Bone Joint Surg* 1950; 32B: 148–60.

6. Nicol EA, Holden NT. Displacement osteotomy in the treatment of osteoarthritis of the hip. *J Bone Joint Surg* 1961; 43B: 50–60.

7. Taylor RG. Pseudarthrosis of the hip joint. *J Bone Joint Surg* 1950; 32B: 161–5.

8. Shepherd MM. A further review of the results of operations on the hip joint. *J Bone Joint Surg* 1960; 42B: 177–204.

9. Law WA. Results of vitallium mold arthroplasty of the hip. *J Bone Joint Surg* 1962; 44A: 1497–517.

10a. Murphy JB. Arthroplasty. *Annals of Surgery* 1913; 5: 593.

10b. Baer WS. Arthroplasty of the Hip. *J Bone Joint Surg* 1926; 769–802.

11. Hey Groves EW. Some contributions to the reconstructive surgery of the hip. *Br J Surg* 1926; 486–517.

12. Smith-Petersen MN. Evolution of mold arthroplasty of the hip joint. *J Bone Joint Surg* 1948; 30B: 59–75.

13. Aufranc OE. *Constructive Surgery of the Hip.* St Louis: CV Mosby Co., 1962.

14. Shepherd MM. A review of 650 hip arthroplasty operations. *J Bone Joint Surg* 1954; 36B: 567–77.

15. Moore AT. The self-locking metal hip prosthesis. *J Bone Joint Surg* 1957; 39A: 81127.

16. Heywood-Waddington MB. Use of the Austin Moore prosthesis for advanced osteoarthritis of the hip. *J Bone Joint Surg* 1966; 48B: 236–44.

17. Thompson FR. Two and a half years' experience with a vitallium intramedullary hip prosthesis. *J Bone Joint Surg* 1954; 36A: 489–500.

18. McBride ED. A femoral head prosthesis for the hip joint. *J Bone Joint Surg* 1952; 34A:989–96.

19. Haboush EJ. A new operation for arthroplasty of the hip based on biomechanics, photoelasticity, fast setting dental acrylic and other considerations. *Bull Hosp J Dis* 1953; 14: 242–77.

20. King DE, Straub LR, Lambert CN. Final report of the Committee for the Study of Femoral Head Prostheses. *J Bone Joint Surg* 1959; 41A: 883–5.

21. McKee GK. Developments in total hip joint replacement. *Proc Inst Mech Eng* 1966; 181: 85–9.

22. McKee GK, Watson-Farrar J. Replacement of arthritic hips by the McKee–Farrar prosthesis. *J Bone Joint Surg* 1966; 48B: 245–59.

23. August AC, Aldam CH, Pynsent PB. The McKee– Farrar hip arthroplasty. *J Bone Joint Surg* 1988; 68B: 520–7.

24a. Charnley J. Arthroplasty of the hip: a new operation. *Lancet* 1961; i: 1129–32.

24b. Ring PA. Uncemented total hip replacement. *J Roy Soc Med* 1981; 74: 719–724.

25. Fitzgerald ER. Post mortem mechanical properties of bone. *Med Phys* 1977; 4: 49–53.

26. Kusleika R, Stupp SI. Mechanical strength of polymethylmethacrylate cement–human bone interfaces. *J Biomed Mater Res* 1983; 17: 441–58.

27. Halawa M, Lee AJC, Ling RSM, Vangala SS. The shear strength of trabecular bone from the femur and some factors affecting the shear strength of the cement-bone interface. *Arch Orthop Traumat Surg* 1978; 92: 19–30.

28. Judet J, Judet R. The use of an artificial femoral head for arthroplasty of the hip joint. *J Bone Joint Surg* 1950; 32B: 166–73.

29. Charnley J. *Acrylic Cement in Orthopaedic Surgery.* Edinburgh: Churchill Livingstone, 1970.

30. Edwards RO, Thomas FGV. Evaluation of acrylic bone cements and their performance standards. *J Biomed Mater Res* 1981; 15: 543–51.

31. Homsy CA, Tullos HS, Anderson MS, King JW. Some physiological aspects of prosthesis stabilization with acrylic polymer. *Clin Orthop Rel Res* 1972; 3: 317–25.

32. Eyerer P, Jin R. Influence of mixing technique on some properties of PMMA bone cement. *J Biomed Mater Res* 1986; 20: 1057–94.

33. Bannister GC, Miles AW. The influence of cementing technique and blood on the strength of the bone–cement interface. *Eng Med* 1988; 17: 131–3.

34. Nelson RC, Hoffman RO, Burton TA. The effect of antibiotic additions on the mechanical properties of acrylic cement. *J Biomed Mater Res* 1978; 12: 473–90.

35. Lee AJC, Ling RSM, Vangara SS. Some clinically relevant variables affecting the mechanical behaviour of bone cement. *Arch Orthop Traumat Surg* 1978; 92: 1–18.

36. Gruen TA, Markolf KL, Amstutz HC. Effects of laminations and blood entrapment on the strength of acrylic bone cement. *Clin Orthop* 1976; 119: 250–5.

37. Lee AJC. The effect of mixing technique and surgical technique on the properties of bone cement. *Aktuel Probl Chir Orthop* 1987; 31: 145–50.

38. Jaffe WL, Rose RM, Radin EL. On the stability of the mechanical properties of self-curing acrylic bone cement. *J Bone Joint Surg* 1974; 56A: 1711–14.

39. Freitag TA, Cannon JL. Fracture characteristics of acrylic bone cements. *J Biomed Mater Res* 1977; 11: 609–24.

40. Sharkey NA, Bargar WL. Properties of retrieved acrylic bone cement. Read at 33rd Annual Meeting, Orthopaedic Research Society, Jan 1987, San Francisco.

41. Stauffer RN. 10 year follow-up study of total hip replacement. *J Bone Joint Surg* 1982; 64A: 983–90.

42. Miller J, Burke DL, Stachiewicz JW *et al*. Pathophysiology of loosening of femoral components in total hip arthroplasty. *Proceedings of the Sixth Open Scientific Meeting of the Hip Society*. St Louis: CV Mosby, 1978; 64–86.

43. Charnley J. *Low Friction Arthroplasty of the Hip*. Berlin: Springer-Verlag, 1979.

44. Malcolm AJ. Pathology of cemented low-friction arthroplasties in autopsy specimens. Chapter 11. In: MJW. Older (ed) *Implant bone interface*. Springer-Verlag, 1990, 77–82.

45. Schneider R. Total prosthetic replacement of the hip, second edition. Toronto, Lewiston NY: Hans Huber, 1987.1987

46. Jasty M, Malowey WJ, Bladon WR *et al*. The initiation of failure in cemented femoral components of hip arthroplasties. *J Bone Joint Surg* 1991; 73B: 551–8.

47. Krause WR, Krug W, Miller J. Strength of the cement bone interface. *Clin Orthop Rel Res* 1982; 163: 290–9.

48. Askew MJ, Steele SW, Lewis JL *et al*. Effect of cement pressure and bone strength on polymethylmethacrylate fixation. *J Orthop Res* 1984; 1: 412–20.

49. Majkowski RS, Miles AW, Bannister GC *et al*. Bone surface preparation in cemented joint replacement. *J Bone Joint Surg* 1993; 75B: 459–63.

50. Bean DJ, Hollis JH, Woo SLY, Convery FR. Sustained pressurization of polymethylmethacrylate: a comparison of low and moderate viscosity bone cements. *J Orthop Res* 1988; 6: 580–4.

51. Markolf KL, Amstutz HC. In vitro measurement of bone–acrylic interface pressure during femoral component insertion. *Clin Orthop Rel Res* 1976; 121: 60–6.

52. Charnley J. Anchorage of the femoral head prosthesis to the shaft of the femur. *J Bone Joint Surg* 1960; 42B: 28–30.

53. Turner RH, Scheller A, McKay WP, van Syckle PB. Cement intrusion as a function of skin design. *Orthop Trans* 1980; 333.

54. Bannister GC, Miles AW, May PC. Properties of bone cement prepared under operating theatre conditions. *Clin Mater* 1989; 4: 343–7.

55. Case CP, Langkamer VG James C *et al*. Widespread dissemination of metal debris from implants. *J Bone Joint Surg* 1994; 76B: 701–12.

56. Gillespie WJ, Frampton CMA, Henderson RJ, Ryan PM. The incidence of cancer following total hip replacement. *J Bone Joint Surg* 1988; 70B: 539–42.

57. Gilbert JL, Buckley CA, Jacobs JJ. *In vivo* corrosion of modular hip prosthesis components in mixed and similar metal combinations. The effect of crevice, stress, motion and alloy coupling. *J Biomed Mater Res* 1993; 27: 1533–44.

CHAPTER 5

Prosthetic design and fixation techniques

G. C. Bannister

Almost all femoral prosthetic designs are variations of the Austin Moore prosthesis (Fig. 5.1). There is a stem of some 15 cm length, an offset, and a head. Within those constraints, there are many variables of shape, thickness, surface finish, offset, and head size. When considering the clinical results, the technique with which the implant was inserted has to be taken into account. The McKee–Farrar had a curved Thompson stem (Fig. 5.2) that often loosened because of excessive strains imposed by increased friction of a failing metal-on-metal joint. Although, in the early days of hip replacements, surgeons wishing to use the Charnley (Fig. 5.3) had to attend a course of training, the curved Muller stem (Fig. 5.4) was available without such a constraint. The curved stem Muller stem was therefore widely used by surgeons undergoing their learning curve in total hip replacement, with cementing techniques that reflected this. Nevertheless, the literature consistently shows a revision rate of between 20% and 50% for curved stems, at between 8 and 15 years. By contrast, the straight-stemmed Charnley implant demonstrates a 9% revision rate after 10 years in multiple centres, maintained by surgeons outside the inventing centre for 13–15 years. The Charnley stem was a relatively narrow prosthesis, polished initially, and capable of insertion with a wide cement mantle. Subsequent experience [1] has shown that broadening the stem (Fig. 5.5) reduces the number of fractures, but increases the rate of aseptic loosening and bone lysis.

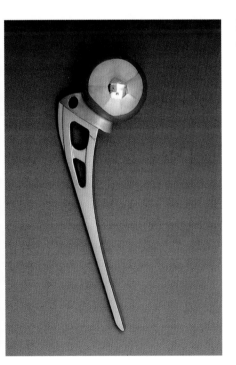

Figure 5.1 – *Austin Moore stem.*

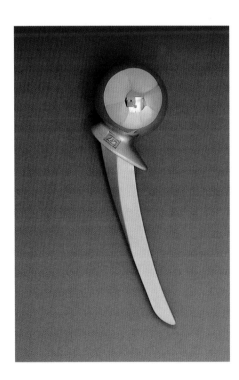

Figure 5.2 – *FR. Thompson stem.*

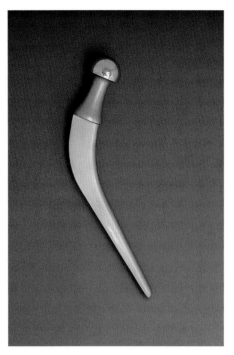

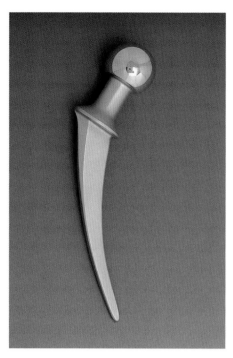

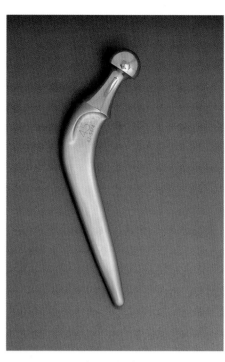

Figure 5.3 – *Charnley flat-back stem.*

Figure 5.4 – *Muller curved stem.*

Figure 5.5 – *Flanged Charnley stem.*

A completely different concept emerged from Exeter (Fig. 5.6). A collarless, tapered stem, originally manufactured in the early 1970s, had a polished finished, as was the custom in prosthetic manufacture at the time. The stem was designed as a wedge to force cement into bone; subsequently, it demonstrated a high level of subsidence at the stem–cement interface. This mechanical

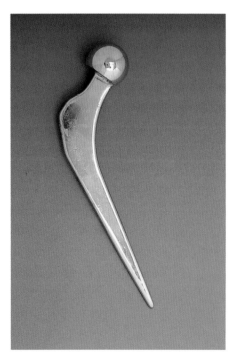

Figure 5.6 –
Exeter stem.

failure, however, spared the cement–bone interface and there was an extremely low incidence of aseptic loosening [2].

It seems that a straight stem is better than a curved one. Beckenbaugh and Ilstrup [3] noted that the best long-term fixation of the Charnley stem occurred when all loose bone had been removed from the medullary cavity and replaced by a prosthesis with an even mantle of 5 mm thickness. There is a fundamental disparity in rigidity between metal and cortical bone; the rigidity of a prosthesis increases by the fourth power of the radius. Thus, broadening a prosthesis both makes it much more rigid and denies the space necessary for cement to act as an elastic decoupler.

The early femoral stem designs fractured. A reaction to this was to broaden the stem and reduce offset. A reduced offset results in a Trendelenberg gait and increased joint reaction. The computer-aided design (CAD) performed significantly less well, at the Hospital for Special Surgery in New York, than the Charnley [4]. It would seem that retaining the normal offset of the hip is the wisest choice.

Using high-density polyethylene cups, head sizes of between 22 mm and 32 mm have been used. The rationale for the larger size is reduced dislocation rates, yet dislocation rates for 32 mm are only marginally lower than those for 22 mm, and polyethylene wear is very much less with the latter. It would, therefore, seem sensible to select a head size nearer 22 mm than 32 mm. Postmortem retrieval studies showed that the flat-back Charnley stem showed osseointegration in successful surviving hips [5]. As a reaction to poor results from early cemented total hip replacements, cementless total hip replacement was revived. Outside the hands of the originators, the results of uncemented total hip replacement have been unreliable. Ring, using his prostheses, achieved results half as good again as other surgeons. Both the Swedish and the Norwegian Arthroplasty Surveys [6] show poorer results with cementless stems. Nevertheless, a number of design principles have emerged. Cementless stems need to be stable and stability is best achieved by a high interference fit at the isthmus. Rotatory stability seems to be achieved best by sharp flutes gripping the cortex. If stems are porous coated to allow bone ingrowth, the porous coating should be circumferential and is better distributed over a longer, rather than a shorter, segment of the prosthesis. Cementless prostheses have a greater tendency to osteolysis than cemented ones.

Acetabular components have been designed from metal, high-density polyethylene, and polyacetyl. Polyacetyl has been uniformly inferior to the other materials. The metal-on-metal Stanmore hip replacement showed a 70% survival rate after 8 years, compared with 88% in metal-on-HDP (high-density polyethylene) prostheses [7]. Likewise, 57% of metal-on-metal Muller stems survived for 10 years [8], compared with 75% of metal-on-HDP [9]. In the German Swiss series, Griss *et al.* [10] reported 10% revision in metal-on-HDP hip replacements after 10 years, compared with 14% in McKee–Farrar metal-on-metal arthroplasties. Overall, HDP appears to be the best choice for acetabular resurfacing at present.

Cups with inside diameter of 22.25 mm last better than those accommodating larger heads. Metal backing does not appear to be an advantage in cemented cups, and equivalent results to cemented cup fixation have been obtained with certain porous coated, hemispherical, uncemented devices. Screw-in cups have tended to be inferior to press-fit hemispheres. Uncemented cups that involve apposition of polyethylene against bone have been fraught with osteolysis.

Fixation techniques

Total hip replacement became a reproducible procedure only after the introduction of bone cement, which

enhanced prosthetic stability. Bone cement remains the most reliable method of implanting a total hip replacement.

Femoral cementing technique

Cementing technique started with finger packing of thick dough into a freshly created intramedullary fracture. The technique was to some extent operator dependent, with wide variation in the pressures achieved [11]. Penetration of cement into bone could be poor using this technique. From an early Swedish series [12], 30% demonstrated radiolucent lines between the cement and bone on the postoperative radiograph. These lines are usually progressive, regressing in only 2% of cases [13]. In an early series from California, 47% of femoral components that progressed to revision for aseptic loosening demonstrated lucent lines between the cement and bone on the postoperative film [14]. Between 1978 and 1980 [15–17], attempts were made to improve cement technique by removing loose bone, cleaning bone surfaces, and enhancing cement pressure through restriction of the distal end of the prepared medullary cavity in the manner advocated by the Exeter group [18]. These changes were combined with alterations in prosthetic design. Curved stems were gradually abandoned, prostheses broadened to avoid fracture, and in North America the addition of a collar became fashionable. The combination of these changes in technique and design became designated second-generation hip replacement.

Harris published a series of stems of mixed geometry, but with a standardized second-generation cementing technique after a mean of 3.3 [15], 6.2 [19], and 11.2 years [20]. Of 234 patients, 63 were lost after 3.3 years, 117 after 6.2, and 129 after 11.2. After 11.2 years, the revision rate of the femoral stem for aseptic loosening was 3%. Three per cent of prostheses had migrated; 24% demonstrated a radiolucent line around 50% of their cement–bone interface and 7% endosteal bone lysis. These results are intermediate between the flat-back Charnley stem and the curved stem Muller inserted by a first-generation technique; there are huge difficulties in the interpretation of these results. The surgical technique may have been an advance, but the stem design was less good than the Charnley. Harris' retrieval rate was 45%, compared with 67% for the accumulated first-generation literature. Seven cases demonstrated a radiolucent line at the cement–bone interface after 3.3 years, but it would appear that these may have been lost to subsequent follow-up because only two cases presented after 6.2 years, and there is general agreement that radiolucent lines persist.

In a further study, Harris [21] selected 50 hip replacements in patients aged under 50 from that series, none of whom was lost to follow-up; he reported that all femoral components had survived for between 10 and 14.8 years. Endosteal bone lysis was present in 12% and lucent lines in over 50% of the cement–bone interface in 18%. This prevalence of lucent lines compares with 2.1% in the Exeter series [2] and 20% in the Charnley stems in New York [22], both inserted with first-generation technique.

Stems were standardized in two other studies comparing first- and second-generation cementing techniques. Roberts *et al.* [16], from Brigham and Women's Hospital, Boston, compared T28 stems inserted by first- and second-generation techniques after 4.3 years. There was a higher incidence of migration, cement mantle inadequacy, and radiolucent defects in the first-generation cases. Paterson *et al.* [17], reviewing Denham's cases from Alton and Portsmouth, compared first- and second-generation techniques in the Charnley and Stanmore stems, and recorded a significantly higher incidence of radiological stem cement loosening in first-generation cases after 6.8 years. At the Mayo Clinic, Russotti *et al.* [23] compared their second-generation experience with their original Charnley series after 5–7 years. The first-generation Charnley stem showed radiological evidence of loosening in 25% of cases, compared with 15% in the second-generation cases. It would appear that second-generation cementing techniques do offer advantages. Adverse radiographic features are rarer in the intermediate term.

The third-generation technique involves curettage of loose bone, pressurized lavage of bone surfaces, proximal and distal restriction, and retrograde insertion of bone cement under pressure. The Swedish Arthroplasty Survey [24] offers the most compelling evidence to support the use of this technique. With a closed population of 8.62 million in a state-run health service, all prostheses inserted are recorded, along with the number of revisions and the cementing technique employed. The importance of the Swedish Arthroplasty Survey is that it represents general orthopaedic practice, rather than the results of the enthusiastic inventor. By applying multivariate analysis to large numbers, it is possible to distinguish the relative effects of individual variables on outcome. Differences

in revision rates of up to 400% between hospitals employing third- and first-generation cementing techniques are reported: the particular advantage is gained from third-generation femoral cementing technique.

Cement mantle

Carlsson and Gentz [12] observed deficient cement in the proximal medial area adjacent to the calcar in 42% of Charnley stems that were revised for femoral loosening, compared with 11% of those still surviving. The same phenomenon was noted in the Stanmore stem [25]. Poor proximal femoral filling with cement was associated with mechanical loosening of the curved stem Muller [26], the Cristiansen [27], and other mixed series [14,28]. Indeed Beckenbaugh and Ilstrup [3] considered that adequate cement packing was more important than avoiding varus alignment when inserting the Charnley stem. The difficulty with this observation is that varus alignment reduces the space for cement in the proximal medial zone of the femur, and varus alignment has been associated directly with aseptic loosening in the curved stem Muller [26,29–31], the McKee–Farrar [32], and the Stanmore [25] prostheses. The flat-back Charnley stem appeared to tolerate varus rather better than curved stem designs, but nevertheless a disproportionate number of cases inserted in varus came to revision [12].

Cement fracture is strongly associated with cement mantle defects in the proximal medial area in both the Muller curved [30] and the Charnley [33], as well as a series of mixed prosthetic designs [34]. A thick, proximal, medial, cement mantle protects against calcar absorption [35], whilst a cement layer of less than 5 mm is associated with endosteal bone lysis [36] and calcar resorption [37]. Bannister [38,39] compared first-generation cementing techniques in a mixed series of cemented Muller and Exeter prostheses. The cement mantle failed to extend beyond the tip of the prosthesis in 20% of cases and, in these, 36% came to revision, compared with 27% in those in which cement was impacted distal to the stem. Proximal femoral filling was 60% or less in 27% of cases; twice as many of these failed than in hip replacements, in which the proximal femur was filled by more than 60%. Proximal cement mantle deficiency was strongly associated with revision. In particular, cement deficiency in the proximal medial Gruen zone 7 was associated with a revision rate of 47%, and an increased relative risk of revision of 2.8. Cement deficiency in zone 7 predisposed to cantilever failure, resulting in stem fracture.

Some 7.4% of femoral components demonstrated lucent lines of 2 mm or more at the cement–bone interface on the postoperative film, and these cases ultimately comprised 17% of all revisions. Two-thirds of all cases that demonstrated postoperative radiolucent lines were revised, compared with a quarter of stems with intact cement–bone interfaces on the postoperative radiograph.

Acetabular cementing technique

The original technique recommended by Charnley was reaming superomedially at 45° and implantation of cement into cancellous bone. This was modified in three ways [5]. Reaming was changed to preserve the subchondral bone of the superior weight-bearing surface of the acetabulum and supplemented the original three 1.25 cm keyholes with multiple small holes. The bone was cleaned by brushing and pressurized lavage, and the shape of the cup changed to include a polyethylene skirt for pressure injection of the cement. This combination of changes was designated second-generation acetabular replacement. The effect of this change of technique was less dramatic than third-generation femoral cementing technique, but it was associated with a lower clinical failure rate in hip replacement for rheumatoid arthritis [38] and with radiographic loosening in other series [2,38].

Surgical technique

Surgical technique should start with preoperative planning, followed by a surgical approach that allows complete visualization of both the socket and femoral neck at implantation of the prosthesis, using second-generation acetabular and third-generation femoral cementing techniques.

Preoperative planning is important, as second-generation acetabular cementing techniques lower the socket in comparison with first, contributing to leg lengthening. The true centre of rotation of the femoral head is slightly inferior to the tip of the greater trochanter and preoperative planning allows adequate resection of femoral neck to avoid leg length discrepancy and to reproduce the anatomical offset. Preoperative planning allows a surgeon to appreciate bone stock deficiency, osteophytes that may project and impinge and identify cysts around the acetabulum and protrusio that require grafting.

Surgical approaches

The original surgical approach proposed by Charnley was trochanteric detachment. McKee and Muller used the modified Watson-Jones anterolateral and Ling and Sarmiento the posterior approach. The transgluteal approach was modified by Hardinge. The posterior approach is most widely used throughout the world, followed by the direct lateral approach. All the surgical approaches have advantages and disadvantages. Trochanteric detachment is complicated by non-union and trochanteric bursitis in between 5% and 10% of cases. The modified Watson-Jones approach affords limited access to the posterior aspect of the femoral neck. As the femur has a natural anterior bow, this tends to result in posterior stem alignment, and few surgeons, during their learning curve of this approach, have failed to penetrate the femur posteriorly. The posterior approach is more extensile than either the Watson-Jones or the direct lateral approach, but it is associated with a higher risk of posterior dislocation, which may become recurrent and effectively negate the benefit of the joint replacement.

The direct lateral approach has very limited proximal extensibility, because, if the muscle is split more than 2.5 cm (1 inch) proximal to the superior tip of the greater trochanter, the superior gluteal nerve is damaged, resulting in a Trendelenberg gait and external rotation deformity. Acute dislocation after the direct lateral approach usually results in breakdown of the repair, and late salvage of a chronically detached anterior half of gluteus medius is rarely successful.

Technique of primary total hip replacement by the posterior approach

The patient is placed in a lateral position with a prop against the sacrum posteriorly and the anterosuperior iliac spine anteriorly. Placement of the posterior prop against the lumbar spine extends the pelvis and confuses acetabular orientation. The anterior prop should allow the hip to flex to at least 90° without impingement (Fig. 5.7).

Incision

A straight, slightly oblique, incision extends from the

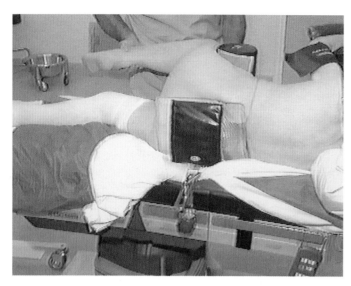

Figure 5.7 – Primary total hip replacement: the anterior prop should allow the hip to flex to at least 90° without impingement.

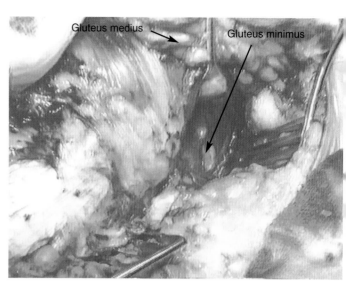

Figure 5.9 – Primary total hip replacement: the gluteal bursa is dissected cleanly from the posterior aspect of the greater trochanter, and a plane developed between gluteus medius and gluteus minimus with retraction of gluteus medius.

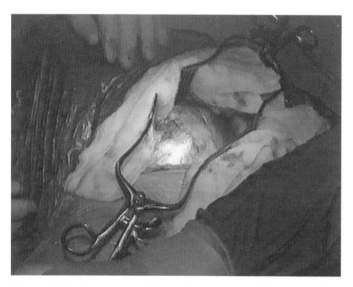

Figure 5.8 – Primary total hip replacement: avoid stripping the fat from the subcutaneous fat.

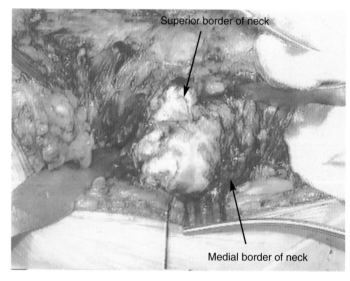

Figure 5.10 – Primary total hip replacement: the inferior capsule is exposed by developing the plane between quadratus femoris and the inferior capsule, and a blunt Homan bone lever is passed inferiorly to expose the area.

mid-femoral shaft, 5 cm distal to the ridge of the vastus lateralis, to transect the skin overlying the anterior two-thirds and distal third of the greater trochanter, extending proximally by a further 10 cm. The incision is deepened to split the fascia lata, which is incised distally with a knife and opened proximally with scissors. Stripping the fat from the subcutaneous fat devascularizes it, can delay healing, and should be avoided (Fig. 5.8). The gluteal bursa is dissected cleanly from the posterior aspect of the greater trochanter and a plane developed

between gluteus medius and minimus with retraction of gluteus medius (Fig. 5.9). The hip is then internally rotated, areolar tissue is swept from the short external rotators and a suture passed through the tendons of obturator internus and its gemelli and piriformis, which are divided as close as possible to the greater trochanter. This reveals capsule, which is then exposed by developing a plane under gluteus minimus superiorly and passing a blunt Homan bone lever horizontally anteriorly. The inferior capsule is exposed by developing the plane between quadratus femoris and the inferior capsule, and a blunt Homan bone lever is passed inferiorly to expose the area (Fig. 5.10). A stay suture is placed in the capsule, which is first resected as close as possible to the femoral neck, then released with two posterior incisions to leave a strip of posterior capsule at least 3 cm wide for repair at the end of the procedure. The hip is then dislocated by flexion and adduction. It is particularly important to avoid vigorous internal rotation in osteoporotic femora, because fracture may occur.

If a hip cannot be internally rotated to a right angle, the following restrainers should be sequentially divided. First the proximal 1 cm of the insertion of gluteus maximus is divided, and the posterior aspect of the femur stripped subperiosteally with a periosteal elevator to allow insertion of a blunt Homan lever. If the hip still does not internally rotate, incision is extended proximally, separating the quadratus femoris from the posterior aspect of the greater trochanter, and sweeping the tissue plane backwards with a periosteal elevator. This reveals the lesser trochanter, where the psoas can be divided, extending on to the anterior capsule. The hip is then flexed to 70°, exposing the medial border of the femoral neck (Fig. 5.11). The head is then resected (Fig. 5.12).

A blunt Homan is placed under this and a sharp Homan over the tip of the greater trochanter from distally to proximally. The stumps of the short external rotators and areolar tissue are dissected sharply from the piriform fossa to the junction of the femoral neck and greater trochanter and excised. The femoral neck is then resected and retracted anteriorly with a bone hook.

The labrum of the acetabulum is excised and, if that fails to give access to the anterior margin of the acetabulum, the superior, anterior, and inferior parts of the capsule are removed. The posterior iliofemoral ligament is rigorously preserved. A self-retaining retractor is placed under the anterior margin of gluteus maximus and the posterior margin of gluteus medius, a blunt Homan is placed anteriorly to retract the femur, a sharp Homan retractor is placed between the posterior capsule and posterior wall of the acetabulum to expose the posterior margin, a sharp Homan retractor is placed under the gluteus minimus 1 cm superior to the superior rim of the acetabulum, and a blunt Homan is placed inferiorly. The entire circumference of the acetabulum is then exposed (Fig. 5.13).

The next task is to find the medial wall of the acetabulum, which is located in the fovea acetabulare. This is obscured by the ligamentum teres. There is a vessel medial to ligamentum teres passing under the transverse ligament of the acetabulum. This retracts if the ligamentum teres, is merely transsected and bleeds. The correct technique is to divide the lateral two-thirds of the ligamentum teres, and then to take a Charnley curette distal to proximal against the roof of the fovea acetabulare. This removes the ligamentum teres, leaving areolar tissue with the vessel visible, emerging under the

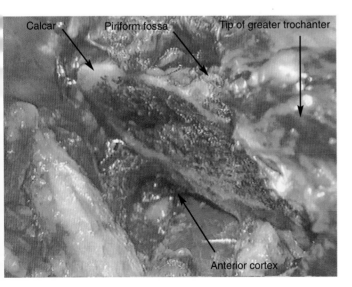

Figure 5.11 – *Primary total hip replacement: the hip is flexed to 70°, exposing the medial border of the femoral neck.*

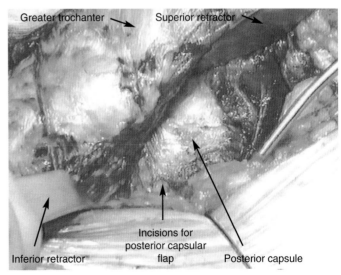

Figure 5.12 – *Primary total hip replacement: the entire circumference of the acetabulum is exposed.*

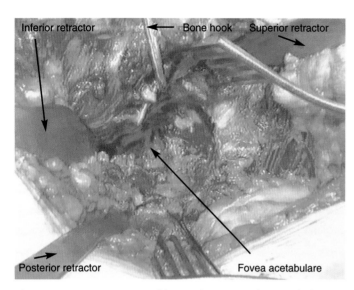

Figure 5.13 – *Primary total hip replacement: the acetabulum is cleared completely of soft tissue.*

transverse ligamentum of the acetabulum. These can be coagulated and resected, clearing the acetabulum completely of soft tissue (Fig. 5.13).

Using hemispherical reamers, the acetabulum is then reamed medially – about 50% of the depth of the fovea, then superiorly, preserving the subchondral plate, but removing cartilage to the point at which punctate haemorrhage appears through the cortical bone. Any cysts are curetted. Multiple small drill holes are placed superiorly and posteriorly, avoiding perforation of the acetabulum. A posterior perforation can allow cement to extrude around the sciatic nerve, giving one of the most devastating complications of total hip replacement.

The acetabulum is then brushed and cleaned by pressurized lavage. A flanged cup at least 4 mm smaller than the size reamed is taken and trimmed, to ensure that it passes freely in and out of the acetabulum. The rim should be left superiorly and a trial insertion without cement from a 90° closed to a 45° open position rehearsed. No specific haemostatic solution has been proved to reduce bleeding in the acetabulum. The acetabulum should be packed with swabs until dry. Once it is completely dry, cement in dough form that does not adhere to the glove is taken, the swab rapidly removed from the acetabulum, and the dough inserted and compressed. It is essential to insert this very quickly to avoid collection of blood between the cement and bone, and consequent weakening of the cement–bone interface. The surface of the cement is then dried of

blood and a cement compressor inserted with a glove overlying it. Use of a compressor without a glove creates a seal between the compressor and the cement, and when the compressor is removed cement may be sheared from the bone, which it has just penetrated.

Four minutes after cement mixing, the cup is inserted closed, pressed medially, and opened to ensure high compressive forces in the acetabular roof. The cup should be anteverted by some 20° so that the anterior rim is level with the anterior margin of the acetabulum. Compression should be maintained until the cement is cured after between 9 and 11 minutes, and loose cement removed from the periphery. A small swab is then placed in the acetabulum to prevent contamination.

Self-retaining retractor and bone levers are removed, and the femur flexed 20° and internally rotated. A blunt Homan retractor is placed medially. The femur is then flexed a further 30°. Another blunt Homan is placed anteriorly and a sharp Homan posterolaterally between gluteus medius and the greater trochanter. The true axis of the femur extends from the tip of the greater trochanter, and reaming of the canal should start lateral to this to ensure not only that the prosthesis can be orientated in neutral, but also that a satisfactory cement mantle can be obtained laterally (Fig. 5.14).

A spiked box osteotome is placed lateral to the tip of the greater trochanter and driven inferiorly, medial and

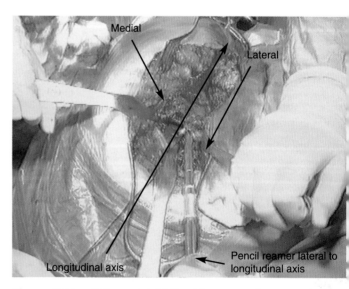

Figure 5.14 – *Primary total hip replacement: the true axis of the femur extends from the tip of the greater trochanter; reaming of the canal should start lateral to this to ensure not only that the prosthesis can be orientated in neutral, but also that a satisfactory cement mantle can be obtained laterally.*

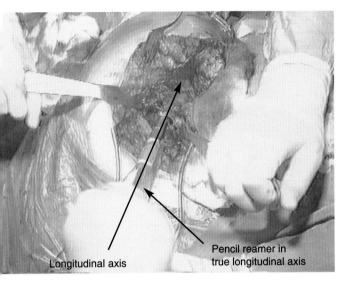

Longitudinal axis

Pencil reamer in
true longitudinal axis

Figure 5.15 – *Primary total hip replacement: the correct axis has been achieved if the reamer engages the medial cortex and straightens from a valgus to a neutral position.*

anteriorly to remove the cancellous bone from the greater trochanter down to the femoral neck. If a box osteotome is not available, an entry point can be made with osteotomes. A pencil reamer is then passed down. The correct axis has been achieved if the reamer engages the medial cortex and straightens from a valgus to a neutral position (Fig. 5.15).

The bone from the proximal femur should be removed by serial curetting, because this produces a lower intra-medullary pressure than broaches. When the bone has been removed to within 3–5 mm of the periphery, broaches can be inserted, leaving adequate space along-side them for marrow to escape. The broaches are inserted to the predetermined level, and a spigot and trial head placed *in situ* and then reduced.

The prosthesis is tested for stability in flexion, ad-duction, and internal rotation, with particular attention to any impingement anteromedially. Leg length is assessed by placing the femur parallel to the one below and palpating the infrapatellar region to ensure that they are level. If the leg is long and the offset correct with a medium-sized head, the neck can be resected further, and the process repeated until leg lengths are equal. When the correct leg length has been determined, the position to which the prosthesis should be inserted is marked on the greater trochanter, the broaches are removed, and the femur further curetted of loose bone, brushed, cleaned by pressurized lavage, restricted 1 cm

distal to the anticipated tip of the prosthesis, and then packed until dry.

Bleeding in the proximal femur occurs predominantly in the distal half of the restricted cavity, the source being the nutrient foramen about 4 cm distal to the greater trochanter. The most critical fixation is proximal and when the cement is gunned retrograde. Blood is usually brought up over the cement–bone interface, weakening it. For this reason, a venting catheter is placed in the prepared cavity distally as far as the restrictor, and a suction tube is applied. Cement is then gunned, beginning about 12 cm distal to the amputated neck, forcing the blood distally on to the venting tube, and leaving the proximal half of the femur dry. Cement is then gunned proximally.

A proximal restrictor is applied and cement continuously compressed until marrow extrudes. The pressure needs to be maintained for at least 10–20 seconds, and the restrictor is withdrawn with gunning continuing to ensure complete canal filling without lamination, which is caused by hand insertion of an additional bolus of cement. The proximal femur is then sealed with a glove and pressure is maintained manually.

After 3–4 minutes of mixing, the femoral component is inserted steadily, maintaining pressure over the medial border of the neck with the thumb of the non-dominant hand, to ensure that the alignment is in anatomical anteversion. The prosthesis is held in place while the cement sets; a trial head is inserted if a modular prosthesis

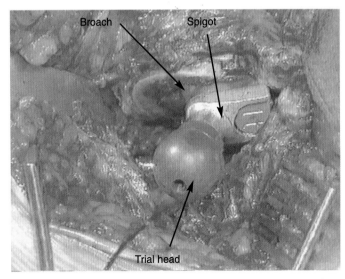

Broach   Spigot

Trial head

Figure 5.16 – *Primary total hip replacement: leg length is assessed and corrected if necessary by a different size modular head checking for stability.*

is used and reduced. Leg length is then assessed and corrected if necessary by a different sized modular head, checking for stability (Fig. 5.16).

Two 3.2-mm drills are placed from the lateral margin of the greater trochanter into the piriform fossa; either the skin hook or a suture passer is placed through these, taking the traction sutures from the capsule and external rotators superiorly and inferiorly. Both of these structures are then repaired with the capsule and the external rotators sutured with the hip extended and externally rotated.

A deep suction drain is inserted and the gluteal fascia repaired. The fat is closed with sutures, apposing the superficial fascia (Sherman's fascia) over another suction drain, and the skin is closed. The postoperative regimen should avoid adduction and internal rotation for 12 weeks to allow repair of the posterior capsule.

References

1. Dall DM, Learmonth ID, Solomon MI *et al.* Fracture and loosening of Charnley femoral stems. Comparison between first-generation and subsequent designs. *J Bone Joint Surg* 1993; 75B: 259–65.

2. Fowler JL Gie GA, Lee AJC, Ling RSM. Experience with the Exeter total hip replacement since 1970. *Orthop Clin N Am* 1988; 19: 477–89.

3. Beckenbaugh RD, Ilstrup DM. Total hip replacement. *J Bone Joint Surg* 1978; 60A: 306–13.

4. Thomas BJ, Salvati EA, Small RD. The CAD hip arthroplasty. *J Bone Joint Surg* 1986; 68A: 640–6.

5. Charnley J. *Low Friction Arthroplasty of the Hip*. Berlin: Springer-Verlag, 1979.

6. Havelin LI, Espehaug B, Vollset JE, Engesaeter LB. Early aseptic loosening of uncemented femoral components in primary total hip replacement. *J Bone Joint Surg* 1995; 77B: 11–17.

7. Dobbs HS. Survivorship of total hip replacements. *J Bone Joint Surg* 1980; 62B: 168–73.

8. Almby B, Hierton T. Total hip replacement. A ten year follow-up of an early series. *Acta Orthop Scand* 1982; 53: 397–406.

9. Reikeras O. Ten year follow-up of Muller hip replacements. *Acta Orthop Scand* 1982; 53: 919–22.

10. Griss P, Hackenbroch MM, Jager M *et al. Findings on Total Hip Replacement after 10 Years*. Bern: Hans Huber, 1982.

11. Markolf KL, Amstutz HC. *In vitro* measurement of bone–acrylic interface pressure during femoral component insertion. *Clin Orthop* 1976; 121: 60–6.

12. Carlsson AS, Gentz CF. Mechanical loosening of the femoral head prosthesis in the Charnley total hip arthroplasty. *Clin Orthop* 1980; 147: 262–70.

13. Cotterill P, Hunter GA, Tile M. A radiographic analysis of 166 Charnley-Muller total hip arthroplasties. *Clin Orthop Rel Res* 1982; 163: 120–6.

14. Tapadiya D, Walker RH, Schurman DJ. Prediction of outcome of total hip arthroplasty based on initial postoperative radiographic analysis. *Clin Orthop* 1984; 186: 5–15.

15. Harris WH, McCarthy JC, O'Neill DA. Femoral component loosening using contemporary techniques of femoral cement fixation. *J Bone Joint Surg* 1982; 64A: 1063–7.

16. Roberts DW, Poss R, Kelley K. Radiographic comparison of cementing techniques in total hip arthroplasty. *J Arthroplasty* 1986; 1: 241–7.

17. Paterson M, Fulford P, Denham R. Loosening of the femoral component after total hip replacement. *J Bone Joint Surg* 1986; 68B: 392–7.

18. Halawa M, Lee AJC, Ling RSM, Vangala SS. The shear strength of trabecular bone from the femur and some factors affecting the shear strength of the cement bone interface. *Arch Orthop Traumat Surg* 1978; 92: 19–30.

19. Harris WH, McGann WA. Loosening of the femoral component after use of the medullary-plug cementing technique. *J Bone Joint Surg* 1986; 68A: 1064–6.

20. Mulroy RD, Harris WH. The effect of improved cementing techniques on component loosening in total hip replacement. *J Bone Joint Surg* 1990; 72B: 757–60.

21. Barrack RL, Mulroy RD, Harris WM. Improved cementing techniques and femoral component loosening in young patients with hip arthroplasty. *J Bone Joint Surg* 1992; 74B: 385–9.

22. McCoy TH, Salvati EA, Ranawat CS, Wilson PD. A fifteen year follow-up of one hundred Charnley low-friction arthroplasties. *Orthop Clin N Am* 1988; 19: 467–76.

23. Russotti GM, Coventry MB, Stauffer RN. Cemented total hip arthroplasty with contemporary techniques. *Clin Orthop* 1988; 233: 141–7.

24. Malchau M, Herberts P. Prognosis of total hip replacement. Surgical and cementing technique in total hip replacement: a revision-risk study of 134,056 primary operations. Presented at the 63rd Annual Meeting of the American Academy of Orthopedic Surgeons, 22–26 February 1996, Atlanta, USA.

25. Kristiansen B, Jensen JS. Biomechanical factors in loosening of the Stanmore hip. *Acta Orthop Scand* 1985; 56: 21–4.

26. Sutherland CJ, Wilde AH, Borden LS, Marks KE. A 10 year follow-up of 100 consecutive Muller curved-stem total hip arthroplasties. *J Bone Joint Surg* 1982; 64A: 970–82.

27. Alho A, Soreide O, Bjers AJ. Mechanical factors in loosening of Christiansen and Charnley arthroplasties. *Acta Orthop Scand* 1984; 55: 261–6.

28. Iannoti JP, Balderston RA, Booth RE *et al.* Aseptic loosening after total hip arthroplasty. *J Arthroplasty* 1986; 1 :99–107.

29. Bosch P, Kriten M, Zweymuller K. An analysis of 119 loosenings in total hip endo prosthesis. *Arch Orthop Traumat Surg* 1980; 96: 83–90.

30. Willert HG, Buchhorn U, Zichner L. Clinical experience with Muller total hip endo prostheses of different design and material. *Arch Orthop Traumat Surg* 1980; 97: 197–205.

31. Brick GW, Poss R. Long-term follow-up of cemented total hip replacement for osteoarthritis. *Rheum Dis Clin N Am* 1988; 14: 565–77.

32. Coudane H, Fery A, Sommelet J *et al.* Aseptic loosening of cemented total arthroplasties of the hip in relation to positioning of the prosthesis. *Acta Orthop Scand* 1981; 52: 201–5.

33. Weber FA, Charnley J. A radiological study of fractures of acrylic cement in relation to the stem of a femoral head prosthesis. *J Bone Joint Surg* 1975; 57B: 297.

34. Chao EYS, Coventry MD. Fracture of the femoral component after total hip replacement. *J Bone Joint Surg* 1981; 63A: 1078-94.

35. Bocco F, Langan P, Charnley J. Changes in the calcar femoris in relation to cement technology in total hip replacement. *Clin Orthop* 1977; 128: 287–95.

36. Huddlestone HD. Femoral lysis after cemented hip arthroplasties. *J Arthroplasty* 1988; 3: 285–97.

38. Bannister GC. Fixation of the femoral component in total hip replacement. MD Thesis, University of Bristol, 1993.

39. Bannister GC. Mechanical failure in the femoral component in total hip replacement. *Orthop Clin N Am* 1988; 19: 567–76.

37. Sarmiento A, Natarajan V, Gruen TA, McMahon M. Radiographic performance of two different total hip arthroplasties of the hip in relation to positioning of the prosthesis. *Orthop Clin N Am* 1988; 19: 505–15.

38. Onsten I, Besjakov J, Carlsson AS. Improved radiographic survival of the Charnley prosthesis in rheumatoid arthritis and osteoarthritis. *J Arthroplasty* 1994; 9: 3–8.

CHAPTER 6

Complications of total hip replacement

G. C. Bannister

In descending order of frequency, the principal complications of total hip replacement are: thromboembolic disease, leg length discrepancy, heterotopic bone formation, dislocation, death, infection and nerve palsy (Table 6.1).

Table 6.1 *Complications of total hip replacement*

Complication	Incidence (%)
Venous thrombosis	40
Leg length discrepancy	27
Heterotopic bone formation	21
Dislocation	3
Death	1.3
Infection	1
Nerve palsy	<1

Thromboembolic disease

Thromboembolic disease causes death, pulmonary embolism, and readmission for venous thrombosis and could theoretically result in a postphlebitic limb; this in turn ulcerates and acts as a potential focus for infection to either the primary joint replacement or any later revision surgery. Of these, death is the most distressing and has been the principal focus of research.

The current incidence of death from pulmonary embolism after total hip replacement is an order of magnitude lower than the level traditionally suggested. Seagroatt et al. [1], using the Oxford Record Linkage Study, attributed death to total hip replacement in 0.6% of cases. Warwick et al. [2] demonstrated a death rate of 0.3% from pulmonary embolism of a consecutive population of 1162 patients undergoing either primary or revision total hip arthroplasty, and receiving antithrombotic medication, only if there had been previous thromboembolic events. Fender et al. [3] recorded four deaths from pulmonary embolism in 2111 consecutive primary hip replacements (0.2%).

Pulmonary emboli are generally preceded by deep venous thromboses. Deep venous thromboses (DVTs) can be investigated by phlebography, ultrasound scan, or radioactive labelled fibrinogen. Phlebography is the reference standard (Fig. 6.1), but gives only a snapshot at whatever point it is performed. Ultrasonography is operator dependent and is reliable for femoral, although less so for calf vein, thrombosis. Studies with radioactively labelled fibrinogen can no longer be performed because of the risk of disease transmission from pooled blood products. Ultrasonography and radioactively labelled fibrinogen studies allow examination of the natural history of DVT but, unless the sensitivity of ultrasonography improves, the state of knowledge will be reliant on historical studies with radioactively labelled fibrinogen.

Using radioactively labelled fibrinogen in a series of almost 500 patients, Sikorski et al. [4] observed a rate of DVT of 42% in patients in whom no attempt at prophylaxis was made. Six per cent of venous thromboses occurred in the first 2 days and 81% between days 3 and 7, and a further 13% over the course of the next 10 days. No venous thromboses developed later than 17 days after hip replacement. The series included a number of randomized prospective control trials, examining the prophylactic effect of heparin, aspirin, hydroxychloroquine, flurbiprofen, and intermittent positive pressure calf

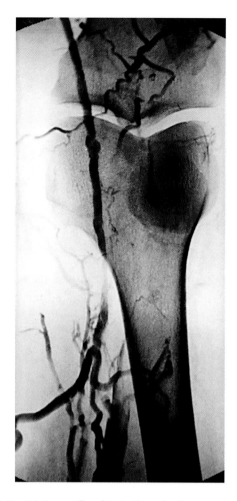

Figure 6.1 – *Major popliteal vein thrombosis.*

compression during and after surgery. None of the interventions significantly reduced the incidence of DVT, but subcutaneous heparin and intermittent positive pressure compression delayed its onset. More than 50% of the venous thromboses occurred 7 days after surgery, when subcutaneous heparin or intermittent positive pressure calf compression was used.

Studies purporting to reduce the incidence of death from thromboembolic disease after total hip replace-

Table 6.2 *Relative risk of venous thrombosis from [56]*

Intervention	Relative risk
Unfractionated heparin	0.86
Warfarin	0.49
Intermittent calf compression	0.43
Low-molecular-weight heparin	0.29
Adjusted dose heparin	0.22
Foot pumps	0.18

ment would ideally measure that variable. As the present death rate is 0.3%, study groups of many tens of thousands would be required to demonstrate any difference; in practice, the surrogate end-point of thrombosis is used. The problem with the surrogate end-point is that the type of venous thrombosis that causes pulmonary embolism is femoral and most DVTs recorded are calf vein, which propagate in only 14% of cases after total hip replacement [5]. The four deaths from pulmonary embolism in Warwick *et al.*'s series [2] of 1162 patients occurred on days 1, 2, and 5, and after 6 weeks in a patient who had been warfarinized. It is extremely unlikely that any venous thrombosis would have formed after total hip replacement on days 1 and 2 or in a warfarinized patient, leaving one patient who potentially would have benefited from thromboprophylaxis (0.09% of cases). Pooling prospective randomized controlled trials, the relative risks of DVT are shown in Table 6.2. In most studies, phlebography is carried out between 7 and 10 days after surgery. These studies inevitably miss between 30% and 50% of venous thromboses because prophylaxis delays their development. Even assuming that the best prophylaxis for DVT is totally representative of the risk of death from pulmonary embolism, the effect is an 80% reduction of death rate from 9 per 1000 to 2 per 1000, but, for reasons detailed above, probably very much lower.

There has been only one prospective randomized controlled trial of pharmacological thromboprophylaxis in total hip replacement using death as the outcome [6]. Patients were anticoagulated with phenindione and death rates in the intervention and control groups were the same, although skewed towards thrombosis in the control group and towards haemorrhage in the intervention group. The Trent Regional Arthroplasty Register [3] showed no difference in death rates between those patients who did and did not receive pharmacological prophylaxis; although the subject is emotive, it may well be that the capacity to influence death as a result of pulmonary embolism after total hip replacement is very limited indeed.

Pulmonary embolism and readmission

The Oxford Linkage Study [1] reported a readmission rate with symptomatic thromboembolic complication of 0.73%. Warwick *et al.* [7] recorded a total incidence of pulmonary embolism of 0.2% and a readmission rate within 28 days of 1.4%, for symptomatic thromboembolic complication.

Postphlebitic limb

McNally *et al.* [8] found that seven of eight patients, who had had phlebographically demonstrated thrombosis in the operated leg after total hip replacement, developed clinical signs of chronic venous insufficiency. Warwick *et al.* [2] reviewed 67 patients a mean of 16 years after studies with radioactively labelled fibrinogen had shown venous thrombosis. There was no difference in chronic venous insufficiency whether or not the limb had had a venous thrombosis demonstrated.

Conclusion

No subject is more emotive or fraught with medicolegal implications than thromboembolic disease. There are a plethora of surrogate data covering the first week and a half, but it is likely that prophylaxis during this period offers very partial protection, if any at all. Foot pumps seem to be the best prophylaxis. In patients who have already had a DVT or pulmonary embolism, anti-coagulation for at least 3 months seems the most sensible intervention.

Leg length discrepancy

It is unusual to obtain perfect equality of leg length after total hip replacement, but two-thirds should be within 5 mm [9]. The literature records discrepancies of about 1 cm up to the 1990s.

Sarangi and Bannister [9] compared true discrepancy, measured from fixed points on the pelvis and femur, with that perceived by patients who had undergone total hip replacement. Lengthening of between 4 mm and 6 mm was perceived by 26% of patients, of 6–10 mm by 53%, and of more than 10 mm by all patients. No patient perceived shortening of 0–5 mm, 50% of those with shortening of between 6 mm and 10 mm noticed a difference, but all patients perceived a difference when shortening exceeded 1 cm.

Techniques for assessment of leg length differential have, for practical reasons, involved measurement of a perpendicular from a horizontal line through the tear-drop, and a fixed point on the femur, and do not take into account pelvic tilt or other differentials within the lower limb. The techniques do, however, either differentiate between pre- and postoperative leg lengths. Leg length differential has become a significantly greater problem in clinical practice, because acetabular components have been fixed in lower, more anatomical, positions increasing leg length. The most vulnerable patient is the one whose leg lengths are absolutely equal before replacement, or whose contralateral hip has been replaced with a high hip centre. The most practical approach to avoidance of excessive leg lengthening is repeated checking of leg length against a fixed point, and a willingness to shorten the femoral neck to accommodate the lower position in which acetabular components are placed in modern practice. The importance of obtaining the closest possible leg length approximation is reflected in the dissatisfaction of patients with shoe raises. In patients provided with a shoe raise in the Sarangi and Bannister series, none with lengthening was satisfied, and only half of those with shortening derived benefit.

Conclusion

The practice of preserving the subchondral plate of the acetabulum, and reproducing the anatomical axis of rotation of the hip, has made patients very much more vulnerable to leg lengthening after total hip arthroplasty. In the early postoperative period, this is compounded by pelvic tilt, which takes several months to correct, even when leg lengths are anatomically correct. Once the leg has been lengthened, it is almost impossible to recover the situation. Shoe raises are unsatisfactory and the decision is whether to revise the femoral component, leaving slacker musculature and the risk of dislocation, or to accept what is often a very substandard hip. Leg length discrepancy is a widespread problem that increasingly presents in medicolegal practice. It behoves the surgeon to establish the closest possible leg length by trial reductions before implanting the femoral component. There should be no hesitation in resecting rather more neck to ensure equal leg length, because most stems transmit forces distally.

The use of short- and long-necked modular femoral heads is only partially helpful because such devices interfere with the offset of the hip and create their own problems. There is no firm proof at present that devices designed to ensure leg length equality are any better than clinical methods or an experienced surgeon. Palpation of the inferior pole of the patella in patients undergoing hip replacement in the lateral position, or of the heels if supine, are the clinical measures available. The patient at risk of lengthening is the one who starts with equal leg lengths; faced with the choice of lengthening or shortening a patient, the surgeon should opt for a little shortening, because that is likely to be much more acceptable.

Table 6.3   *Brooker classification*

Class	
I	Islands of bone in soft tissues
II	Bone spurs arising from pelvis or femur with 1 cm between
III	As II with less than 1 cm between
IV	Apparent ankylosis

Heterotopic bone formation

Heterotopic bone formation was found in 14.6% of the 2000 cases of hip arthroplasty performed at the Centre for Hip Surgery at Wrightington between 1970 and 1971. The complication was invariably seen if a previous hip arthroplasty had developed new bone; otherwise it was more common in patients with osteoarthritis and in men [10]. Increasing heterotopic bone formation was associated with a decrease in hip movement.

Brooker *et al.* [11] noted heterotopic bone formation in 21% of 100 consecutive total hip replacements, classifying the complication to four groups (Table 6.3). Only class IV was associated with deterioration of function, as measured by Harris' Hip Score. Experimental data suggest that pluripotential mesenchymal cells released from marrow initiate new bone formation in the first 10 days after hip arthroplasty. Thus, interventions during this period are likely to reduce heterotopic bone formation, and indeed do. Non-steroidal anti-inflammatory drugs and low-dose irradiation have both been used. There seems to be little difference between indomethacin administered for the first 3 days postoperatively and indomethacin administered for 7 days [12]. Diclofenac is equally effective [13], but ibuprofen slightly less so [14]. Irradiation is only practical in units with radiotherapy centres; in the postoperative period, it presents practical difficulties, because patients have to be moved from their ward to the radiation centre quite soon after surgery, at a time when they are in maximum pain and at greatest risk of dislocation. Preoperative radiation has been tried [15] but is less good than postoperative radiation [16]; it is approximately as effective as ibuprofen.

Conclusion

Overall, it would appear that all patients who have previously formed heterotopic bone should have at least

a 3-day postoperative course of a strong non-steroidal anti-inflammatory drug, or postoperative radiation. Males with hypertrophic osteoarthritis are also at high risk and should be treated by the same regimen. If patients have ankylosed one total hip arthroplasty and irradiation facilities are available, four doses of irradiation of 3 Gy is the most effective regimen reported in the literature [17].

Dislocation after total hip replacement

Although dislocation occurs less frequently in the hands of experienced surgeons [18], the incidence is rising. Modern series have great difficulty in rivalling the 0.4% recorded by Etienne *et al.* (1978) [19] from Wrightington in the 1970s.

Natural history

If dislocations are going to occur, they tend to do so early. Khan *et al.* [20] recorded that 66% of dislocations of cemented primary total hip replacements occurred within 5 weeks of surgery, whereas Williams *et al.* [21] recorded 70% in the first 30 days. The natural history of dislocation is that the majority stabilize after the first event. Khan *et al.* [20] found that 81% of patients who dislocated within 5 weeks of surgery stabilized, as did 73% of those whose first dislocation was after that time. Most patients are unable to recollect the mechanism of dislocation. A small proportion occur in the operating room, 27% on rotation, and 21% on flexion. The direction of dislocation depends on the surgical approach employed. The most stable is the anterolateral approach, followed by trochanteric detachment. The least stable is the posterior approach. In dislocations in series in which trochanteric detachment has been employed, non-union is a major cause [19,22,23]. The only dissenter from this premise is Khan *et al.*, who found comparable rates of dislocation, regardless of approach, in a series of 142 cases.

Factors affecting dislocation

Factors affecting dislocation after total hip replacement may be either within or outside the surgeon's influence. Woo and Morrey [24] found that dislocation rates quadrupled when total hip replacement was performed after non-union of femoral neck fracture, Girdlestone arthroplasty, or septic arthritis. Newington *et al.* [25]

recorded similar levels in primary total hip replacements in patients aged 80 years or over. Woo and Morrey [24] found that primary total hip replacement for displaced intracapsular fracture, after previous arthrodesis, or congenital dislocation more than doubled the risk of dislocation. Lindberg *et al.* [26] associated dislocation with alcoholism in men and Khan *et al.* [20] associated it with dementia or Parkinson's disease.

Hip arthroplasty surgery is at greatest risk of dislocation if it is carried out for recurrent dislocators or after previous hip surgery, with dislocation rates in excess of 25% and 10%, respectively, being regularly recorded.

A number of factors can be influenced by the surgeon, and in general these involve restoring hip anatomy as closely as possible. Thus, Khan *et al.* [20] found that 48% of acetabular components in hips that had dislocated were malaligned, along with 25% of stems. Daly and Morrey [27] found 28% of acetabular components were retroverted in a series of re-explorations and Williams *et al.* [21] noted that open cups were associated with a higher dislocation rate. Lewinnek *et al.* [28] recorded a narrow range of cup orientation, in which hips were relatively protected from dislocation. Cup orientation depends on the position of the patient on the table. Ease of cup orientation was a major factor that led Charnley [29] to prefer to place patients in the supine position. If hip arthroplasty is carried out in the lateral position, placement of the posterior prop against the sacrum may antevert the pelvis, thus placing the cup at risk of retroversion.

Abductor function

Abductor function can be disrupted by surgical detachment of the glutei, reducing either their power by shortening the hip or their lever arm by failing to restore anatomical offset. Detachment of the greater trochanter is strongly associated with dislocation. Shortening of the hip by placing a high hip centre or resecting too much femoral neck [23], and reducing the distance from the centre of the head to the greater trochanter [18,19], are all associated with a higher dislocation rate. Non-trochanteric detaching approaches, horizontal reaming in preparing the acetabulum for cup insertion, and pre-operative planning to restore femoral offset make these complications avoidable.

Head size and neck impingement exert some influence over dislocation. Woo and Morrey [24] recorded a dislocation rate of 2.6% in 22.25-mm heads, which fell to 1.3% when the head size increased to 28 mm. Dislocation in the 22.25-mm Charnley head was halved when the long posterior wall cup was introduced, presumably converting full dislocation to recoverable subluxations.

Ligamentous balance about the hip has attracted relatively little interest compared with the knee. Charnley originally preserved the capsule to maintain stability [19], but it is axiomatic that, unless the entire capsule is excised, it will be damaged at the site of approach and anteroposterior balance will be lost. The natural hip has the constraining effect of the ligamentum teres, which cannot be replaced at arthroplasty, and capsular balance must be considered. Woo and Morrey [24] were the first to point out the higher dislocation rate that follows the posterior approach. They repaired the short external rotators, but not the capsule. In contrast to their dislocation rate of 5.8%, Hedley *et al.* [30] were able to report 0.8% after repairing the posterior capsule and short external rotators. These results have been widely reproduced and are currently at the report stage.

The captive cup has long since been an option for patients likely to dislocate. Khan *et al.* [20] showed that the Howse had only a slightly lower dislocation rate than the Charnley. The Howse had a larger head and a cup that was held captive by a rim in the polyethylene cup. Fackler and Poss [18] recorded dislocations despite a constrained cup and Anderson *et al.* [31] recorded a 27% dislocation rate after using the S-Rom device. Goetz *et al.* [32] have recorded a promising 96% stability after salvage surgery for dislocation, using the Omnifit constrained cup; if these results are reproduced, there is a place for this device not only in the salvage of dislocation, but in revision arthroplasty in vulnerable groups.

Conclusion

In all total hip replacements, the surgeon should endeavour to orientate components in anatomical anteversion and avoid closed position of the cup. Regardless of the surgical approach used, muscle and capsule layers should be carefully repaired to restore ligamentous balance. Groups at risk of dislocation include those undergoing revision hip arthroplasty, patients with neurological deficit, or octogenarians. In these groups of patients, long posterior wall acetabular components should be used at the very least, and a 28-mm head if polyethylene thickness allows; if the Omnifit constrained cup proves as successful as its initial report, it would seem sensible to use it routinely.

Prevention of infection

Deep infection rates of the order of 10% were reported in the early series of cemented hip arthroplasties [33]. Indirect studies on operating room air by Charnley and Eftekhar [33], and experimental studies by Southwood *et al.* [34], indicate that it takes as little as 10 organisms to infect a cemented arthroplasty in human and animal models, whereas it takes of the order of 500 000 organisms to infect sequestrum. The potential to influence infection in total hip arthroplasty involves reducing the inoculum of bacteria, wearing occlusive clothing, using antibiotic prophylaxis, washing the wound, using antiseptics, and general operating room discipline. In conventional operating rooms, some 2000 colony-forming units per square metre per hour (CFU/m^2 per h) are isolated on settle plates [35]. This can be reduced by thick operating room clothing [36], but dramatic reductions come only with laminar flow [33] or ultraviolet light [37].

The laminar flow systems employed in operating rooms enjoyed their first use as prophylaxis against infection in top fermenting beer at the Friary Meux Brewery in south London. At this particular brewery, bacteria were infecting the wort of the top fermenting beer and laminar flow was extremely effective in eliminating this. It is less effective in operating rooms because of interposition of operating room personnel.

Salvati *et al.* (1982) [38a] examined infection rates after hip and knee arthroplasty in conventional and ultra-clean air operating rooms. In conventional ones, infection rates for both hip and knee arthroplasty were 1.4% and, in ultra-clean air, this fell to 0.9% for hip arthroplasty but rose to 3.9% in knee replacement. The reason for this was interposition of operating personnel, bacteria from whom were blown into the wound. Charnley [38b] had anticipated this problem and combined ultra-clean air with occlusive clothing, which removed all bacteria from the surgeon out of the operating room enclosure. Taylor and Bannister [39] reproduced the Salvati experience experimentally, showing that interposition of operating room personnel increased shedding of bacteria onto settle plates by a factor of 27.

Hubble *et al.* [35] repeated this work, testing the effects of mask, hat, and modern closely woven polyester clothing with elasticated sleeves, ankles, and necks. Failure to wear a mask in an ultra-clean air environment increased shedding of bacteria 22-fold, balloon cotton clothing sixfold, but a hat, a mask, and polyester gowns by only 1.4-fold, indicating that it is possible with existing clothing to approach the standard of cleanliness achieved by the much more cumbersome Charnley 'space suit'.

The standard method for testing operating room technique is air sampling. It is of interest that, in this study, air sampling failed to detect organisms that were found on settle plates underneath the surgeon's head in 57% of experiments.

Comments on clothing

Conventional operating rooms are so contaminated that clothing is unlikely to make a significant difference to infection rates. Reliance should instead be placed on antibiotic prophylaxis and antiseptics. In laminar flow operating rooms, clothing is critical in personnel interposed between the clean air source and the patient. It would appear that closely woven polyester with elasticated sleeves and well-covered hair matches space suits and should suffice. It is axiomatic that operating room gowns, worn by personnel who have contact with the wound, should be absolutely waterproof, because bacteria permeate wet clothing and migrate from surgeon to wound.

Antibiotic prophylaxis

The principle of antibiotic prophylaxis was established by Burke on guinea-pig skin [40]. Regardless of the antibiotic, the greatest effect was achieved when prophylaxis was given 1 hour before introduction of bacteria and ceased after 4 hours. The principle was rapidly reproduced in both hip fracture and replacement surgery by Ericson *et al.* [41] and in joint replacement by Hill *et al.* [42]. The duration of antibiotic prophylaxis in the early studies was 14 days in Ericson's, and 5 days in Hill's. Pollard *et al.* [43] examined 12 hours prophylaxis, showing no difference, but the study was powered to show a 30% difference and rather better evidence in implant surgery was provided by Gatell *et al.* [44], who showed that one dose of cefamandole was less effective than five doses. It would appear that at least 24 hours of antibiotic prophylaxis is necessary to be effective in bone and joint surgery.

The type of antibiotic has to reflect the protean nature of bacterial contamination. Some 40% of contamination is staphylococcal. In early series coagulase-positive staphylococci dominated, but, with increasing use of antibiotics and the development of resistance, the coagulase-negative *staphylococcus* is now the most common contaminant. The remaining organisms are a mixture of streptococci, and skin and faecal bacteria.

Lidwell *et al.* [45], in a prospective randomized controlled trial comparing laminar flow operating rooms with conventional ones, also prospectively studied the use of antibiotics and found that the cephalosporins had half the infection rate of cloxacillin alone. Joseffson *et al.* [46] carried out a prospective randomized controlled trial comparing gentamicin cement with narrow-spectrum, anti-staphylococcal, systemic antibiotics. Superficial infection rates were slightly greater in the gentamicin group, but deep infection fell to 0.4% in the gentamicin cement group, compared with 1.6% in those receiving systemic antibiotics.

Conclusion

As a third of major skin infections spread to deep tissues, it would appear sensible to use antibiotics both in the cement and systemically for maximum effect.

Combination of interventions

Lidwell [47] reviewed his cases 5 years later, examining the additive effects of ultra-clean air, systemic antibiotics, and body exhaust suits. A baseline infection rate of 3.4% in conventional operating rooms, with balloon cotton clothing and no antibiotics, reduced to 1.6% with ultra-clean air, conventional clothing, and no antibiotics, and to between 0.9% and 0.7% with ultra-clean air and body exhaust suits, conventional operating rooms, conventional clothing, and antibiotics, and ultra-clean air, conventional clothing, and antibiotics. The real advantage came when ultra-clean air, body exhaust suits, and anti-biotics were combined, at which point infection rates fell by an order of magnitude to 0.06%. It would appear that there are huge potential advantages from combining ultra-clean air, occlusive clothing, and antibiotics in the prevention of infection.

The surgeon can influence wound contamination and infection by technique. Taylor *et al.* [39] modelled wounds using irradiated ovine muscle, fat and agar, and standardized distribution of air-borne bacteria; they

Table 6.4 *Reduction of bacteria on ovine muscle model*

Intervention	Reduction (%)
Pulsed jet lavage with chlorhexidine 0.05%	100
Chlorhexidine 0.05%	90
Pulsed jet lavage (Hartmann's)	79
Povidone-iodine 1%	67
Hydrogen peroxide 3%	−25

were able to examine the effects of lavage and antiseptics (Table 6.4). Pulsed jet lavage cleared 79% of organisms, 1% povidone-iodine (the highest concentration permissible in human tissue) killed 67%, and 0.05% chlorhexidine 90%. Hydrogen peroxide 3%, which is widely used, in fact increased the colony count because it broke colony-forming units off from the squames that had transported them to the model wounds.

Operating room discipline

Operating room discipline applies to surgeons and support staff. Pavel [48] examined the effect of length of surgery on infection rates. Operations between 0 and 1 hours had an infection rate of 2.6%, rising to 4.6% between 1 and 2 hours, 8.5% between 2 and 3 hours, and 8.6% at over 3 hours. It would appear that surgeons would be wise to restrict their operative endeavours to no more than 1 hour in a primary joint replacement, and certainly no more than 2 hours. This is achieved by preoperative planning to minimize time wasted while the wound is open.

In operating rooms, the greater the number of personnel, the greater the risk. A maximum of four personnel should be allowed and movement within a clean air enclosure minimized.

Conclusion

A combination of ultra-clean operating room, occlusive clothing, local and systemic antibiotics, pulsed lavage, antiseptics, and operating room discipline should enable surgeons to achieve infection rates of a fraction of a percentage in primary total hip replacement.

Nerve palsy

Nerve palsy is a rare complication of total hip replacement and recovery is usually incomplete. The mean incidence is 1.2% [49], being tripled in revision hip arthroplasty and at least doubled in total hip replacement for developmental dysplasia [50]. By far the most frequently injured nerve is the common peroneal component of the sciatic and, overall, sciatic palsies account for 79% of reported cases [51]. The femoral (13%) and obturator nerve (1.6%) are injured less frequently.

As the motor end-plates fibrose after 18 months, recovery from sciatic palsy is rarely complete: 41% recover virtually fully, 44% require orthotics, and the remainder are severely handicapped. If recovery has not occurred by 21 months, it is unlikely to do so [51].

Although clinical nerve palsy is rare, electrophysiological evidence is more widespread. Weber *et al.* [51] identified subclinical nerve injury in almost 70% of cases, and Weale *et al.* [52] observed five lesions in four patients whose hips had been replaced by the direct lateral approach. No electrophysiological disturbance was found in patients whose hip had been approached posterolaterally.

Superior gluteal injury via the direct lateral approach affects some 17% of patients, most of whom have a long-term Trendelenberg gait [53,54]. It would appear that taking an anterior sliver of the greater trochanter in the course of a direct lateral approach reduces this significantly [53].

Conclusion: prevention of nerve palsy

Although no specific cause can be identified in the vast majority of cases, some nerve palsy resulting from extrusion of cement through acetabular defects can clearly be avoided by retaining the integrity of the acetabulum in preparation before cementing. Lengthening by more than 4 cm [55] has been associated with nerve palsy and, in cases of developmental dysplasia or revision, it would seem sensible to identify, dissect, and free the sciatic nerve from adhesions before lengthening significantly. The logical general advice would be to ensure that sufficient soft tissue releases are carried out to allow access to the hip without undue force, giving adequate exposure to place retractors accurately.

References

1. Seagroatt V, Tan HS, Goldacre M *et al.* Elective total hip replacement, incidence, emergency re-admission rate and postoperative probability. *Brit Med J* 1991; 303: 1431–5.

2. Warwick D, Perez J, Vickery C, Bannister GC. Does total hip arthroplasty predispose to chronic venous insufficiency? *J Arthroplasty* 1996; 11: 529–33.

3. Fender D, Harper WM, Thompson JR, Gregg PJ. Mortality and fatal pulmonary embolism after primary total hip replacement. *J Bone Joint Surg* 1997; 79B: 896–9.

4. Sikorski JM, Hampson WG, Staddon GE. The natural history and aetiology of deep vein thrombosis after total hip replacement. *J Bone Joint Surg* 1981; 63B: 171–7.

5. Oishi CS, Grady-Benson JC, Otis SM *et al.* The clinical course of distal deep venous thrombosis after total hip replacement and total knee arthroplasty as determined with duplex ultrasonography. *J Bone Joint Surg* 1994; 76A: 1658–62.

6. Crawford WJ, Hillman F, Charnley J. *A clinical trial of prophylactic anticoagulant therapy in elective hip surgery.* Centre for Hip Surgery, Wrightington Hospital, Internal Publication 14: 1968.

7. Warwick DJ, Williams M, Bannister GC. Death and thrombo-embolic disease after total hip replacement. A series of 1162 cases with no routine chemical prophylaxis. *J Bone Joint Surg* 1995; 77B: 6–10.

8. McNally M, McAlden MG, O'Connell ECL, Mollan RAB. Post phlebitic syndrome after hip arthroplasty. *Acta Orthop Scand* 1994; 65: 595–8.

9. Sarangi PP, Bannister GC. Leg length discrepancy after total hip replacement. *Hip Int* 1997; 7: 121–4.

10. De Lee J, Ferrari A, Charnley J. Ectopic bone formation following low friction arthroplasty. *Clin Orthop* 1976; 121: 53–9.

11. Brooker AF, Bowerman JW, Robinson RA, Riley LH. Ectopic ossification following total hip replacement. *J Bone Joint Surg* 1973; 55A: 1629–32.

12. Dorn U, Grethan C, Effenburger H *et al.* Indomethacin for prevention of heterotopic ossification after hip arthroplasty. *Acta Orthop Scand* 1998; 69: 107–10.

13. Wahlstrom O, Risto O, Djer K, Hammerby S. Heterotopic bone formation prevented by diclofenac. *Acta Orthop Scand* 1991; 62: 419–21.

14. Persson PE, Sopemman B, Wilsson OS. Preventative effects of ibuprofen on periarticular heterotopic ossification after total hip replacement. *Acta Orthop Scand* 1998; 69: 111–15.

15. Van Leuwen WM, Deckers P, De Lannge WJ. Preoperative irradiation for prophylaxis of ectopic ossification after hip arthroplasty. *Acta Orthop Scand* 1998; 62: 116–18.

16. Pellegrini VD, Gregoritch SJ. Preoperative irradiation for prevention of heterotopic ossification following total hip arthroplasty. *J Bone Joint Surg* 1996; 78A: 870–81.

17. Knelles D, Barthel T, Karrer A *et al.* Prevention of heterotopic ossification after total hip replacement. *J Bone Joint Surg* 1997; 79B: 596–602.

18. Fackler CD, Poss R. Dislocation in total hip arthroplasties. *Clin Orthop* 1980; 151: 169–78.

19. Etienne A, Cupic Z, Charnley J. Postoperative dislocation after Charnley low-friction arthroplasty. *Clin Orthop* 1978; 132: 19–23.

20. Khan MAA, Brakenbury PH, Reynolds ISR. Dislocation following total hip replacement. *J Bone Joint Surg* 1981; 63B: 214–18.

21. Williams JF, Gottesman MJ. Dislocation after total hip arthroplasty. *Clin Orthop* 1982; 171: 53–8.

22. Eftekhar NS. Dislocation and instability complicating low friction arthroplasty of the hip. *Clin Orthop* 1976; 121: 120–5.

23. Framer GA, Wroblewski BM. Revision of the Charnley low-friction arthroplasty for recurrent or irreducible dislocation. *J Bone Joint Surg* 181; 63B: 552–5.

24. Woo RVG, Morrey BF. Dislocation after total hip arthroplasty. *J Bone Joint Surg* 1982; 64A: 1295–306

25. Newington DP, Bannister GC, Fordyce M. Primary total hip replacement in patients over 80 years of age. *J Bone Joint Surg* 1990; 72B: 450–2.

26. Lindberg HO, Carlsson AJ, Clentz C, Pettersson H. Recurrent and non recurrent dislocation following total hip arthroplasty. *Acta Orthop Scand* 1982; 53: 947–52.

27. Daly PJ, Morrey BF. Operative correction of an unstable total hip arthroplasty. *J Bone Joint Surg* 1992; 74A: 1334–43.

28. Lewinnek GE, Lewis JL, Tarr R *et al.* Dislocations after total hip replacement arthroplasties. *J Bone Joint Surg* 1978; 60A: 217–20.

29. Charnley J. *Low Friction Arthroplasty of the Hip: Theory and practice.* Berlin: Springer-Verlag, 1979.

30. Hedley AK, Hendren DH, Mead LP. A posterior approach to the hip joint with complete posterior capsular and muscular repair. *J Arthroplasty* 1990; 5(suppl): 57-66.

31. Anderson MJ, Murray WR, Skinner HB. Constrained acetabular components. *J Arthroplasty* 1994; 9: 17–23.

32. Goetz DD, Capello WN, Callaghan JJ *et al.* Salvage of a recurrently dislocating total hip prosthesis with use of a constrained acetabular component. *J Bone Joint Surg* 1998; 80A: 502–9.

33. Charnley J, Eftekhar N. Postoperative infection in total prosthetic replacement arthroplasty of the hip joint. *Br J Surg* 1969; 56: 641–9.

34. Southwood RT, Rice JL, McDonald PJ *et al.* Infection in

experimental hip arthroplasties. *J Bone Joint Surg* 1985; 67B: 229–31.

35. Hubble MJ, Weale AE, Perez JV *et al.* Clothing in laminar flow operating theatres. *J Hosp Infect* 1996; 32: 1–7.

36. Taylor GJS, Bannister GC. Infection and interposition between ultra clean air source and wound. *J Bone Joint Surg* 1993; 75B: 503–4.

37. Berg M, Bergman BR, Hoborn J. Ultraviolet radiation compared to an ultraclean air enclosure. Comparison of air bacteria counts in operating rooms. *J Bone Joint Surg* 1991; 73B: 811–15.

38. Salvati EA, Robinson RP, Zeno SM *et al.* Infection rates after 3175 total hip and total knee replacements performed with and without horizontal unidirectional air-flow system. *J Bone Joint Surg* 1982; 64A: 525–35.

39. Taylor GJS, Leeming JP, Bannister GC. Effect of antiseptics, ultraviolet light and lavage on airborne bacteria in a model wound. *J Bone Joint Surg* 1993; 75B: 724–30.

40. Burke JF. The effective period of preventive antibiotic action in experimental incisions and dermal lesions. *Surgery* 1961; 50: 161–8.

41. Ericson C, Lidgren L, Lindberg L. Cloxacillin in prophylaxis of postoperative infections of the hip. *J Bone Joint Surg* 1973; 55A: 808–13.

42. Hill C, Mazas F, Flamant R, Evrard J. Prophylactic cefazolin versus placebo in total hip replacement. *Lancet* 1981; i: 795–7.

43. Pollard JP, Hughes SPF, Scott JE *et al.* Antibiotic prophylaxis in total hip replacement. *Brit Med J* 1979; 1: 707–9.

44. Gatell JM, Garcia S, Lozano L *et al.* Perioperative cefamandole prophylaxis against infections. *J Bone Joint Surg* 1987; 69A: 1189–93.

45. Lidwell OM, Lowbury EJL, Whyte W *et al.* Effect of ultraclean air in operating rooms on deep sepsis of the joint after total hip or knee replacement: A randomised study. *Brit Med J* 1982; 285: 10–14.

46. Joseffson G, Lindberg L, Wiklander B. Systemic antibiotics and gentamicin-containing bone cement in total hip arthroplasty. *Clin Orthop* 1981; 159: 194–200.

47. Lidwell OM. Air, antibiotics and sepsis in replacement joints. *J Hosp Inf* 1998; 11(suppl C): 18–40.

48. Pavel A, Smith RL, Ballard A, Larsen IJ. Prosphylactic antibiotics in clean orthopaedic surgery. *J Bone Joint Surg* 1974; 56A: 777–782.

49. Schmalzried TP, Amstutz HC, Dorey FJ. Nerve palsies associated with total hip replacement. *J Bone Joint Surg* 1991; 73A: 1074–81.

50. Schmalzried TP, Noordin J, Amstrutz HC. Update on nerve palsy associated with total hip replacement. *Clin Orthop* 1997; 344: 188–206.

51. Weber ER, Daube JR, Coventry MB. Peripheral neuropathies associated with total hip arthroplasty. *J Bone Joint Surg* 1976; 58: 66–9.

52. Weale AE, Newman P, Ferguson IT, Bannister GC. Nerve injury after posterior and lateral approaches for hip replacement. *J Bone Joint Surg* 1996; 78B: 899–902.

53. Baker AS, Bitounis VC. Abductor function after total hip replacement. *J Bone Joint Surg* 1989; 71B: 47–50.

54. Ramesh M, G Byne JM, McCarthy N *et al.* Damage to the superior gluteal nerve after the Hardinge approach to the hip. *J Bone Joint Surg* 1996; 78B: 903–6.

55. Edwards BN, Tullos MS, Noble PC. Contributory factors and aetiology of sciatic nerve palsy in total hip arthroplasty. *Clin Orthop* 1987; 218: 136–41.

56. Warwick D, Harrison J, Whitehouse S. The prevention of thrombo embolism in orthopaedic surgery. *Clin Risk* 1997; 3: 103–8.

CHAPTER 7

Total hip replacement in special circumstances

D. C. Mears, S. M. Durbhakula, and G. Slowik

At the time of a primary total hip arthroplasty, a diverse spectrum of complicating factors may be encountered that immeasurably increase the potential magnitude of the technical difficulty. Some examples include prior trauma or surgery to the hip, the aftermath of a fracture, osteotomy, or fusion with alteration of the proximal femur, the acetabulum, or both. Other factors that may compromise the anatomical structures include infection and irradiation therapy. Alternatively, congenital malformation or metabolic derangement may profoundly influence the anatomical size, shape, and density of the bone. Other complicating factors may include the presence of dense scar tissue or heterotopic bone, or the predilection for a deep wound infection.

Representative examples of these conditions are reviewed with a focus on the recommendations for appropriate technical modifications for each situation. Irrespective of the nature of the complicating factors, initially a thorough history and physical evaluation are needed. Certain potential complicating factors have a direct impact on the anatomy of the relevant hip joint. Others of relevance may affect the ipsilateral or contralateral hip or knee or the lower back, or the functional capabilities of extremities, in a way that compromises the feasibility of a reconstructive procedure on the involved hip. High-quality radiographs of the hip and pelvis of known magnification are needed, along with suitable templates of proposed implants. Supplementary

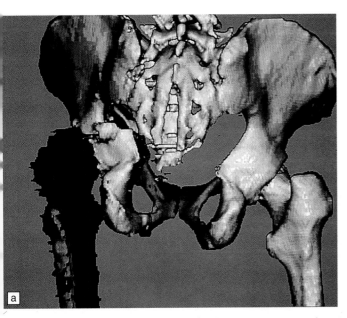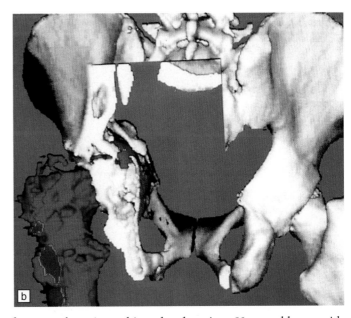

Figure 7.1 – *Specialized imaging to facilitate preoperative planning for a complex primary hip arthroplasty in a 60-year-old man with post-traumatic arthritis of the left hip after a peritrochanteric fracture and a malunited both-column acetabular fracture. (a) Posterior three-dimensional CT; (b) posterior three-dimensional CT re-formatted through the centre of the femoral head;*

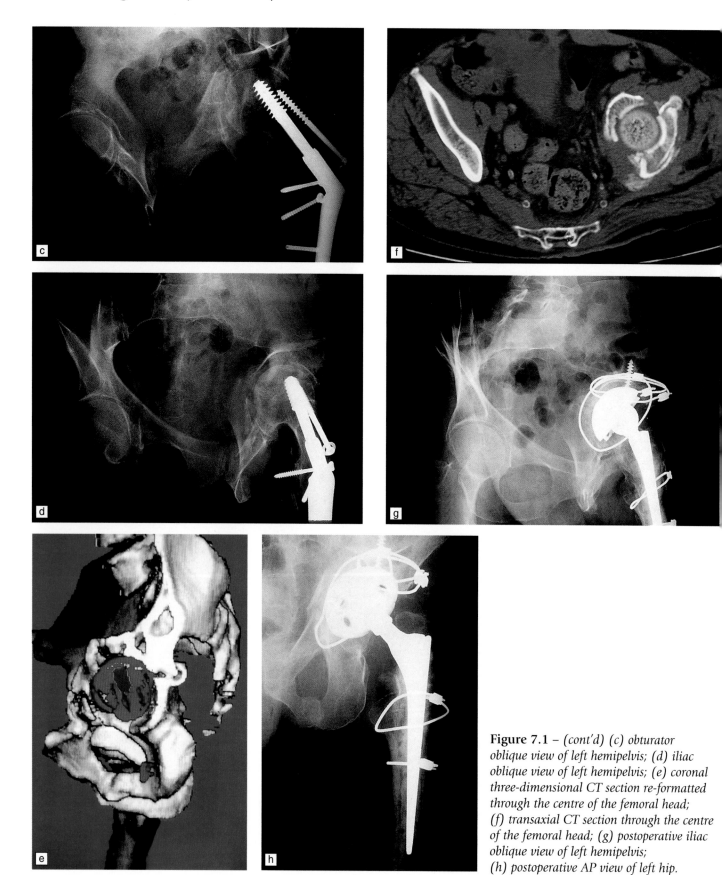

Figure 7.1 – *(cont'd) (c) obturator oblique view of left hemipelvis; (d) iliac oblique view of left hemipelvis; (e) coronal three-dimensional CT section re-formatted through the centre of the femoral head; (f) transaxial CT section through the centre of the femoral head; (g) postoperative iliac oblique view of left hemipelvis; (h) postoperative AP view of left hip.*

images such as the obturator and iliac oblique views, and scanograms for limb length, may be necessary. In the presence of marked distortion of the hip, after prior trauma, surgical reconstruction, congenital abnormality, or other provocation, three-dimensional computed tomography (CT) scans of the hip and pelvis may be helpful (Fig. 7.1).

In the presence of a significant femoral bow, possibly to evaluate Paget's disease, multiple lateral radiographic projections, taken at slightly differing degrees of rotation, facilitate an assessment for the optional configuration and alignment of a femoral stem. On a review of the radiographs, a surgeon can define the optimal size and type and alignment of implants. In the presence of a bony deformity or defect, an appropriate strategy can be identified. In certain instances, a corrective osteotomy for realignment of the pelvis or femur may be necessary. In other cases, augmentation of the bone with allograft or occasionally autograft may be necessary. The appropriate type of morselized or structural graft needs to be planned, possibly in combination with suitable techniques of internal fixation. Specialized implants such as an acetabular cage may be required. The surgeon is strongly encouraged to devise one or more alternative strategies to cope with potential problems or complicating factors. The necessary supplies should be organized so that, at the time of surgery, the surgeon can respond to the intraoperative recognition of an anticipated problem by a timely modification of the procedure in an orderly way. For some unusual problems, the surgeon should consider a preoperative consultation by a hip specialist, at least for a review of the radiographs.

With respect to the role for cementless and cemented implants, the prior training and clinical experience of the surgeon are major factors that heavily dictate the selection process. Nevertheless, some additional considerations are necessary, particularly to limit the use of cementless devices where they are likely to experience premature failure with loosening or subsidence. Representative examples include the presence of mostly allograft around a cup, a significant dose of prior irradiation therapy, and a markedly distorted and osteopenic bone. As a general rule, the authors strongly discourage the use of 'custom'-made implants, except for highly unusual circumstances. Not only is such a device extraordinarily costly, it also does not favour a ready adaptability and versatility during a complex procedure,

which is a crucial attribute for any preferred surgical strategy.

Another typical objective of total hip arthroplasty is restoration of limb length equality. Nevertheless, with the diverse array of conditions that culminate in a complex arthroplasty, enthusiasm for equalization of limb length needs to be tempered by anatomical realities. These include the site(s) and magnitude of deformity, the quality of the bone, and the potential for injury to the lumbosacral plexus and sciatic nerve with excessive lengthening. The use of intraoperative neurological monitoring with continuous EMGs (i.e. electromyographic studies) or SSEPs (i.e. somatosensory evoked potentials) is helpful where lengthening beyond a length of 3 cm is anticipated.

Before embarking on a complex arthroplasty, the potential for significant complications needs to be carefully analysed. The general health of the patient and the documentation of significant co-morbidities need to be evaluated. Certain psychological or psychiatric conditions or dementia may significantly compromise the outlook for satisfactory prolonged function of the reconstructed hip joint. The potential for alternative surgical strategies such as an osteotomy with preservation of the relevant joint needs to be examined. In summary, surgeons should satisfy themselves that the arthroplasty is the best therapeutic alternative and a realistic undertaking.

History of prior surgery to the hip

A wide variety of specialized arthroplasties follows prior surgical procedures that initiate a diverse array of potential complicating factors. After a fusion, osteotomy, prior open reduction and internal fixation of a fracture, or resectional arthroplasty, a subsequent total hip arthroplasty may be hampered for any number of reasons. These include architectural changes in the hip, altered quality of the bone, heterotopic bone formation, the presence of diverse hardware, devascularization of bone, and occult infection [1–3]. Preoperative radiographs may be compromised by the presence of existing hardware or by the occasional presence of bone cement. At the time of the procedure, the presence of dense scar tissue, possibly permeated with heterotopic bone, may thwart the approach. As a general rule, such a total hip arthroplasty is unlikely to achieve the functional quality that typifies a conventional arthroplasty. The heterotopic bone is a radiographic marker that is usually indicative of compromised abductor musculature with scar formation and devascularization of the entire surgical field, including the acetabulum.

Also, when a surgical fusion is performed for post-traumatic arthritis, concomitant traumatically involved deformities and other forms of compromise to the musculoskeletal system may hamper the anticipated outcome of the arthroplasty. Perhaps the highest failure rate for the arthroplasty is when an acetabular fracture, which was initially managed surgically, culminated in massive heterotopic bone formation, with the belated onset of post-traumatic arthritis. In this scenario, the secondary arthroplasty is likely to culminate in a refusion with further heterotopic bone formation, despite the application of irradiation therapy. Typical causes of spontaneous ankylosis include septic arthritis during childhood and adolescence, inflammatory arthritis, and occasionally degenerative disease. In the following sections, specific recommendations for total hip arthroplasty after diverse surgical procedures are given, which are summarized in Table 7.1. In a similar way, Table 7.2 outlines the preferred reconstructive techniques for a variety of other special circumstances.

The ankylosed hip

A fused hip may become symptomatic in widely differing ways. Secondary painful degenerative change and/or instability may develop in the ipsilateral knee or contralateral hip or the low back. Where the fused hip possesses a considerable intrinsic deformity or malposition, the adjacent or contralateral weight-bearing joints are especially vulnerable to symptomatic deterioration. Reversing the hip deformity may reduce significantly the magnitude of pain in the other symptomatic joints, although it cannot lead to a reversal of an established degenerative process. Another source of symptoms after a surgical fusion is a painful pseudarthrosis (Fig. 7.2). In this case, the relative merits of refusion versus a conversion to an arthroplasty need to be evaluated. Typically, the surgical challenge for an attempted refusion is the relative limitations associated with the available pelvic bone stock. At the time of a refusion, disuse osteoporosis of the pelvis is likely to impede any technique of internal fixation significantly.

A patient with a painless fusion may present clinically in the hope of mobilizing a stiff joint. At a total hip arthroplasty, a previously strong supportive, stiff hip may be replaced by a mobile but significantly weaker one, possibly without demonstrable improvement in global function. A patient who walked independently before the arthroplasty possesses a more than 50% likelihood of progressing to the need for a cane. Although such a patient may be grateful for his or her improved mobility, manoeuvrability, and ability to sit comfortably, his or her presurgical expectations need nevertheless to reflect accurately the anticipated functional capabilities.

For many patients, as part of a conversion of a hip fusion to an arthroplasty, the most beneficial result of surgery is the frequent severe impairment of gait as a result of a long-standing discrepancy of limb length (Fig. 7.3). Limb length discrepancy is generally greatest where a fusion followed pyogenic sepsis or tuberculosis and is usually least in a patient who had osteoarthritis. Where a limb length discrepancy arises as a result of a fixed pelvic obliquity or a marked distortion of the bony anatomy, the patient should be cautioned about the likelihood for persistent discrepancy, despite the arthroplasty. In the presence of a fusion with an apparent discrepancy that accompanies flexion and adduction contractures, restoration of limb length equality can be anticipated after the arthroplasty. In the presence of a limb length discrepancy of multifactoral origin, ultimately at the time of the arthroplasty the tension in the soft tissues and the potential for excessive stretching of the sciatic nerve are the limiting factors that dictate the degree of lengthening. In most series, a maximum average restoration of limb length approximates 4 cm.

After a conversion of a fused hip to an arthroplasty, usually the range of motion that is recorded is less than that documented for hip replacement after degenerative arthritis. In the presence of heterotopic bone, marked soft tissue contractures, and significant malposition of the fusion, greater postoperative restriction of mobility can be anticipated.

From all of the previous perspectives, the functional outcome for a conversion of a hip fusion to an arthroplasty, including assessments for activities of daily living and work status, is likely to be modest. Nevertheless, the patient who possesses accurate expectations, especially if the fusion is accompanied by pain in the ipsilateral or contralateral extremity or the lower back, may be highly grateful for the arthroplasty [1–3].

Table 7.1 *Guidelines for performing a total hip arthroplasty after a previous surgical procedure to the hip*

Prior surgery	Unique circumstances	Selection of the components	Bone grafting	Fixational devices
Hip fusion	Correct marked gait-restricting limb length discrepancy Release marked flexion/adduction contracture Resect scar tissue Remove heterotopic bone Assess hip abductor strength	Restore weakened abductor-lever arm with medialized acetabular cup and long femoral stem Correct flexion contracture with shortened femoral neck length Augment exposure with trochanteric osteotomy	Augment acetabular bone stock with morselized autograft	Use braided cables to anchor trochanteric bone block
Femoral osteotomy	Correct femoral neck-shaft angle or alignment of proximal femur	Use custom femoral stem for marked angulation/displacement Consider single-/two-staged corrective femoral osteotomy	Augment femoral defects with primary impaction grafting/strut allografts	Use cerclage wires for femur Removal of existing hardware as necessary
Acetabular osteotomy	Release appropriate contractures, soft tissues, and capsule Resect scar tissue Remove heterotopic bone	Use specialized 'CDH' stem with miniature cemented/cementless cup May need to derotate stem considerably Insert cup into true acetabulum	Anchor structural autograft to high posterior wall to enlarge acetabular recess	Use screws to secure autograft
ORIF (open reduction and internal fixation) of a femoral fracture		Consider corrective femoral osteotomy Use straight femoral stem to minimize risk of perforation Use long femoral stem, either cemented/cementless	Use impaction grafting/strut allografts for widened and irregular femoral canal Use cancellous autograft to obliterate deficient femoral cortex	Use cerclage wires to augment proximal femur Consider heavy stainless steel mesh to support osteotomy site Consider special plate to augment fixation
Closed treatment of an acetabular fracture	Correct acetabular displacement/defect/incongruity/non-union/malunion	Use corrective acetabular osteotomy for realignment Consider cemented cup for non-union with large gap Use elevated wall of acetabular liner	Pack small non-union gap with cancellous autograft Pack larger non-union gap with morselized or bulk allograft	Use fine stainless steel/titanium mesh to buttress acetabulum Use cage or ring for moderate gap Use supplementary lag screw, plate, or cable to augment fixation
ORIF of an acetabular fracture	Remove necrotic acetabular bone Remove marked heterotopic bone Excise dense scar tissue with impregnated bone Rule out infection with cultures	Use cemented cup on non-viable bone	Impaction grafting with morselized cancellous allograft to obliterate a persistent fracture gap Augment a large defect with anchored segment of autograft	Leave hardware intact if possible Immobilize fracture with cables Plate, lag screw, or cable to augment fixation/bone graft

Table 7.2 *Guidelines for performing a total hip arthroplasty in special circumstances*

Medical condition	Unique circumstances	Selection of the components	Bone grafting	Fixational devices
Previous irradiation therapy	Resect dense scar tissue Remove markedly necrotic bone and tissue	Use cemented cup Avoid trochanteric osteotomy	Minimize use of bone graft	Buttress acetabulum with threaded rods/pins/ring Use titanium/steel mesh for deficient medial acetabular wall Use extensile cage for deficient acetabular roof/walls
Quiescent sepsis	Resect scar tissue Release contracture Correct limb length discrepancy Consider flap coverage of defect Send intraoperative cultures	Selection rests on preservation or loss of bone	Consider impaction grafting/strut allografts to augment femur	Use prophylactic cerclage wires for femoral defects
Quiescent tuberculosis	Assess for pseudarthrosis Send intraoperative cultures Resect scar tissue Osteotomize ankylosed femoral head/neck	Selection rests on preservation or loss of bone and degree of osteopenia		
Sickle-cell disease	Give prophylactic antibiotics Expect major blood loss Expect densely sclerotic bone	Use cementless cup and stem Cement may provoke component loosening	Obliterate widened femoral medullary canal with impaction grafting	Use prophylactic cerclage wires for femoral defects
Paget's disease	Expect major blood loss Premedicate with calcitonin/bisphosphonate therapy Expect densely sclerotic bone	Cement/restrictor can help fill widened femoral canal	Obliterate widened femoral medullary canal with impaction grafting	
Gaucher's disease	Gaucher cells compromise quality of cement–bone interface	Consider hybrid arthroplasty	Use primary impaction grafting	
Dwarfism and bone dysplasia	Consider markedly distorted anatomy/biomechanics Consider concomitant TKR (total knee replacement)	Use miniature custom components May need longer stem for markedly narrow femoral canal	Augment dysplastic acetabulum with femoral head autograft	Use screws to anchor femoral head autograft
Fibrous dysplasia	Curettage dysplastic segment Correct limb length discrepancy to within reason	Long femoral stem Cemented/non-cemented stem Corrective femoral osteotomy	Augment proximal femur with impaction grafting/strut allografts	Use cerclage wires to augment femur
Down's syndrome	Release flexion/adduction contractures Immobilize postoperatively	Use cemented cup Use custom components	Usually unnecessary	Usually unnecessary

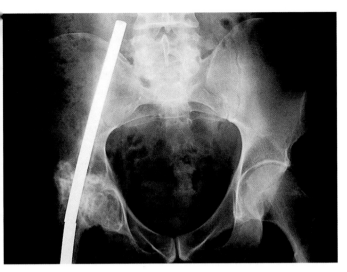

Figure 7.2 – *A painful pseudarthrosis developed in the right hip of this 42-year-old man after sustaining a fall with subsequent fracture of the immobilizing rod 18 years after the primary fusion.*

In addition to the availability of sufficient bone stock for insertion of the components with appropriate alignment and stability, another crucial preoperative criterion is the provision of effective hip abductors. The determination of 'sufficient' strength of the abductors after a hip fusion remains problematic. Inadequate strength of the abductor muscles results in a Trendelenburg gait, a feeling of instability of the hip, the need for a supplementary walking aid, and an inability to stand on one leg. Unless the patient is adequately informed of these problems before the conversion arthroplasty, he or she may be dissatisfied with the outcome. Of the several methods available to assess the abductor function before surgery, palpation of the contracting muscles remains the best technique. For an assessment of the tensor fascia lata and a means to distinguish the gluteal abductors, during an abduction lift, the knee is extended to document the former and flexed to assess the latter. If the contracted abductors cannot be palpated, a conversion arthroplasty is likely to culminate in an unstable hip. Although magnetic resonance imaging (MRI), EMGs, and muscle biopsies have been used sporadically to assess abductor muscle function, none of the techniques has achieved an established role. Where immobilization of the hip was achieved by the use of a Cobra plate, the relationship between the plate and the greater trochanteric insertion of the glutei needs to be carefully examined (Fig. 7.4). If the plate were applied to an intact trochanteric region without a careful osteotomy and reflection of the glutei, in all likelihood, on surgical removal of the plate, marked destruction of the gluteal tendinous insertion would be encountered. This provides a devastating permanent compromise to the hip abductors.

Where the greater trochanteric insertion was surgically released as part of the fusion, a failure to reattach the tendons to the approximate anatomical site is likely to

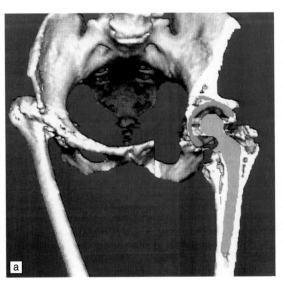
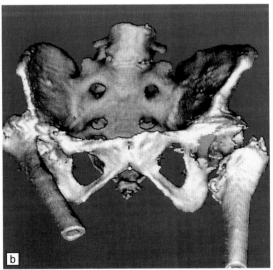

Figure 7.3 – *Three-dimensional CT views displaying a right hip fusion in a 65-year-old woman who underwent the procedure at 3 years of age for TB sepsis. Although she desires mobility and apparent limb lengthening and lessening of chronic low back pain, the limited bone stock compromises the feasibility of the arthroplasty. (a) Anterior three-dimensional CT view, re-formatted through the left total hip arthroplasty; (b) outlet three-dimensional CT view.*

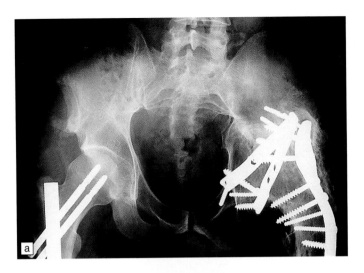

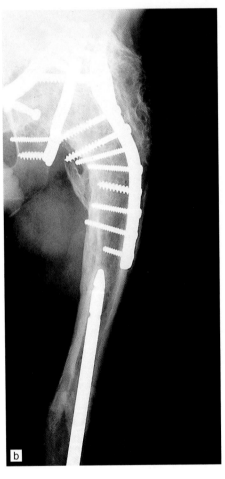

Figure 7.4 – *This 22-year-old man would like a conversion of his left hip fusion to an arthroplasty to manage limb shortening, a fixed external rotation deformity secondary to a malunited femoral fracture, and secondary low back pain. The surgical concern is whether the gluteal hip abductor function would be sufficient to provide a stable hip. (a) AP view of pelvis; (b) AP view of left hip.*

represented as the distance from the tip of the trochanter to the centre of the femoral head, divided by the distance from the symphysis pubis to the centre of the head. A ratio of less than 0.5 is undesirable and potentially consistent with a subsequent positive Trendelenburg test. To increase the abductor : lever arm ratio, at least in certain cases with suitable bone stock, the position of the socket is medialized while, concomitantly, the femoral component is selected with a longer neck.

The abductor muscle mass can be expected gradually to strengthen for up to 5 years after the conversion arthroplasty. Such a strengthening plan rests on the presence of healthy, unscarified, and innervated gluteal muscles, a sound biomechanical position of the hip, and the implementation of an appropriate regimen of exercise. During the assembly of a preoperative plan, a few special preparations are needed. Certain fixation devices require unusual tools for their removal, for which appropriate arrangements are needed. With the difficulty of identifying critical bony landmarks around the hip, preoperative radiographs merit meticulous evaluation. Unless a rigorous identification of predictable landmarks is feasible, the provision for intraoperative image intensification may be necessary. The relative merit of a greater trochanteric osteotomy is assessed. The assets include an augmented exposure, whereas the liability is the need for effective reattachment of a trochanteric bone block to the proximal femur. The selection of a suitable incision depends on focal anatomical features, the presence of prior surgical scars, and the familiarity of the surgeon with anterior, posterior, or transtrochanteric lateral exposures, as well as the triradiate extensile approach.

Once the proximal femur is exposed, the femoral neck is provisionally osteotomized at an unusually high level. Afterwards, the femur is isolated for the application of a standard proximal femoral cutting guide. With a power saw, the definitive cut of the femoral neck is made. Once the proximal femur is mobilized, scarified remnants of hip capsule, short external rotators, and heterotopic bone are removed. Release of a muscular contracture, particularly iliopsoas, may be necessary. After an appropriate development of the exposure to the acetabular rim, the remainder of the femoral neck is osteotomized with the power saw. For identification of the appropriate level and inclination for this cut, image intensification is helpful. A large portion of femoral

culminate in marked shortening and effective weakening of the musculotendinous unit, so that, belatedly, it cannot be anchored to the trochanteric region.

Where the preoperative assessment of the abductor strength is marginal, another intraoperative strategy is to restore anatomically the proper abductor : lever arm ratio. The abductor : lever arm ratio is a radiographic measurement on an anteroposterior (AP) view. It is head obliterates the normal acetabular recess. Initially such bone can be removed by resort to a power burr, gouge, or curved osteotome. Further enlargement of the recess is achieved by the use of standard acetabular reamers to the predetermined size. If the thickness of the acetabulum is limited or marginally adequate, a central drill hole of 2 mm in diameter permits a confirmation of the optimal depth for reaming. The anteroinferior spine is a helpful anatomical landmark. In certain cases, augmentation of the acetabulum may require the use of a structural bone graft, which is harvested from the excised portion of the femoral head and neck (Fig. 7.5).

In the authors' experience, usually a cementless multiple-screwed cup is used. A contained acetabular defect is obliterated with morselized autograft [4–8]. With the potential for marked alteration of normal anatomical relationships, the direction and length of the drill holes, which allow the insertion of anchorage screws, need to respect the risk zones for possible impalement of neighbouring vessels, especially the external iliac artery and vein.

The preparation of the proximal femur with appropriate reamers and broaches needs to respect potential weakened sites, such as screw holes where internal

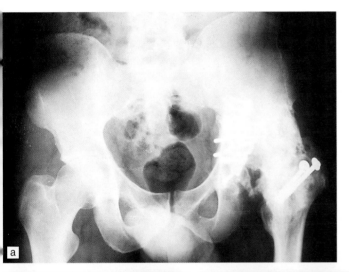

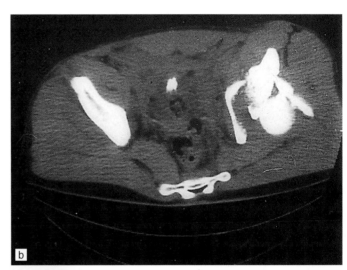

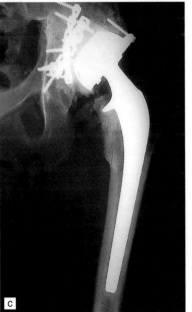

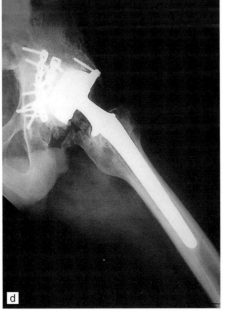

Figure 7.5 – *An open reduction of a T-type left acetabular fracture in this 28-year-old man culminated in a painful arthritis and the presence of massive heterotopic bone. In view of the markedly deficient posterior column, the use of a structural autograft combined with the use of a cage was necessary. (a) Preoperative AP view of pelvis; (b) transverse CT scan demonstrating the deficient posterior column; (c) postoperative AP view of left hip; (d) postoperative lateral view of left hip.*

fixation devices were removed. Once a trial stem or a corresponding broach is fully seated, the neck length and offset for the prosthesis are assessed by a combination of the preoperative radiographic templating with the tension in the neighbouring soft tissues [9–14]. The latter factor varies considerably with respect to the intrinsic scarification of the hip musculature. As a realistic standard, a stable reduction of the hip accompanied by less than 3 mm, with a 'push-pull' test on the located hip, is a suitable guideline. A trial reduction should display full extension with at least 70° of flexion and 30° of abduction and adduction. A minor flexion contracture may be corrected by the selection of a shorter

neck length. A larger contracture may require a further soft tissue release. Where greater length is desired, an additional soft tissue release may be necessary. After liberation of the capsule, short external rotators, and iliopsoas, release of the subperiosteal plane of scarified glutei and tensor muscles on the lateral ilium may be helpful, along with the indirect head of rectus femoris. While the lengthening stage is under way and subsequently, the knee is maintained in a flexed position beyond 100° to relieve the tension on the sciatic nerve.

During the assessment for stability of the hip, a careful consideration is given to impingement with dislocation. This type of case possesses a high likelihood of

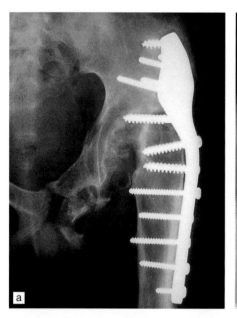
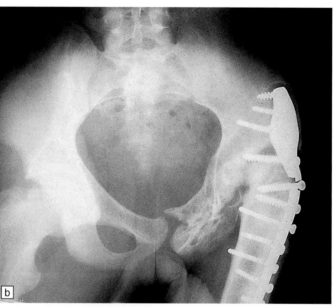
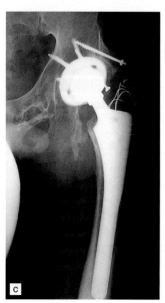
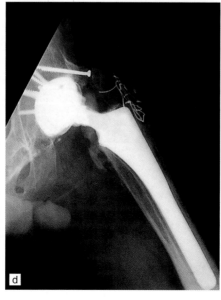

Figure 7.6 – *Radiographs of a 15-year-old man who underwent a left hip fusion for avascular necrosis of the left hip after a femoral neck fracture that was complicated by sepsis. When a pseudarthrosis with implant failure ensued, a cementless arthroplasty followed. A tenuous repair of the gluteal insertion necessitated bracing for 8 weeks after the surgery. (a) AP view of the left hip 2 months after the fusion; (b) AP view of the pelvis 6 months later with a broken plate; (c) AP view of the left hip 4 years later; (d) lateral view of the left hip 4 years later.*

a bony prominence around the residual acetabulum and proximal femur, which greatly enhances the risk for dislocation. If identified, such a prominence is removed. Before closure of the wound, an osteotomized trochanter is reattached in a conventional manner, typically by the use of braided cables.

For the early postoperative period, the structural integrity of the abductor muscles dictates the rate of initiation of the corresponding resistance exercises. In the presence either of a trochanteric osteotomy or of mechanically weakened gluteal insertions into the greater trochanter, abductor strengthening may need to be deferred for about 6 weeks (Fig. 7.6). Otherwise a conventional rehabilitation programme is undertaken.

Prior proximal femoral osteotomy

In a younger patient, an intertrochanteric osteotomy may retard the progression or temporarily arrest the symptoms of painful degenerative arthritis of the hip. Many of these patients ultimately do progress to a total hip replacement [2]. Ironically, although a proximal femoral osteotomy holds considerable potential to relieve the arthritic pain temporarily, nevertheless the procedure jeopardizes the outcome of a subsequent total hip arthroplasty, with respect to both the intraoperative complication rate and the durability of the arthroplasty. Reported complications include intraoperative fractures of the femoral shaft, calcar, and greater trochanter, along with technical difficulties that accompany the removal of screws and hardware, or broaching and reaming the femoral shaft and inserting the femoral prosthesis. A progressively greater displacement of the osteotomy culminates in a correspondingly greater risk of intra-operative technical problems and of premature failure of the arthroplasty [15–18].

Detailed preoperative planning is essential to document the anticipated distortion of the proximal femur, particularly with respect to the neck-shaft angle after a valgus or varus derotational osteotomy (Fig. 7.7). Other relevant features of the femoral component include its size, the head/neck offset, and the presence of a collar. In the presence of marked angulation or displacement of the osteotomy site, a special component may be necessary. A double-curved stem, a small straight stem, or a custom-made component may be required. If marked displacement of the osteotomy site is documented, a correction of the deformity by the use of an osteotomy is necessary as either a single- or a two-staged procedure. If

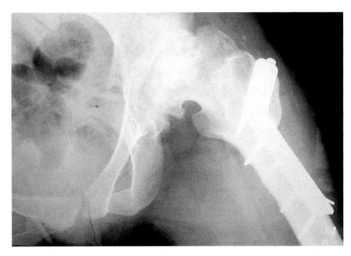

Figure 7.7 – *In this lateral view of this severely arthritic left hip, the distortion of the upper femur secondary to an osteotomy is evident, along with the presence of typical hardware.*

a single-staged osteotomy is planned and a cementless prosthesis is intended, preoperative measurements should ensure a precise and stable fit of the stem across both fragments. A stable fixation must be obtained, in order to achieve union of the bone in a timely manner.

When an arthroplasty is planned, it remains contro-versial whether the device for immobilization of the osteotomy should be removed by the use of a separate preliminary procedure [16,17]. Certainly, the liabilities that accompany staged procedures include the extra cost and time and, frequently after metal removal, an additional period of protected weight-bearing activity. Nevertheless, when the fixation device is removed at the time of the conversion to an arthroplasty, the potential problems associated with the combined procedure include a predilection for a spiral fracture through weakened bone and empty screw holes, extravasation of cement during pressurization, and suboptimal pressur-ization of the cement. In selected cases, prophylactic cerclage wiring of the femur may be a prudent consider-ation, along with a primary impaction grafting. The last measure facilitates an obliteration of holes in the bone and the preparation of a generally cylindrical pathway within an irregularly shaped bone.

After a prior varus osteotomy, the optimal preparation of the femoral neck may include a horizontal cut for the preservation of bone and the elimination of the need for a special component with a long neck. Where the upper femoral shaft and subtrochanteric region possess a significant deformity, reaming and broaching of the femur are vulnerable to penetration of the cortex, with the creation of a defect or initiation of a fracture. A corrective osteotomy may be necessary to achieve an adequate realignment of the bone. The precise determination of the direction of the osteotomy is needed, so that both accurate realignment and a complete fit of the osteotomy line are achieved.

In the presence of a prior osteotomy that alters femoral anteversion, the standard landmarks for insertion of the femoral prosthesis may be altered. Various types of prior osteotomy may alter the position of the greater trochanter so that it blocks the access to the medullary canal, thereby inhibiting the insertion of the femoral component. In such a case, a trochanteric osteotomy may be necessary. A trochanteric osteotomy may also be required to augment the surgical exposure or to adjust the tension in the abductor muscles [17]. After an osteotomy, a distortion of the bone may become the source of a residual femoral cortical defect during a conversion to an arthroplasty. The use of a strut allograft and supplementary cerclage wire fixation provides a realistic means to augment the corresponding region of the femur. The method can also be used in conjunction with impaction grafting.

When an arthroplasty follows a prior proximal femoral osteotomy, the postoperative management is similar to a conventional primary total hip arthroplasty. Likewise the management of postoperative complications is similar in the two clinical situations.

Prior acetabular osteotomy

An acetabular osteotomy is a reconstructive procedure that permits a redirection of the acetabulum or a relative enlargement or diminution in its size. The principal indication is developmental dysplasia of the hip (DDH), although exceptional cases of Legg–Perthes disease, prior acetabular trauma, and rarely other conditions progress to an acetabular osteotomy. A wide variety of triplane osteotomies redirect the acetabulum by the preparation of cuts across the ilium, ischium, and pubis, which are somewhat distant from the articular surface. A peri-acetabular osteotomy achieves the same end by resorting to a cut that is in juxtaposition with the articular portion. A Salter osteotomy, with its transiliac cut, displaces the acetabulum by hinging at the symphysis, which thereby limits the degrees of freedom of the displacement. A Chiari osteotomy provides an

enlargement whereas a Pemberton osteotomy achieves a reduction in acetabular volume. With respect to a belated total hip arthroplasty, all of the procedures culminate in the formation of scar tissue, potentially with heterotopic bone and a distortion of the normal acetabular landmarks [1].

In clinical practice, the diverse family of osteotomies may restore the normal anatomical alignment and the size of the acetabulum to a highly variable degree. In such a complex case as a DDH of late presentation in a 3- or 5-year-old child, supplementary procedures may have included an acetabular shelf or a proximal femoral osteotomy, so that the initial dysplastic acetabular anatomy is further altered. If secondary degenerative arthritis or avascular necrosis of hip ensues, meticulous preoperative planning is needed to prepare for a total hip arthroplasty. Special small sizes of so-called developmental dysplasia of the hip (DDH) femoral stems may be needed, possibly with small cemented or cementless cups, for head sizes of 22 or 26 mm. If a cementless cup with screws is used, after a triplane or periacetabular osteotomy, the size of the potentially hazardous zone for insertion of the screws, in the vicinity of the external iliac vessels, is enlarged. This unsafe region of the high anterior wall should not be breached by a drill bit or any other sharp tool. Similarly, a Homan type of pointed retractor should not be placed around the anterior wall, next to the antero-inferior spine, where the proximity of the vessels provides a considerable risk for impalement or other type of vascular injury.

In some of the DDH cases, despite the prior completion of an acetabular osteotomy with or without other procedures, the true acetabulum may be highly deficient. Occasionally, the femoral head remains subluxed or dislocated adjacent to a false acetabulum. In the authors' experience, for most cases the preferred reconstructive strategy is to insert the cup into the true acetabulum. Usually a structural bone graft harvested from the femoral head and neck has to be anchored to the high posterior wall with screws, to enlarge the acetabular recess adequately for appropriate coverage of the cup. If the position of the femoral head is substantially lowered from the false to the true acetabulum, an extensive soft tissue release may be necessary to achieve that realignment. The preferred sequence for the releases is the hip capsule, the short external rotators, the iliopsoas, and gluteus maximus insertion into the proximal femur and the indirect head of rectus femoris.

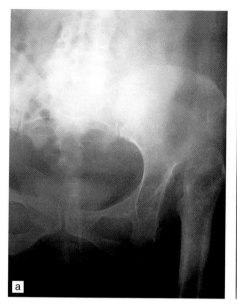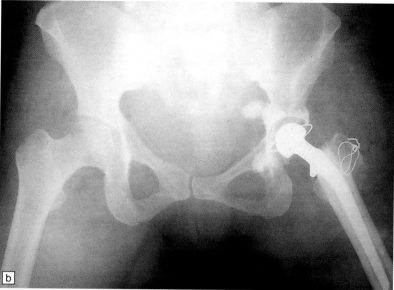

Figure 7.8 – This 37-year-old woman progressed to a cemented total hip replacement for a painful left hip, for which she underwent a shelf procedure as a child. (a) Preoperative AP view of left hip; (b) postoperative AP view of pelvis taken 12 years later.

If a prior surgical dissection was performed on the lateral ilium, notably with the creation of a shelf, a sharp release of the corresponding scarified origins of the tensor fascia lata muscle, along with the gluteus medius and gluteus minimus on the lateral ilium, may be necessary (Fig. 7.8). Nevertheless, every attempt is made to preserve the origins of these muscles on the iliac crest.

During the distal displacement of the proximal femur and in the early postoperative period, the ipsilateral knee joint is maintained in a flexed position of more than 100°, for protection of the sciatic nerve. If the proximal femur cannot be adequately lowered to the true acetabulum, two alternative techniques merit consideration. Either a proximal femoral osteotomy can be performed to shorten the bone or a superior displacement of the cup, nominally to the false acetabulum, can be considered. Unless the false acetabulum was significantly enlarged by a prior shelf procedure, usually it affords far less bone stock than might seem to be evident by a review of the AP pelvic radiograph.

During the preparation of the proximal femur, the potential for marked femoral anteversion is borne in mind. The femoral stem may require considerable rotation with respect to the position of the base of the femoral neck. From this perspective, along with the potential for supplementary femoral deformities and the anticipated small size of the bone, the authors prefer the use of a cemented stem.

Prior proximal femoral fracture

After a proximal femoral fracture, most of the cases that progress to a total hip arthroplasty pertain to a femoral neck fracture that culminates in avascular necrosis with secondary degenerative arthritis [2]. With respect to this last group, no significant distortion of the proximal femoral anatomy is encountered at the time of a total hip arthroplasty. Admittedly, if a hip screw or other device is removed at the time of the arthroplasty, vacant holes need to be obliterated as part of the procedure, usually by the application of a cancellous bone graft, which is harvested from the femoral head. Otherwise, the holes provide a series of stress risers that serve to weaken the bone. If a cementless stem is selected, particular care is needed during the use of the reamer and rasp, so that the risk of creating a fracture is minimized. Alternatively, a cerclage cable or heavy wire can be anchored prophylactically around the proximal femur. Intertrochanteric and subtrochanteric fractures, managed operatively or conservatively, may culminate in considerable deformity of the bone. Again, at the time of a belated arthroplasty with a concomitant removal of hardware, various stress risers may be created at the sites of vacant holes. A careful preoperative templating on the AP and lateral projections is needed to determine whether a conventional stem can be inserted. With the widely differing geometries of available stems, the procurement of a particular model, such as an exceptionally straight stem, minimizes the risk of intra-operative perforation of the bone. In the presence of a marked deformity, a surgical correction is necessary.

Although, historically, this measure was frequently undertaken as a separate surgical procedure, currently the prevailing financial pressures and considerations of the duration of the global recovery period favour a combined procedure that includes the arthroplasty. Once the site and extent of the deformity are documented, the geometry of the corrective osteotomy is determined. Several different strategies for fixation of the osteotomy are feasible [19–21]. If a cemented stem is selected, external support of the osteotomy site can be achieved by the use of cerclage cables, combined with strut allografts or heavy stainless steel mesh. With the potential for a markedly irregular or unduly capacious intramedullary canal, an impaction grafting with the use of cancellous allograft chips merits serious consideration. Another option is the use of special plates that use cables for proximal fixation and conventional screws for distal fixation. Still another possibility is the use of an implant with a long stem either as a cementless or a cemented device.

Patterson *et al.* [19] described a technique of hip arthroplasty that can be used for certain complications of an intertrochanteric hip fracture, such as a non-union of the fracture, post-traumatic arthritis, perforation of the acetabulum by an internal fixation device, and avascular necrosis of the femoral head. The nailplate that was used originally to stabilize the intertrochanteric fracture is removed through a lateral approach. The removed screws are shortened to a length that is about the width of the lateral femoral cortex and reinserted into the screw holes, flush with the endosteal surface. A dowel-shaped bone graft from the femoral head is used to fill the cortical defect caused by the removed nail. The cemented femoral component is then placed in the usual fashion. After the cement has polymerized, the screws are removed without difficulty and grafts of cancellous bone are inserted into the cortical voids. The authors reported no complications from the procedure.

Prior acetabular fracture

After a displaced acetabular fracture, a patient has a considerable likelihood of progressing to a total hip arthroplasty, irrespective of the method of definitive management [1,22,23a]. Generally, the specific indication for the secondary arthroplasty is the onset of symptomatic post-traumatic arthritis or avascular necrosis of the femoral head. The predilection for progression to an arthroplasty is related to the initial type of fracture, the magnitude of the provocation force, the age of the patient, and, where an open reduction and internal fixation are undertaken, the time from the injury to the surgical procedure. When such an arthroplasty is performed, frequently one or more complicating factors are encountered. After the use of conservative treatment of the acetabular fracture, residual displacement and incongruity of the acetabulum, possibly combined with a non-union, are likely to ensue. Where, initially, surgical management is employed, secondary problems may include the presence of dense scar tissue, heterotopic bone, avascularity of the hip muscles or the acetabulum, obstructive hardware and occult infection (Fig. 7.9). From a review of prior studies, the prognosis for a total hip arthroplasty that follows an acetabular fracture is markedly worse than one that is undertaken for primary degenerative arthritis. The following account addresses the principal concerns, where the initial management of the acetabular fracture was closed or open respectively, followed by a review of a new and somewhat controversial solution – an acute total hip arthroplasty.

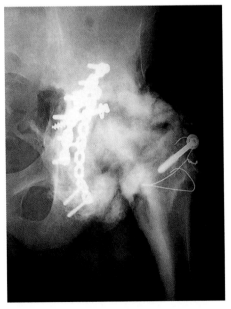

Figure 7.9 – *This AP view of the left hip highlights the anticipated problems for a total hip arthroplasty after an open acetabular reconstruction, including abundant heterotopic bone, retained metal, and avascularity of the femoral head and acetabulum.*

Prior closed treatment of an acetabular fracture

Before the arthroplasty, the preoperative assessment attempts to characterize fully the potential for a non-union or malunion of the acetabulum. When such a case is accompanied by a pelvic ring disruption, the potential for a significant deformity of the entire pelvis needs to be borne in mind. In the latter case, conceivably a reconstructive hip procedure may require a concomitant or preliminary osteotomy and realignment of the pelvic ring (Fig. 7.10). The details of such a procedure are beyond the scope of this chapter although they have been presented elsewhere [1,22].

At the time of a total hip arthroplasty for post-traumatic arthritis after an acetabular fracture, a non-union is particularly likely to be encountered after a posterior wall or column injury. After a transverse, both column, or other injury pattern, a non-union ensues infrequently when florid displacement is uncorrected. Preoperative multiplanar imaging of the acetabulum is particularly helpful to characterize the magnitude, site, and vector of displacement of a non-union. The degree of malalignment of an acetabular non-union can be broadly subdivided into three categories. Where the gap at the non-union is less than 10 mm, obliteration of the gap is readily achieved by packing it with autograft, which is harvested from the femoral head. Occasionally, the fracture fragments are sufficiently mobile to approximate the fracture surfaces by the use of suitable bone-holding forceps. Where the gap at the non-union is 10–25 mm, usually scar tissue and the presence of heterotopic bone or fracture callus considerably impede an attempted open reduction. The gap can be obliterated with morselized or bulk autograft (Fig. 7.11). For structural augmentation, one of several strategies may be considered. Fine stainless steel or titanium mesh can be used to buttress the acetabulum to facilitate an impaction grafting. Alternatively, a multi-screwed cup can be used. For the larger defects, a cage or ring can be used in combination with a cemented cup.

Once the gap exceeds 25 mm, there needs to be serious consideration for realignment and reapproximation of the acetabulum. Otherwise, a technical failure with a persistent non-union, premature loosening of the cup, or other complication related to the florid deformity is highly likely to occur. In the last situation, a preoperative, three-dimensional computed tomography (CT) scan is helpful for the optimal characterization of the deformity. An extensile exposure, notably the triradiate or the extended iliofemoral, may be necessary to visualize fully the complete non-union, as well as the hip joint. The use of large pelvic bone-holding forceps may be necessary to achieve the reduction. To obtain adequate mobilization of the non-union, extensive removal of callus along the non-union site can be anticipated. Fixation of the hemipelvis can be realized by a variety of techniques, depending on the geometry of the fracture lines, the degree of osteoporosis, and other factors. A multiscrewed cup that is anchored with screws can be perceived as a hemispherical plate. Supplementary lag screws, reconstruction plates, or cables are effective means of augmenting the fixation.

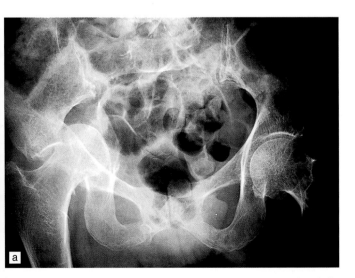 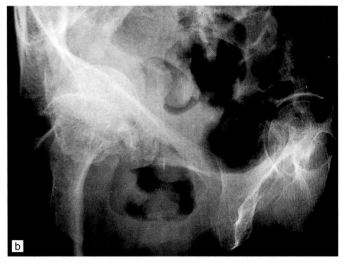

Figure 7.10 – *Radiographs displaying a marked acetabular deformity with a defect of 6 cm, where an attempted arthroplasty merits an osteotomy and correction of the defect. (a) AP view of the pelvis; (b) obturator oblique view of the right hemipelvis.*

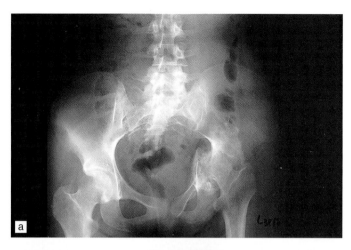

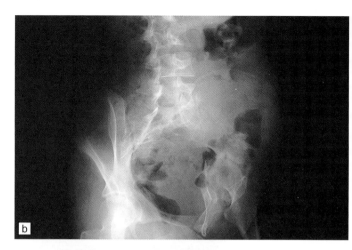

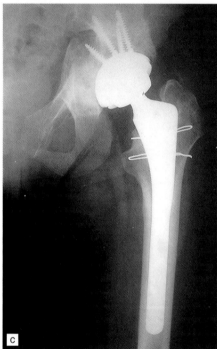

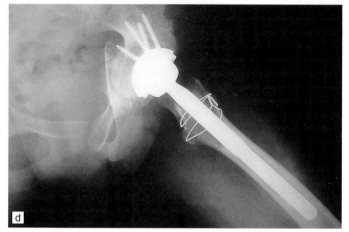

Figure 7.11 – *Radiographs with features of a non-united and displaced right T-type fracture in a 34-year-old woman, where painful erosion of the femoral head was managed with a cementless total hip arthroplasty and the use of a large structural autograft of femoral head. (a) Preoperative AP view of the pelvis; (b) preoperative iliac oblique view of the right hemipelvis demonstrating an extensive posterior defect; (c) postoperative AP view of the right hip taken 2 years later; (d) postoperative lateral view of the right hip taken 2 years later.*

On completion of the fixation and insertion of a metal backing, it is advisable to have an elevated wall of acetabular liner available. In the presence of such a deformed acetabulum, the orientation of the metal backing may be suboptimal. The use of the elevated wall may allow the optimal degree of stability of the hip joint to be realized. After insertion of the femoral broach, a trial acetabular liner can be inserted, with adjustment of its rotation until the optimal stability is documented.

Prior operative treatment of an acetabular fracture

Clearly, a broad spectrum of acetabular fractures is managed surgically. The complexity of a subsequent arthroplasty may vary enormously. As a general rule, the

technical difficulty anticipated for the arthroplasty corresponds with the magnitude of the initial fracture, the extent of the open reduction, and the amount of heterotopic bone formation. The most challenging cases are those that pertain to a fracture that involved both columns, where an extensile approach or multiple approaches were used, along with those in which massive heterotopic bone is documented radiographically. In the authors' experience, several general guidelines have evolved which provide the basis for the subsequent observations.

After a posterior fracture dislocation that was managed operatively, usually the sciatic nerve becomes scarified to the site of the posterior fixation. For the arthroplasty, generally an anterolateral or a modified

Hardinge approach is preferred. In this way, the need for a posterior dissection is minimized. In many of these cases, some degree of contusion of the sciatic nerve accompanies the initial traumatic injury. At the time of the arthroplasty, the sciatic nerve is particularly vulnerable to clinically significant aggravation, merely by a seemingly trivial retraction. The posterior fixation is left in situ apart from a limited portion, such as a single screw that traverses the site, which is needed to insert a cup. If a non-union of a fracture line is encountered, it is débrided and obliterated with bone graft, before insertion of a multiscrewed cup (Fig. 7.12).

Heterotopic ossification

In a case where an initial lateral exposure was performed,

especially if an extended lateral approach was used, the presence of some degree of heterotopic bone is typical. Although the amount of heterotopic bone may be limited, the radiographically demonstrable area is usually surrounded by an extensive region of dense scar tissue. The latter may be impregnated with multiple small deposits of bone that are radiographically invisible. Such tissue has to be excised to permit a dislocation of the hip and subsequent completion of the procedure. If the preoperative radiographs display extensive Brooker grade 3 or 4 heterotopic bone, vigorous characterization of the extent of the problem is essential before the surgery. Both supplementary iliac and obturator oblique radiographs, and a CT scan, are suggested. Considerations for the essential removal of

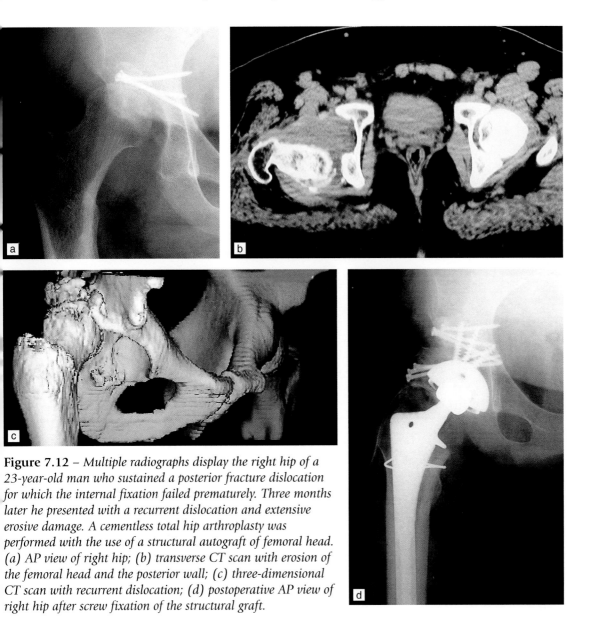

Figure 7.12 – *Multiple radiographs display the right hip of a 23-year-old man who sustained a posterior fracture dislocation for which the internal fixation failed prematurely. Three months later he presented with a recurrent dislocation and extensive erosive damage. A cementless total hip arthroplasty was performed with the use of a structural autograft of femoral head. (a) AP view of right hip; (b) transverse CT scan with erosion of the femoral head and the posterior wall; (c) three-dimensional CT scan with recurrent dislocation; (d) postoperative AP view of right hip after screw fixation of the structural graft.*

the heterotopic bone include the optimal approaches to the sites, the potential anatomical hazards, and the precise distribution of the bone.

One typical pattern is where the heterotopic bone is limited to the site of the prior capsule, with preservation of the adjacent hip muscles and the femoral head. The opposite extreme is where circumferential heterotopic bone around the hip joint extends radially from the femoral head to pervade the capsule and the adjacent musculature, with associated osseous bars that anchor the entire proximal femur to the pelvis. Almost all of the more florid cases are encountered in the closed head injury population, particularly in young obese adult men. Despite the application of postoperative irradiation therapy, the likelihood for recurrent formation of massive heterotopic ossification is great. With the loss of the normal tissue planes and mobile interfaces, the resection of heterotopic bone in such a heavily involved case is a formidable undertaking. After the extensive procedure, the risk for a serious deep wound infection is considerable.

Once the amount and site of distribution of the heterotopic ossification have been characterized, the optimal surgical approach can be selected. Whereas the presence of grade 1 or 2 heterotopic bone does not materially influence the approach, the presence of grade 3 or 4 heterotopic bone does lead to a preference by the authors to use a triradiate incision, although with preservation of an intact greater trochanter. This technique permits direct visualization and removal of the anterior and posterior portions of the heterotopic bone. The insertion of the gluteal tendons into the trochanteric region defines a crucial lateral landmark. The exposure of a fixation plate on the posterior column or an isolated screw is a valuable landmark for the surface of the intact pelvis. In the most extensive cases, the anteroinferior spine is a useful anterior landmark. Supplementary image intensification can be used to delineate the position of the acetabular rim. With a power saw, the femoral neck is provisionally divided in its midportion. Sufficient heterotopic bone is removed so that the hip can be placed in approximately 90° of external rotation. Afterwards, the standard cut at the base of the femoral neck is made with the proper orientation. Once the heterotopic bone has been completely removed, the remainder of the procedure continues in a conventional fashion.

Another potential complicating factor is avascular necrosis of the acetabulum. After an extensile approach or two approaches for the acute reconstruction of an acetabular fracture, the blood supply to the acetabular bone may be heavily compromised for a prolonged period of years. At the time of a belated arthroplasty necrotic acetabular bone may thwart the insertion of the cup and predispose the arthroplasty to premature acetabular loosening (Fig. 7.13). A helpful radiographic sign of acetabular necrosis is a radio-opacity of the acetabulum, especially in the region of the dome.

The optimal method to address acetabular necrosis is prevention by minimizing the use of extended lateral approaches and by maintaining the blood supply of all major acetabular fragments at the time of the open reduction. Once a case is identified, at the time of the arthroplasty, a cementless cup needs to be placed on viable bone. Even if a cemented cup is selected, a viable bony bed markedly improves the likelihood for durability.

Occult infection

Occult infection is another consideration when a total hip arthroplasty is undertaken after an initial open reduction of an acetabular fracture. Although clinical, radiographic, or other features of sepsis may be demonstrable, more typically clear evidence of sepsis is not available until the arthroplasty is performed. With the anticipated presence of dense scar tissue or heterotopic bone, a preoperative aspiration or even trephine biopsy of the hip may be difficult or impossible. At the time of the arthroplasty, specimens of joint fluid are sent to the laboratory for analysis including the use of a Gram stain and a histological scrutiny for white blood cells (WBCs). The presence of 10 WBCs per high power field is presumptive evidence of an infection. If the hip is infected, the preferred method by the authors is to débride the hip thoroughly, including a resection of the femoral head and neck. After pulsatile jet lavage and antibiotic irrigation, a cement spacer impregnated with antibiotic, typically gentamicin, is inserted into the acetabulum. The wound is closed in layers over a suction drain. Postoperatively, after identification of the pathogen, appropriate intravenous antibiotics are given for at least 6 weeks. On cessation of the antibiotics, a trephine biopsy of the hip under image intensification is performed. If the specimen is sterile, insertion of the total hip arthroplasty is arranged. If the specimen is consistent with persistent infection, another débridement with replacement of the cement spacer is undertaken, along with further antibiotic therapy.

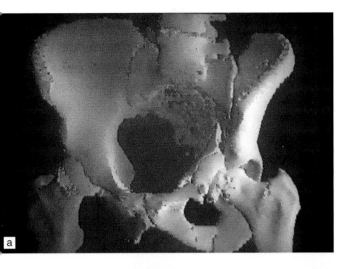

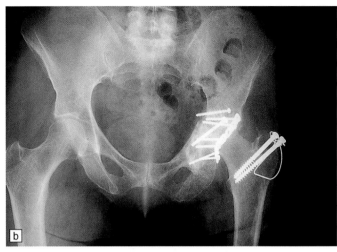

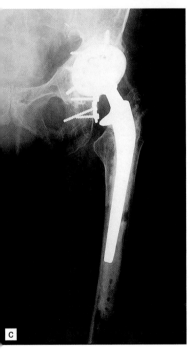

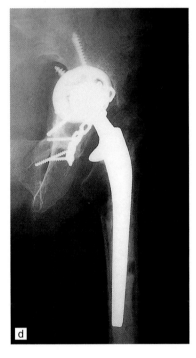

Figure 7.13 – *A radiographic example of avascular necrosis of the left acetabulum in a 64-year-old woman who initially underwent an open reduction and internal fixation (ORIF) of an anterior-wall, posterior-hemitransverse fracture by resort to a triradiate incision (in view of a belated presentation, one month after the injury). Eighteen months later she progressed to a total hip arthroplasty (THA) for painful arthritic changes. Within one year the cup migrated through the avascular acetabulum. (a) Three-dimensional CT view of the acute injury; (b) AP view of pelvis taken 10 months after the injury; (c) AP view of left hip taken 12 months after the THA; (d) AP view of left hip taken 24 months after the THA.*

Acetabular fractures in elderly people

Acetabular fractures in elderly people represent the most rapidly growing spectrum of acetabular trauma. Furthermore, an elderly patient with an acetabular fracture may possess one of a broad spectrum of predisposing factors and co-morbidities, which may complicate the management and rehabilitation. Certain acetabular fractures in elderly people constitute wholly traumatic events in which the provocative blow imposed on relatively normal bone accounts for the injury (Fig. 7.14). As a general rule, an elderly victim who sustains a significant acetabular fracture along with trauma to multi-organ systems possesses a much less favourable prognosis for survival and recovery, primarily as a result of decreased compensatory mechanisms in the setting of excessive metabolic derangements.

Many or most of the fractures that occur in elderly people are the result of a simple fall on osteoporotic bone. Although classically a simple fall in elderly people is best recognized as a provocation for a femoral neck or intertrochanteric fracture, a significant and rapidly increasing number of such cases are presenting clinically as acetabular fractures. The classic injury pattern follows an injury where the patient lands on his or her side to provoke an anterior column, wall, and quadrilateral surface fracture (Fig. 7.15). This area of the acetabulum is the weakest portion and the most vulnerable to pathological fracture. Another common pattern in elderly

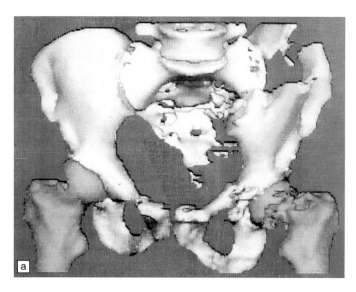

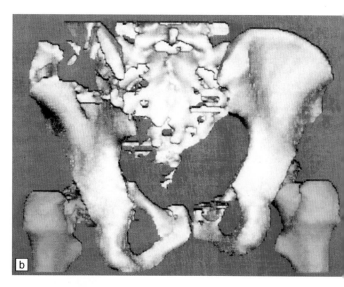

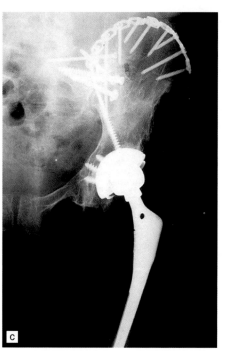

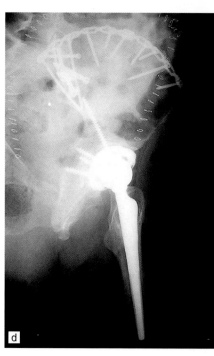

Figure 7.14 – *Multiple images displaying a complex fracture-dislocation of the left sacroiliac joint with a left anterior column fracture and a completely displaced left femoral neck fracture in a 60-year-old woman who sustained multiple injuries after a motor accident. One month later, when pelvic reconstruction was feasible, avascularity of the femoral head was documented. An open reduction of the left hemipelvis and a hybrid total hip arthroplasty were performed through an extended iliofemoral approach. (a) Initial anterior three-dimensional CT view; (b) initial posterior three-dimensional CT view; (c) postoperative AP view of left hip; (d) postoperative iliac oblique view of left hemipelvis.*

people is a posterior fracture dislocation, typically as a result of a motor vehicle accident. Many of these are posterior wall injuries with a marked degree of impaction of both the acetabulum and the femoral head. In an analysis of his results, LeTournel and Judet [23b] commented on their least favourable results after anterior and posterior wall injuries as a manifestation of trauma to elderly people, where the presence of osteopenia accounts for marked impaction or comminution. Superimposed on the fracture, degenerative arthritis of a moderate or severe degree complicates the reconstructive options available to the surgeon.

During the initial clinical evaluation of the elderly patient, a thorough history of the patient focuses on the magnitude of the provocative blow and the potential comorbidities that may prevail. The activity level and lifestyle of the patient, and the anticipated life expectancy, are significant factors. Radiographically, in addition to the conventional acetabular views, the transaxial CT scan is particularly helpful to characterize acetabular impaction involving the posterior wall or the femoral head. Unless the slice thickness of the scan is 3 mm or less, large impacted lesions involving the femoral head may be undetected. Once a single or

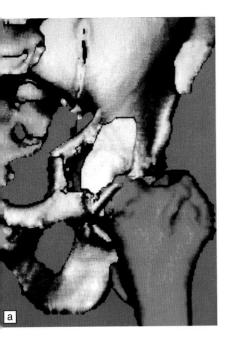

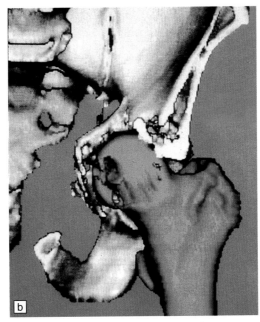

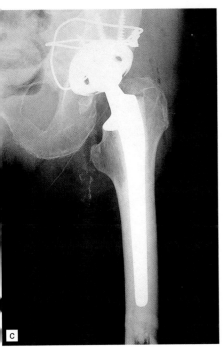

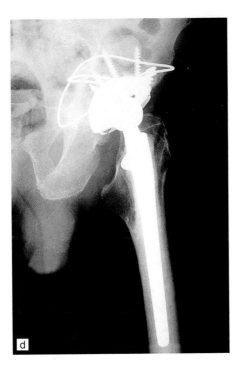

Figure 7.15 – *Multiple images of a left anterior column, wall and quadrilateral surface fracture in an 81-year-old man in which an acute total hip arthroplasty was undertaken in view of the comminution, osteopenia and impaction. Cables were used to immobilize the quadrilateral surface acutely. (a) Anterior three-dimensional CT view of left hip; (b) re-formatted anterior three-dimensional CT view through the centre of the femoral head; (c) postoperative AP view of left hip; (d) postoperative iliac oblique view of left hemipelvis.*

multiple images define the presence of a femoral head lesion, usually at the time of surgery, a surprisingly large lesion involving at least 20% of the surface area of the femoral head can be anticipated. Central acetabular impaction is optimally visualized on sagittal or coronal re-formatted computed images or corresponding tomograms. Comminution is underestimated by a scrutiny of a plain radiograph and over-emphasized by a review of a CT scan. An insufficiency fracture may become a source of pain before its visualization on a standard radiograph. Either a technetium bone scan or a magnetic resonance imaging (MRI) scan is a much more sensitive assessment. With the diverse clinical spectrum of presentations in elderly people, not surprisingly a correspondingly diverse array of therapeutic options arises.

Certain acetabular fractures can be anticipated to progress to an arthroplasty in view of the overwhelming predilection for post-traumatic arthritis. Currently, a controversy exists with respect to the optimal therapeutic option in such cases. Examples include the presence

111

of marked comminution, impaction or abrasion of the articular surfaces, an associated displaced femoral head or neck fracture, or the presence of severe degenerative arthritis. The therapeutic alternatives include a conventional acute open reduction and internal fixation, followed by a belated arthroplasty, initial conservative treatment and belated arthroplasty, or an acute arthroplasty with limited internal fixation. Where the initial conservative treatment is followed by a secondary total hip replacement, the arthroplasty may be complicated by the presence of malalignment or non-united acetabular fracture fragments [24,25]. Where an initial open reduction is followed by a belated arthroplasty, the scar tissue and presence of hardware may hamper the secondary procedure. Also the multiple surgeries may contribute to a somewhat greater predilection for an infected arthroplasty. Whether primary operative or conservative treatment is followed by an arthroplasty, the latter procedure possesses a marked increase in premature failure within a few years, i.e. at least five- to 20-fold greater than would be anticipated for a total hip replacement for a virgin degenerative hip.

These problems have culminated in another therapeutic alternative, in the form of an acute arthroplasty with minimal internal fixation. This is not a new concept. Historically, the earlier experience was complicated by acute loosening of a cemented cup in an unstable acetabular bed. More recent studies have focused on techniques that would permit the assembly of stable acetabular bone stock with a minimally invasive surgical dissection. Currently, this method appears to merit serious consideration especially for elderly people in whom a functional intact hip after either acute conservative treatment or an open reduction of a complex fracture is a remote possibility.

Technique for acute total hip arthroplasty

The procedure can be undertaken by resort to a posterolateral or an anterolateral (Hardinge) exposure [24]. The authors' personal preference is the posterolateral if the indication for the total hip arthroplasty is unclear before the arthrotomy, and the Hardinge when the preoperative indication for the arthroplasty is defined. The latter method of exposure provides a better view of the acetabular recess, with a somewhat more limited dissection. The osteotomized femoral head and neck are used as a morselized or structural graft. The

method for fixation and bone grafting depends on the specific fracture pattern. For a posterior wall fracture with extensive marginal impaction, typically involving 50% of the acetabulum, a segment of femoral head is anchored to the defect with the use of 3.5-mm screws (see Fig. 7.12). Then the acetabulum is reamed for insertion of a cementless cup and two or three anchoring screws. Before insertion of the cup, morselized reamings of bone are packed into any gaps that persist between the intact acetabulum and the structural graft. Reverse reaming is followed by the insertion of a slightly oversized cup, typically by 2 mm.

For a transverse, T-type fracture or for one with involvement of the quadrilateral surface (see Fig. 7.15), the inferior half of the acetabulum is immobilized by resort to a 2-mm cable. The cable is passed along the inner pelvis wall by resort to a Statinski cardiothoracic clamp. One end of the cable is brought out of the greater sciatic notch, whereas the other end gains access to the outer pelvic table between the anterosuperior and anteroinferior spines. For a high transverse fracture, the use of one cable suffices. If the transverse fracture is below the mid-tectal level or in the presence of a T-type fracture, a second cable is used. The second cable also passes along the quadrilateral surface, so that one end exits the lesser sciatic notch. The other end of the cable passes anterior to the superior pubic ramus, into the obturator foramen, where it gains access to the outer pelvic surface. That end passes anterior to the hip joint and through a drill hole in the anteroinferior spine. The free ends of the cable are connected in the supra-acetabular region. The two cables buttress the quadrilateral region in a criss-crossing fashion.

In the presence of a both-column fracture, initially the high anterior column fragment is reduced with forceps and immobilized by the use of a 4.5-mm cortical lag screw, which is inserted through a small stab wound superficial to the anteroinferior spine. Then the cable technique is employed to immobilize the remainder of the acetabulum. As an arthroplasty will follow in all these cases, a moderately accurate reduction can be accepted, provided that stable bone contact is achieved. For cases with central displacement, it is critical that the acetabular protrusion is corrected sufficiently, so that the cup will be centred in a conventional fashion, directly below the iliac wing.

Once the acetabulum is stable, conventional reaming is performed in the acetabular recess. Persistent fracture gaps or defects are obliterated with morselized cancellous autograft. Reverse reaming is undertaken to achieve a regular hemispherical depression. The acetabular cup is inserted with two to four cancellous screws. The orientation of each screw corresponds to the planes of the fracture lines, so that the optimal fixation is achieved. The remainder of the arthroplastic procedure follows in a typical fashion.

In the most typical scenario an acute total hip arthroplasty is undertaken to manage an elderly patient, who possesses somewhat compromised strength, agility, and balance compared to that in a younger adult. A partial weight-bearing or weight-bearing to tolerance gait becomes almost essential or the risk of a fall becomes excessive. The acetabular repair requires sufficient structural integrity so that some degree of immediate weight-bearing is feasible. Whenever practical, vigorous progressive resistance exercises of the hip abductors, quadriceps, and hamstrings, and active motion exercises are encouraged. At 6–8 weeks after an acute arthro-plasty, full weight-bearing activity generally can be encouraged.

Irradiation therapy

Osteonecrosis of the femoral head and the acetabulum is a well-recognized complication of pelvic irradiation. Radiation-induced changes such as osteopenic or necrotic bone and fibrotic bone marrow can predispose the bone to subchondral collapse, protrusio acetabulum, and subsequent pathological fracture [1,26]. Many of the patients in this population develop a markedly symptomatic hip, so that a total hip replacement merits serious consideration.

In many instances, the subtle radiographic features are indicative of extensive irradiation necrosis to the hip joint, and the adjacent bone and soft tissues (Fig. 7.16). Formidable technical problems may be encountered, including a surgical approach through dense scar tissue with the absence of normal intervals and planes, hazard to neighbouring neurovascular structures, and insufficient anchorage of the components into the structurally deficient bone. In the postoperative period, a florid wound infection may culminate in persistent drainage, which necessitates the removal of the components, despite aggressive antibiotic therapy and multiple surgical débridements.

The optimal surgical approach depends on the degree of structural compromise and alteration to the

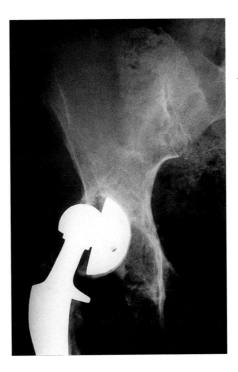

Figure 7.16 – *This AP view of the right hip with a failed cup displays irradiation necrosis of the pelvis in a 52-year-old woman. Careful scrutiny provides evidence of marked avascularity and osteopenia above the roof of the greater sciatic notch and extending to the anterior ilium.*

acetabulum, as well as the familiarity of the surgeon. A trochanteric osteotomy is discouraged in view of the predilection for a non-union. If the acetabulum requires an extensive degree of augmentation, a triradiate approach with preservation of the acetabulum may be necessary. Nevertheless, with the risk of a wound infection after an extensile exposure, a more conventional and limited approach is preferred whenever possible. A modified Hardinge exposure with elevation of the origin of the indirect head of rectus femoris and the tensor fascia lata muscle permits a considerable degree of acetabular exposure. Once the femoral head has been removed and the acetabulum exposed, the extent of acetabular compromise becomes evident. In the most florid case, with a curette, the markedly necrotic and softened acetabular roof or walls can be peeled away. This tissue has to be removed before initiation of buttressing or structural augmentation.

Several strategies for reconstruction of the acetabulum have been assessed (see Table 7.2) [27]. As a general rule, the use of any method that relies on the incorporation of bone graft or the ingrowth of bone into an acetabular cup is absolutely doomed. The ischaemic bed does not favour the necessary biological response. Alternative methods have relied on buttressing of the acetabulum with the use of threaded rods, mesh, or a cage, in combination with the use of methylmethacrylate cement and cemented cups. Alternatively, large threaded pins or rods can be driven from the ilium into the ischium or pubis. Subsequently, a cup is cemented into the acetabular recess.

Where the medial acetabular wall is thin or wholly deficient, metallic mesh can be used for augmentation. Titanium mesh is most readily contoured, although stiffer stainless steel, which is purchased in the form of a hemispherical configuration, is suitable. Once the acetabular roof and walls are lost, the use of a cage merits consideration [27,28]. If a cage is selected, one of the more extensile ones, such as a Bursch-Schneider design, with proximal and distal plate extenders is needed. For anchorage of the corresponding screws into the ilium and ischium, augmentation of the bone with cement may be necessary. Typically, a conventional technique for the insertion of a cemented femoral implant can be followed.

Several reports of total hip arthroplasty after irradiation therapy to the pelvis and hip have documented the exceptionally high complication rates (up to 52%) that may be anticipated [29,30]. Clearly, the role for total hip replacement after significant irradiation therapy to the pelvis is limited. In the patient who presents with severe destruction of the acetabulum, multiple pathological fractures of the pelvis, or an irradiation-induced soft tissue vascular injury such as stenosis of an iliac vessel, a Girdlestone procedure may be a more practical alternative to a total hip replacement. After a thorough review of the high likelihood for major postoperative complications and premature arthroplastic failure, the patient needs to be adequately counselled with respect to realistic expectations for a surgical reconstruction.

Quiescent sepsis

It is well recognized that recrudescence of infection may occur in a previously infected joint that has been quiescent for many years [3]. After a total hip arthroplasty, the exacerbation of a previously quiescent infection may culminate in prosthetic failure. The most typical sources of provocation of the initial pyogenic arthritis of the hip include a septic hip in infancy, reconstructive surgery to manage developmental dysplasia, Legg–Calve–Perthes disease, slipped capital femoral epiphysis, or a surgically managed acetabular fracture. To manage the infection, such a patient may undergo numerous procedures to the affected hip, including

drainage and sequestrectomy, resectional arthroplasty, or occasionally an arthrodesis. In other instances, the hip may have ankylosed spontaneously or formed a painless pseudarthrosis. At the time of clinical presentation of a previously septic hip, the strategy for management depends on the symptoms, the virulence of the prior infection, the nature of the original treatment and the subsequent management. There may be complete destruction of the femoral head and neck, with a high riding greater trochanter and severe acetabular dysplasia. The hip may be nearly or completely fused, frequently with a poor functional alignment. Alternatively, the hip may be dysplastic or hypoplastic or the proximal femur may display a proximal migration. The soft tissues may be severely scarred whereas the anatomy may be markedly distorted from previous multiple drainage procedures. Frequently, the ipsilateral limb is shortened, with the potential for a fixed flexion, adduction, and internal rotation contracture of the hip.

When considering a total hip arthroplasty in a patient who previously had a septic hip, the relevant factors include the duration of the quiescent period, the absence of clinical and radiographic findings, or the results of laboratory tests that might be indicative of the potential for an occult infection. In questionable cases, an aspiration arthrogram or a trephine biopsy under image intensification can be undertaken. Certain clinical findings merit particular concern about a potential recurrence of a prior infection. Rapid progression of symptoms may be consistent with a reactivation of the primary infection. Marked pain on weight-bearing is another clinical feature of concern. If the patient is immunocompromised by a concomitant illness, long-term steroid dependency, or another cause, a more critical assessment merits consideration, such as a percutaneous biopsy.

With the potential for marked anatomical distortion, a meticulous preoperative templating is necessary. Where dysplasia of the acetabulum is documented on an AP pelvis radiograph, supplementary oblique projections or a CT scan may be helpful to determine the need for acetabular reconstruction. Despite a thorough mobilization of the hip at the time of the arthroplasty, the patient should be aware that further scar tissue formation may limit the postoperative range of motion.

In the presence of a deficient proximal femur, prophylactic cerclage wiring or the use of strut allografts or impaction grafting may merit consideration. In the unusual case where the soft tissue is markedly deficient or scarified, a consideration for plastic coverage may be necessary. Consultation with a plastic surgeon is advisable before initiation of such a procedure. The plastic reconstruction may be staged as a preliminary event or it may accompany the arthroplasty. Intra-operative smears and excised specimens are sent for appropriate cultures for aerobic, anaerobic, tuberculous, and histological preparations. If a focus of active infection is encountered, it is prudent to débride the hip

thoroughly, to resect the femoral head, and to insert a cement spacer into the acetabulum (Fig. 7.17). After a course of intravenous antibiotics and a sterile trephine biopsy, a secondary procedure for the arthroplasty can be considered.

After a total hip replacement for a previously infected hip, several perioperative complications have been reported. Examples include an intraoperative femoral fracture during the reaming process, a sciatic nerve or femoral nerve palsy primarily in association with mobilization of an ankylosed hip, postoperative heterotopic

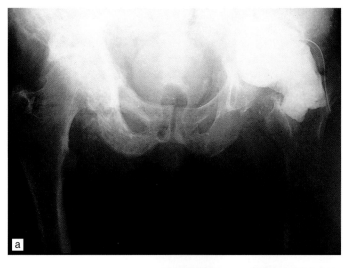
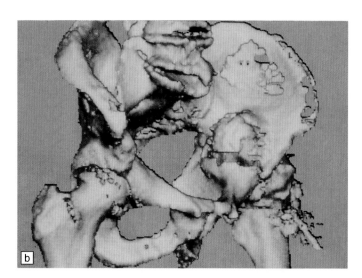
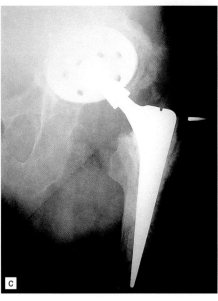
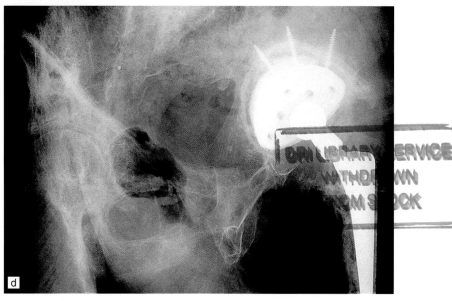

Figure 7.17 – *Multiple images display the left hip of a 74-year-old man who was managed for a long-standing septic hip with débridement, insertion of a cement spacer and antibiotic therapy. Four months later, after confirmation from a sterile trephine biopsy, a hybrid total hip arthroplasty with impaction grafting was performed, which included the use of a large cup. (a) AP view of pelvis with cement spacer; (b) anterior, iliac, oblique, three-dimensional CT with medial defect around spacer; (c) postoperative AP view of right hip; (d) postoperative iliac oblique view of right hemipelvis.*

ossification, and premature loosening of a component. Nevertheless, the low incidence of recurrent hip infection documented in several prior studies is a confirmation of the therapeutic role for such an arthroplasty [31–33].

Quiescent tuberculosis

In under-developed countries, skeletal tuberculosis continues be a significant medical problem [34]. In well-developed countries, tuberculosis of the hip may present in immigrant populations or in the susceptible population, especially individuals with a prior history of tuberculosis or those with immune suppression. In such a susceptible individual, upon primary arthroplasty for apparent degenerative arthritis, occasionally the recurrence of hip pain and stiffness with radiographic lucency of the acetabulum and proximal femur may be indicative of a reactivation of a previously quiescent tuberculous infection [3,34–37].

The procedure may be hampered by the presence of a fibrous or bony ankylosis. Once the deep exposure is completed, a provisional osteotomy through the mid-portion of the femoral neck is undertaken. Subsequently, the proximal femur is rotated so that the conventional resection of the femoral neck can be performed. In the presence of a fibrous ankylosis with tenacious intra-articular adhesions, the femoral head may be morselized in situ to facilitate its removal. Alternatively, in the presence of a bony ankylosis, a third osteotomy of the femoral neck is made at the periphery of the femoral head and at the level of the acetabular rim. Then an acetabular reamer is placed on the base of the femoral head to create an acetabular recess. A small drill hole is made through the medial acetabular wall to judge the thickness of the residual bone. Once the appropriate depth of the acetabular recess is achieved, enlargement is undertaken with progressively larger reamers. The remainder of the procedure is undertaken in a conventional manner.

If reactivation of a tuberculous infection follows a primary arthroplasty, the débridement of the hip with implant and cement removal is undertaken. A complete synovectomy is performed. This may require an extensive dissection, extending superior to the iliac crest and distal to the midshaft femur, for removal of the anticipated voluminous infected tissue.

Sickle-cell haemoglobinopathy

Osteonecrosis of the femoral head as a unilateral or bilateral clinical presentation is a frequent and significant complication of a sickle-cell haemoglobinopathy [38–40]. In the scenario of a painful collapse of the femoral head with marked incongruity and secondary degenerative changes of the hip joint, a total hip arthroplasty merits serious consideration. Technically, the procedure is liable to a potential weakening of the subchondral acetabular bone and the anticipated thin proximal femoral cortex, with an associated widened femoral canal. In some circumstances, prophylactic cerclage wiring of the proximal femur merits consideration.

Occasionally, reaming of the femoral canal is hampered by the presence of sclerotic bone, which obliterates the medullary canal. This problem further predisposes the bone to perforation, fracture, and a susceptibility to premature loosening of the femoral component [38–40]. Generally, the use of cementless components is strongly recommended for such a primary or revision total hip arthroplasty.

The arthroplastic procedure can be associated with a significant surgical blood loss, which contributes to the presentation of complications such as a sickle-cell crisis and the formation of a wound haematoma. A blood transfusion may be needed to optimize oxygenation and perfusion of the tissues, and thereby to minimize the risk of a perioperative sickle-cell crisis. In view of the extraordinary susceptibility of such a patient to bacteraemia with haematogenous spread to the hip, the use of perioperative prophylactic antibiotics is essential [41]. Despite the implementation of these precautionary measures, a high incidence of postoperative complications, including prosthetic failure, has been documented in the previous series of sickle-cell patients who underwent a total hip arthroplasty [41–44].

Paget's disease

Paget's disease is a common metabolic bone disease that subsequently affects the proximal femur, hip, and pelvis [44,45]. In the later stages of the disease, the involved bone becomes enlarged, dense, and sclerotic, with an irregular trabecular pattern, obliterated medullary canal and thickened cortices. The poor structural integrity of the bone renders it prone to either a major pathological fracture or to repetitive stress fractures [46,47]. A patient with Paget's disease of the hip can develop severe pain secondary to degenerative hip disease, a pathological hip fracture, or rarely as part of a sarcomatous change [48]. For Paget's disease that involves the hip, with secondary degenerative changes, operative intervention is indicated to manage significant pain, joint stiffness, deformity, or a pathological fracture of the femoral neck.

Preoperative treatment with bisphosphonates or calcitonin has been used to reduce the incidence of intraoperative bleeding, heterotopic ossification, and loosening, although the efficacy of these agents remains unproven. Also, preoperative planning is necessary to ascertain the size of the enlarged medullary canal, and to determine the proper amount of cement and the proper size of the components. Ready availability of blood is needed, in view of the potential for significant intraoperative haemorrhage from hypervascular and osteoporotic bone [3].

Nevertheless, certain features of pagetoid bone technically complicate a total hip arthroplasty. A broad spectrum of deformities of the proximal femur or acetabulum may hamper dislocation of the hip, exposure of the bone, or alignment of the components. In the presence of a protrusio acetabuli, dislocation of the hip may require morselization of the femoral head. In the presence of a marked coxa vara deformity or an anterolateral bowing of the femoral shaft, an osteotomy with realignment may be necessary to align the femoral component properly. Immobilization of the osteotomy can be achieved by the use of a strut allograft or a plate with cables, or a long-stemmed femoral component. In the presence of dense sclerotic bone, exceptionally sharp reamers may be necessary to shape the femoral canal. In contrast, if a widened medullary canal is encountered, a primary impaction grafting with cancellous allograft chips is recommended. In the authors' experience, obliteration of the canal with bone, as opposed to bone cement, culminates in a much more durable anchorage of the stem. Where the stem is capacious, a particularly large cement restrictor or cement plug is needed. Despite the potential for intraoperative complications and prolongation of the operative time, generally the long-term results after a cemented hip replacement in a pagetoid patient have been encouraging [47,48].

Gaucher's disease

Gaucher's disease is an inherited, autosomal recessive, systemic disorder of lipid metabolism, which frequently culminates in avascular necrosis of the femoral head, and renders the femoral neck and upper shaft vulnerable to a pathological fracture or deformity. The involved bone becomes osteopenic, with progressive widening of the medullary canal [3,38,49]. A total hip arthroplasty is indicated to manage painful avascular necrosis of the femoral head or a pathological fracture of the femoral neck. Complicating factors include intraoperative haemorrhage, along with the associated osteopenia and the presence of residual Gaucher cells within the bone, which compromise the quality of the cement–bone interface and potentially lead to premature loosening of the stem [50–52]. Although a cemented or hybrid total hip arthroplasty may be considered, in the presence of a capacious, thin-walled, proximal femur, the authors recommend primary impaction grafting with allograft cancellous bone. This method serves as an effective way to optimize the anchorage and potential longevity of the femoral stem, and to restore the bone stock.

Dwarfism and bony dysplasia

Achondroplasia is a common form of disproportionate dwarfism, which is associated with an abnormality of endochondral bone formation. Typically, such patients display broad, short iliac wings, coxa valga, markedly shortened femora, and genu varum, in addition to other characteristic features. The altered anatomy and biomechanical properties of the achondroplastic hip joint predispose to the development of early symptomatic degenerative hip disease, which may progress to a consideration for a total hip replacement. Typically, special miniaturized components (Fig. 7.18) are necessary for the procedure [53–55]. A particularly small femoral stem is needed to permit its insertion into the markedly narrowed femoral canal. Similarly, an acetabular cup with a small outside diameter is necessary to achieve a fit into the diminutive acetabular recess. With the small size of the femoral head component, the risk for a postoperative dislocation is increased. A preoperative CT scan of the pelvis and femur may be helpful for the determination of the optimal acetabular and femoral implant [3]. At the time of the surgical procedure, particular attention to the alignment of the components is necessary. The use of a cemented stem markedly decreases the difficulty to prepare the femoral canal with the minimal risk of fracture. With the small size of the canal, effective pressurization of the cement is particularly easy to achieve.

Multiple epiphyseal dysplasia is a common form of osteochondrodysplasia that is characterized by irregular or delayed ossification at multiple epiphyses. The frequent involvement of the hips may be manifest as bilateral and symmetrical coxa vara, irregular femora, recurrent subluxation of the hip, and the onset of

premature arthritis. The acetabular changes vary from a markedly dysplastic hip to protrusio acetabulum. Another manifestation, unilateral osteonecrosis, may culminate in significant asymmetrical hip disease [38]. Spondylo-epiphyseal dysplasia constitutes a group of disorders in which the formation of articular cartilage is compromised. Frequently, such a patient displays fractures that pertain to the hip, as well as dwarfism and kyphoscoliosis. The manifestations of the hip may include a marked coxa vara, subluxation, dislocation, or the premature onset of arthritis [38]. Symptomatic degenerative changes in the hip of a dysplastic patient

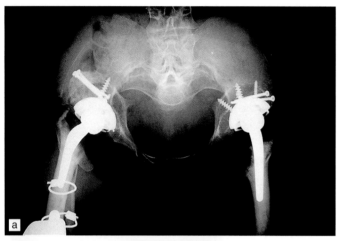

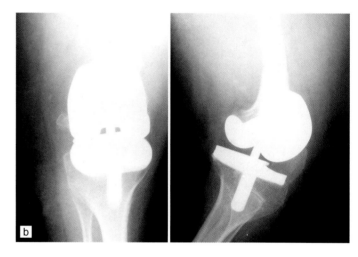

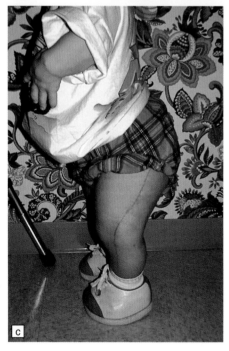

Figure 7.18 – *Radiographs of a 34-year-old achondroplastic dwarf of height 37 inches (94 cm) who underwent sequential ipsilateral total hip and knee replacements for marked bilateral degenerative changes, using custom cemented femoral implants apart from the small but conventional cementless cups. (a) AP view of pelvis; (b) AP and lateral views of right knee; (c) postoperative photograph of patient.*

warrant consideration for an osteotomy or a total hip replacement.

It is essential to have a meticulous preoperative plan with respect to selection of the implants. Custom implants may be necessary to account for the extraordinarily small size of the proximal femur. If such a patient displays marked degenerative and symptomatic changes in the ipsilateral knee, a concomitant total knee replacement merits consideration. Both arthroplasties can be undertaken through an incision, which is not materially longer than that required for an isolated arthroplasty of the hip or knee. At the time of such a total hip replacement, a fastidious preparation of the femoral canal, with the possible use of small, cannulated reamers, is necessary. With the bizarre configuration of the proximal femur, particular attention to the alignment of the femoral stem is needed, especially with respect to rotation. Although cementless or cemented cups appear to be comparable for this application, the use of a cemented stem greatly simplifies the preparation of the femur.

Fibrous dysplasia

Fibrous dysplasia is an osseous developmental disorder of unknown aetiology, characterized by the appearance of abnormal fibrous tissue in bone. Typically, fibrous dysplasia affects the proximal femur, with the potential initiation of a deformity secondary to repetitive minor fractures or a single major pathological fracture. The problem may be complicated by the presence of a leg length discrepancy or a limited and asymmetrical range of motion of the hip [56]. If symptomatic degenerative joint disease ensues secondarily, a total hip arthroplasty may be indicated.

As part of the reconstructive procedure, a meticulous curettage of the dysplastic segment is necessary. Technically, the procedure is complicated by the potential for marked deformity, thinning of the relevant cortical wall, and an enlargement of the corresponding marrow cavity. Two different strategies for effective immobilization of the femoral component may be considered. Where the disease is restricted to a segment of the proximal femur, a large-stemmed device, either of a cemented or a non-cemented type, may be used. As an alternative measure, impaction grafting with the use of a polished stem and cement is highly attractive (Fig. 7.19). Where the upper femur is precariously fragile, or so deformed that an osteotomy is needed to realign it, the use of supplementary strut allografts and cerclage cables may be necessary. Where foreshortening of the involved segment of the femur is documented, elevation of the stem and augmentation of the neck length can achieve moderate lengthening of the limb. Enthusiasm for lengthening needs to be tempered by the other clinical complexities that may be encountered in such a case.

Down's syndrome

A patient with Down's syndrome is vulnerable to generalized ligamentous laxity, which serves as a predilection for an inherently unstable hip joint [3]. With the variable degree of mental handicap, such a patient is limited in his or her ability to comply with physiotherapy or postoperative restrictions of activity. Occasionally, the severely afflicted Down's syndrome patient who becomes bedridden presents clinically with a marked contracture of the hip and profound wasting of muscle. To complicate matters, the assessment of pain in a severely handicapped patient is challenging. Frequently, a family member or nurse will have observed a recent decrease in activity level or an alteration in mood or behaviour.

For the preoperative planning, the radiographic templating may identify the need for small components. At the time of surgery, meticulous alignment of the components is needed to optimize the stability of the hip joint [57,58]. Particular attention must be paid to the alignment of the cup, including a recognition of and compensation for the anticipated exaggeration of the degree of lumbar lordosis. From the experience of the authors, a hybrid arthroplasty appears to be a generally satisfactory technique for this patient population. Immediate unlimited weight-bearing can be anticipated.

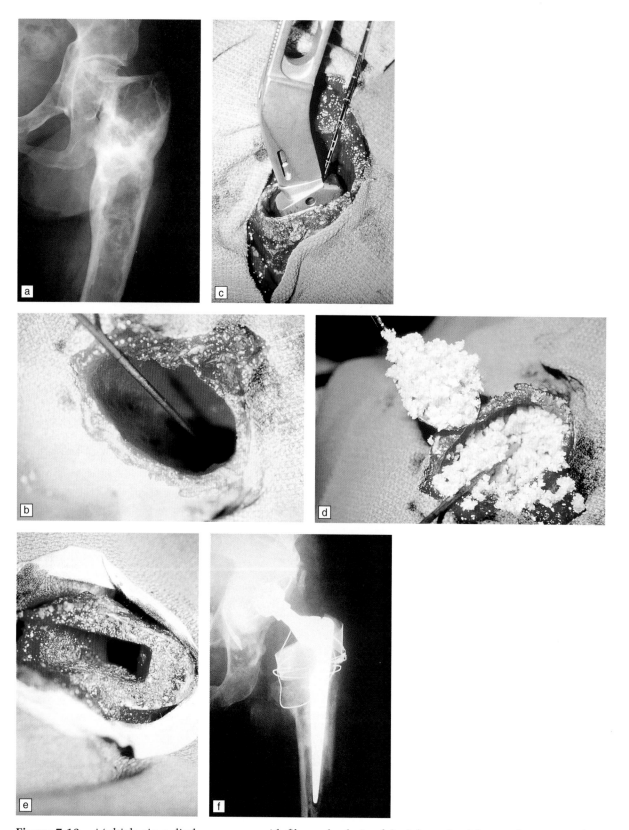

Figure 7.19 – *Multiple views display a woman with fibrous dysplasia of the left proximal femur who progressed to a cemented total hip arthroplasty for avascular necrosis of the hip secondary to a pathological fracture. A primary impaction grafting of the femur with proximal mesh augmentation was undertaken. (a) Preoperative AP view of left hip; (b) intraoperative view after femoral curettage; (c) insertion of a smooth broach over a guide wire; (d) impaction of cancellous allograft chips; (e) appearance of the augmented femur before cementation; (f) postoperative AP view of left hip.*

References

1. Vail TP, McCollum DE. Complex primary acetabular replacement. In: Callaghan JJ, Rosenberg AG, Rubash HE, eds. *The Adult Hip*. Philadelphia: Lippincott-Raven, 1998; 1183–200.

2. Glassman AH. Complex primary femoral replacement. In: Callaghan JJ, Rosenberg AG, Rubash HE, eds. *The Adult Hip*. Philadelphia: Lippincott-Raven, 1998; 1201–20.

3. Harkess JW. Arthroplasty of hip. In: Crenshaw AH, ed. *Campbell's Operative Orthopaedics*, 9th edn. St. Louis: Mosby-Year Book, Inc., 1998; 296–472.

4. Gie GA, Linder L, Ling RS *et al.* Contained morselized allograft in revision total hip arthroplasty: surgical technique. *Orthop Clin North Am* 1993; 24: 717–25.

5. Gie GA, Linder L, Ling RS *et al.* Impacted cancellous allografts and cement for revision total hip arthroplasty. *J Bone Joint Surg* 1993; 75B: 14–21.

6. Ling RSM, Timperley AJ, Linder L. History of cancellous impaction grafting in the femur. *J Bone Joint Surg* 1993; 75B: 693–6.

7. Paprosky WG, Magrus RE. Principles of bone grafting in revision total hip arthroplasty: acetabular techniques. *Clin Orthop* 1994; 298: 147–55.

8. Slooff TJ, Huiskes R, van Horn J *et al.* Bone grafting in total hip replacement for acetabular protrusion. *Acta Orthop Scand* 1984; 55: 593–6.

9. Amstutz HC, Sakai DN. Total joint replacement for ankylosed hips: indications, technique, and preliminary results. *J Bone Joint Surg* 1975; 57A: 619.

10. Brewster RC, Coventry MB, Johnson EW Jr. Conversion of the arthrodesed hip to a total hip arthroplasty. *J Bone Joint Surg* 1975; 57A: 27.

11. Lubahn JD, Evarts CM, Feltner JB. Conversion of ankylosed hips to total arthroplasty. *Clin Orthop* 1980; 153: 146.

12. Hardinge K, Murphy JCM, Frenyo S. Conversion of hip fusion to Charnley low-friction arthroplasty. *Clin Orthop* 1986; 211: 173–9.

13. Kilgus DJ, Amstutz HC, Wolgin MA *et al.* Joint replacement for ankylosed hips. *J Bone Joint Surg* 1990; 72A: 45.

14. Strathy GM, Fitzgerald RH Jr. Total hip arthroplasty in the ankylosed hip. *J Bone Joint Surg* 1988; 70A: 963.

15. Soballe K, Boll KL, Kofod S *et al.* Total hip replacement after medial-displacement osteotomy of the proximal part of the femur. *J Bone Joint Surg* 1989; 71A: 692–7.

16. Ferguson GM, Cabanela ME, Ilstrup DM. Total hip arthroplasty after failed intertrochanteric osteotomy. *J Bone Joint Surg* 1994; 76B: 252.

17. Boos N, Krushell R, Ganz R *et al.* Total hip arthroplasty after previous proximal femoral osteotomy. *J Bone Joint Surg* 1997; 79B: 247–53.

18. Benke GJ, Baker AS, Dounis E. Total hip replacement after upper femoral osteotomy: a clinical review. *J Bone Joint Surg* 1982; 64B: 570.

19. Patterson BM, Salvati EA, Huo MH. Total hip arthroplasty for complications of intertrochanteric fracture. *J Bone Joint Surg* 1990; 72A: 776–7.

20. Franzen H, Nilsson LT, Stromqvist B *et al.* Secondary total hip replacement after fractures of the femoral neck. *J Bone Joint Surg* 1990; 72B: 784–7.

21. Boardman KP, Charnley J. Low-friction arthroplasty after fracture-dislocations of the hip. *J Bone Joint Surg* 1978; 60B: 495.

22. Joly JM, Mears DC. The role of total hip arthroplasty in acetabular fracture management. *Oper Techniques Orthop* 1993; 3: 80–102.

23a. Mears DC, Shirahama M. Stabilization of an acetabular fracture with cables for acute total hip arthroplasty. *J Arthroplasty* 1998; 13: 104–7.

23b. Le Tournel E, Judet R. Fractures of the Acetabolum. New York: Springer, 1993, 392.

24. Soni RK. An anterolateral approach to the hip joint. *Acta Orthop Scand* 1997; 68: 490–4.

25. Romness DW, Lewallen DG. Total hip arthroplasty after fracture of the acetabulum. Long term results. *J Bone Joint Surg* 1990; 72B: 761–4

26. Deleeuw HW, Pottenger LA. Osteonecrosis of the acetabulum following radiation therapy. A report of two cases. *J Bone Joint Surg* 1988; 70A: 293–9.

27. O'Conner MI, Sim FH, Chao EYS. Special implants for massive bone loss about the hip. In: Morrey BF, ed. *Joint Reconstructive Surgery*. New York: Churchill Livingstone Inc., 1996.

28. Gross AE, Allen DG, Catre *et al.* Bone grafts in hip replacement surgery: the pelvic side. *Orthop Clin N Am* 1993; 24: 679–96.

29. Massin P, Duparc J. Total hip replacement in irradiated hips: a retrospective review of 71 cases. *J Bone Joint Surg* 1995; 77B: 847–52.

30. Jacobs JJ, Kull LR, Frey GA *et al.* Early failure of acetabular components without cement after previous pelvic irradiation. *J Bone Joint Surg* 1995; 77A: 1829–35.

31. Kim YH. Total arthroplasty of the hip after childhood sepsis. *J Bone Joint Surg* 1991;73B: 783.

32. Hardinge K, Cleary J, Charnley J. Low-friction arthroplasty for healed septic and tuberculous hips. *J Bone Joint Surg* 1979; 61B: 144–7.

33. Cherney DL, Amstutz HC. Total hip replacement in the previously septic hip. *J Bone Joint Surg* 1983; 65A: 1256.

34. Kim YH, Han DY, Park BM. Total hip arthroplasty for tuberculous coxarthrosis. *J Bone Joint Surg* 1987; 69A: 718.

35. Johnson R, Barnes KL, Owen R. Reactivation of tuberculosis after total hip replacement. *J Bone Joint Surg* 1979; 61B: 148–50.

36. Jupiter JB, Karchmer AW, Lowell JD. Total hip arthroplasty in the treatment of adult hips with current or quiescent sepsis. *J Bone Joint Surg* 1981; 63A: 194–200.

37. Kim YY, Ko CU, Ahn JY *et al.* Charnley low friction arthroplasty in tuberculosis of the hip. *J Bone Joint Surg* 1988; 70B: 756.

38. Lachiewicz PF, Kelley SS. Systemic diseases resulting in hip pathology. In: Callaghan JJ, Rosenberg AG, Rubash HE, eds. *The Adult Hip*. Philadelphia: Lippincott-Raven, 1998; 437–50.

39. Hanker GJ, Amstutz HC. Sickle cell disease and the hip. In: Amstutz HC, ed. *Hip Arthroplasty*. New York: Churchill Livingstone Inc., 1991; 677–92.

40. Chung SM, Ralston EL. Necrosis of the femoral head associated with sickle cell anemia and its genetic variants: a review of the literature and study of thirteen cases. *J Bone Joint Surg* 1969; 51A: 33–58.

41. Gunderson C, D'Ambrosia RD, Shoji H. Total hip replacement in patients with Sickle-Cell disease. *J Bone Joint Surg* 1977; 59A: 760–2.

42. Bishop AR, Roberson JR, Eckman JR *et al.* Total hip arthroplasty in patients who have sickle-cell hemoglobinopathy. *J Bone Joint Surg* 1988; 70A: 853.

43. Acurio MT, Friedman RJ. Hip arthroplasty in patients with sickle-cell haemoglobinopathy. *J Bone Joint Surg* 1992; 74B: 367.

44. Moran MC, Huo MH, Garvin KL *et al.* Total hip arthroplasty in sickle cell hemoglobinopathy. *Clin Orthop* 1993; 294: 140.

45. Mirsky EC, Einhorn TA. Metabolic bone disease. In: Callaghan JJ, Rosenberg AG, Rubash HE, eds. *The Adult Hip*. Philadelphia: Lippincott-Raven, 1998; 507–26.

46. Johnston KS, Chow GH, Finerman GAM. Paget's disease and total hip arthroplasty. In: Amstutz HC, ed. *Hip Arthroplasty*. New York: Churchill Livingstone Inc., 1991; 787–98.

47. Merkow RL, Pellicci PM, Hely DP *et al.* Total hip replacement for Paget's disease of the hip. *J Bone Joint Surg* 1984; 66A: 752.

48. Stauffer RN, Sim FH. Total hip arthroplasty in Paget's disease of the hip. *J Bone Joint Surg* 1976; 58A: 476.

49. Amstutz HC. Gaucher's disease and total hip arthroplasty. In: Amstutz HC, ed. *Hip Arthroplasty*. New York: Churchill Livingstone Inc., 1991; 693–9.

50. Lachiewicz PF, Lane JM, Wilson PD Jr. Total hip replacement in Gaucher's disease. *J Bone Joint Surg* 1981; 63A: 602.

51. Lau MM, Lichtman DM, Hamati YI *et al.* Hip arthroplasties in Gaucher's disease. *J Bone Joint Surg* 1981; 63: 591–601.

52. Goldblatt J, Sacks S, Dall D, Beighton P. Total hip arthroplasty in Gaucher's disease: long-term prognosis. *Clin Orthop* 1988; 228: 94.

53. Peterson LAF. Little people. In: Morrey B, ed. *Joint Replacement Arthroplasty*. New York: Churchill Livingstone, 1991; 749–58.

54. Huo MH, Salvati ER, Lieberman JR *et al.* Custom designed femoral prostheses in total hip arthroplasty done with cement for severe dysplasia of the hip. *J Bone Joint Surg* 1993; 75A: 1497–1504.

55. Woolson ST, Harris WH. Complex total hip replacement for dysplastic or hypoplastic hips using miniature or microminiature components. *J Bone Joint Surg* 1983; 63A: 1099.

56. Wirganowicz PZ, Lane JM, Eckardt JJ. Primary tumors and tumorous conditions. In: Callaghan JJ, Rosenberg AG, Rubash HE, eds. *The Adult Hip*. Philadelphia: Lippincott-Raven, 1998; 527–46.

57. Skoff HD, Keggi K. Total hip replacement in Down's syndrome. *Orthopedics* 1987; 10: 185–489.

58. Skoff HD. Total hip replacement in the neuromuscularly impaired. *Orthop Rev* 1986; 15: 154–9.

SECTION III
Revision

CHAPTER 8

Assessment of the unsatisfactory or failed total hip replacement

M. D. Northmore-Ball

The determination of whether something is wrong with a total hip replacement (THR), and what the problems are, is by no means straightforward. Revision, if appropriate however, is very much more likely to work if an accurate analysis of the presenting problem, preferably with a complete understanding of why the problem arose, is made. A correct analysis depends on a very careful analysis of all the evidence available rather than dependence on any one test. The history, physical examination, plain radiographs, and special tests need to be looked at as a whole. Only then is it likely that the correct diagnosis will be made and a good result, if revision is required, obtained.

Presenting complaints

These include, singly or in combination:
- Group 1: the hip is painful.
- Group 2: the patient's walking distance has become less and/or walking aids have become necessary or their requirement has increased.
- Group 3: an obvious infection is present with a discharging sinus.
- Group 4: the hip is stiff or does not move at all.
- Group 5: the hip recurrently dislocates, probably such that repeated hospital admissions have been required.
- Group 6: the hip may click or the patient may feel a clunking sensation (often described as its being loose), but the hip does not actually dislocate.
- Group 7: less common symptoms may be present – the leg has been too long ever since the replacement or is short or becoming shorter, the first of these being the most significant.

These presentations are discussed below.

Group 1: painful hip

The *possible causes* for pain are as follows:
- Group 1A: the hip, in fact, has nothing wrong with it and the pain comes from somewhere else, e.g. the lumbar spine.
- Group 1B: aseptic loosening is present of one or both components.
- Group 1C: infection is present without loosening.
- Group 1D: a combination of infection and loosening is present.
- Group 1E: there is a fracture of the stem.
- Group 1F: there are broken trochanteric wires or another failed fixation device with or without trochanteric escape.
- Group 1G: some genuine, but difficult to pin down, cause is present, such as psoas tendon irritation or trochanteric bursitis.

Group 1A: nothing wrong with the hip
This may be because either the hip was never the pain source or there is a new one.

Group 1A(i): hip never a source of pain
The author has, on a number of occasions, observed the following sequence. A hip replacement has been done; the hip is subsequently painful; the hip is then revised; pain continues and the patient is referred, the symptoms after revision being considered to result from possible infection. The sequence may often be longer and very frequently includes partial removal of unbroken

trochanteric wires in the presence of sound trochanteric union. Perusal of the case notes and radiographs of such patients not infrequently shows that the original hip before replacement was hardly, if at all, arthritic, so that with the 'retrospectoscope' it is clear that the original symptoms did not come from the hip.

The salient features of these patients are that pain, whatever its distribution, was not relieved by the original replacement. The distribution of the pain may also suggest another cause, particularly, if in the buttock, that it is derived from the lumbosacral spine. Sometimes such patients have had a very definite history of back problems, perhaps associated with spinal surgery, such as discectomy. The hip may have been moderately arthritic, but again there is failure of pain relief, or extremely early recurrence of pain after non-specific postoperative pain relief for a few weeks. The question of correct initial treatment in the case of a patient with an arthritic back and an arthritic hip is discussed elsewhere in this book. Not infrequently, patients with an apparently failed THR, in whom the original symptoms did not come from the hip, are found to have had pain at a number of different sites with only a relatively minor underlying organic problem. Examination may show features suggestive of a problem with the THR, such as a limp, some limitation of motion, and some limitation of active straight leg raising, but, nevertheless, none of these signs is likely to be gross.

The essential point, however, is that the plain radiograph will either show good appearances or have quite minor abnormalities only (such as a very thin peri-acetabular radiolucent line). The erythrocyte sedimentation rate (ESR) is low and bone scanning will either be normal or show only very minor increase in activity. It is vitally important not to over-interpret such test results. The true pain source must be found; if this is elusive, the patient should simply be reassured and observed.

Group 1A(ii): new pain source

In this case, the pain (radiating from the hip to the groin and/or thigh) was relieved in a convincing fashion by the original THR and remained in abeyance for a considerable period. Pain then started again, probably insidiously. This may be noted in a follow-up clinic or be sufficient for the patient to be re-referred by the GP if already discharged. It is common for it to be assumed that such pain is caused by something being amiss with the THR. An accurate history is vital. The pain may be similar to one that the patient had before, but is more likely to be felt by the patient as somewhat different, e.g. in the buttock or associated with pain across the low back. The pain may be worse after being still, then gradually improving with activity, but unfortunately this can also be the case with a THR. Examination may well be completely unhelpful, but there could be a suggestion of reproduction of the pain on lateral spinal flexion or spinal extension, suggesting, for example, that the pain is in fact derived from facet arthritis. The patient may unfortunately limp to some degree even if the hip is not at fault. There is probably no neurological deficit and, if such deficit is present, it is probably irrelevant. In a clear-cut case, active movement of the hip may be excellent, but there is usually some reluctance on the part of the patient.

Radiography

In the simplest type of case, the hip radiograph is clearly excellent, but unfortunately there are likely to be imperfections, most of which may not, however, be of any consequence. Notable among these is a trochanteric non-union as described below. There may, however, also be radiolucent lines. If previous radiographs are available (and every attempt should be made to locate these), comparison will show that any such radiolucencies are either non-progressive or else have progressed only to a minor degree. Radiographs of the lumbosacral spine may show degenerative change and it is important to note that pain in the anterior thigh may be referred from the hip, but also from the upper lumbar spine; thigh pain with bad degenerative change, particularly in the upper lumbar levels, suggested that the new pain is derived from the lumbar spine. The author has found that hip blocks, with confirmation of needle placement by arthrography, although very useful in confirmation of the arthritic hip as a pain source, seem unfortunately of less value in the identification of pain resulting from a THR, perhaps through lack of full dispersal of the local anaesthetic to the true pain sources within the joint. Others, however, have found the technique useful in this situation.

Figure 8.1 shows an anteroposterior (AP) pelvic radiograph of a patient with a lumbosacral fusion and bilateral THRs. The patient complained of pain in the left leg. The hip radiographs are unremarkable, although there are minor radiolucencies. Analysis by the method indicated above showed that the level of the disc above

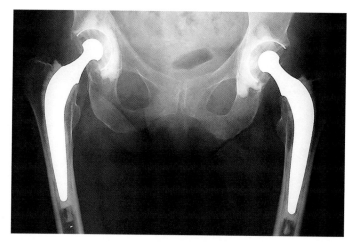

Figure 8.1 – *Group 1A(ii) case with pain apparently after total hip replacement, but resulting from a new problem in the lumbosacral spine (see text).*

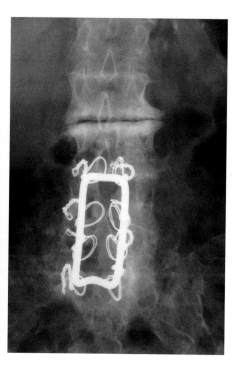

Figure 8.2 – *Same patient as in Figure 8.1.*

the fused level had become severely degenerate (Fig. 8.2), and further investigation by a spinal surgeon demonstrated that the new problem was derived from this level.

Much the most common cause of diagnostic confusion is of course pain derived from the lumbosacral spine (which may indeed often coexist with pain derived from the hip), but there are a number of rare causes, such as stress fractures of the pelvis and tumours.

It is vitally important to consider the above possibilities. All too often patients are seen who have had completely unnecessary and unhelpful further hip

surgery, sometimes including a full revision. Such revisions undertaken for hips that have nothing wrong with them and well-fixed components not infrequently produce complications of their own. If in doubt such a patient should certainly be referred, at least for an opinion.

There are frequently cases of considerable clinical doubt. The better plan is to do nothing and await events. This may, however, be quite difficult to do, particularly with patients who have pain that does not originate from the hip, because sometimes such patients can be very demanding. Doing nothing, however, even if it comes to the point that patients look as if they are about to make a complaint because of apparent refusal to believe them, is hugely better than to embark on further valueless surgery with no real prospect of symptom relief.

Groups 1B-1D: differential diagnosis

Infection (the third presentation) is sometimes obvious, with a discharging sinus, but usually the question is whether a loose hip is also infected.

Some question the value of trying to distinguish between mechanical and infective loosening. The author's view is that this is vital. It is perfectly possible to eradicate an infection by appropriate revision surgery, but only by the use of other measures that are not necessary in the aseptic case, as discussed in Chapter 12.

The history

In all the above, there is pain, frequently radiating to the groin and/or thigh, together with additional limitations in terms of walking distance and the use of walking aids.

Aseptic loosening

In aseptic loosening, in the great majority of cases, the hip will have been functionally extremely well for some time (usually several years) after replacement, and symptoms start insidiously. They then steadily worsen. If the hip is cementless and of an early uncoated design, in which some degree of pain has always been present, this pain increases. It is perfectly possible initially to believe that such patients are in group 1A(ii); changes on radiographs at first minimal, but worsening symptoms with obvious radiological loosening will clarify the diagnosis after a sometimes substantial period of expectant management.

Infection

If infection is present (and assuming that this has been present since the original THR, as is most common), pain will have been improved or perhaps altered in quality, but never completely relieved, after THR. Sometimes an extremely brief period (a few weeks) of symptomatic relief is reported. Pain then continues unremittingly. The patient may have moved on to the use of one stick, but has probably never got rid of it and may later have had recourse to increased use of walking aids. Uncommonly, a true haematogenous infection occurs, producing infection in a previously perfectly satisfactory THR. All too often, such a mode of infection is proposed when in fact the infection was introduced at the time of surgery. Such an explanation is of course a considerably more attractive one to the operating surgeon. Nevertheless, clear-cut cases are seen. In Figure 8.3, the patient's hip function had been extremely good until she developed pneumonia with septicaemia caused by *Staphylococcus aureus*. Subsequently, a deep infection of the hip developed. The shorter the time after THR at which symptoms that cause concern occur, the higher the likelihood that the problem is infection. If very early, the hip is probably not loose and the pain derives from the increased joint hydrostatic pressure. Later, loosening, either resulting directly from the infection or as a consequence of mechanical imperfections in the THR, occurs as a secondary effect and the pain caused by the increased fluid pressure is then compounded by the loosening.

The timing of the pain's onset ought to correspond to the known lifetime of the type of replacement used. Thus, a number of designs are now known to have fundamentally unsound features, such as a thin-walled plastic socket or a curved stem with a sharp edge in the calcar region (e.g. McKee–Arden or early Muller), in comparison with numerous other more modern implants. The principle of 'Ocham's razor' is of importance. This principle states that if, on the one hand, there are several combinations of possible causes for a set of observations but, on the other, there is one single cause that can explain all of them together, then the latter is correct. In the present context, it is, of course, possible that infection as well as mechanical factors could be responsible for loosening of a given hip. If the design of the hip is, however, such that very long-term function is rather unlikely, it is almost certain, in the absence of other indicators, that loosening at 7 or 8 years from the

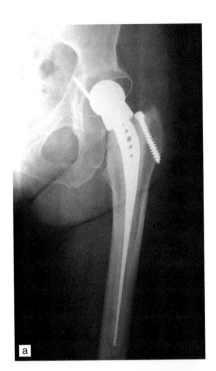

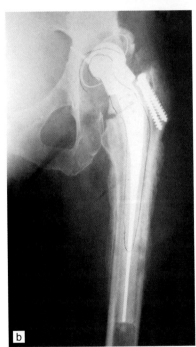

Figure 8.3 – *(a) Postoperative appearance after total hip replacement with RM-Isoelastic. After several years of very good function the patient had a serious staphylococcal pneumonia and septicaemia, and the left hip became painful. (b) The striking radiograph finding is the obvious osteomyelitis of the upper femur.*

THR is solely aseptic. If, on the other hand, the hip is of good design and apparently well inserted, then loosening at this stage might be more difficult to explain on mechanical grounds alone, and an element of infection would have to be suspected.

Sometimes, patients refer to a lump in the wound which may disappear spontaneously. This is very suggestive of deep infection. In the case shown in Figure 8.4,

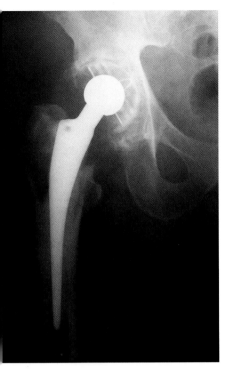

Figure 8.4 – *The transient appearance of a small lump in this patient's wound was highly suggestive of deep infection, and this was later confirmed.*

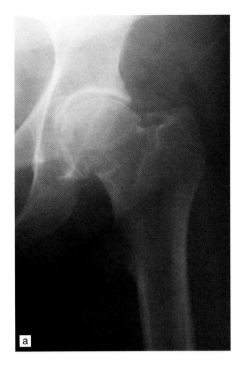

Figure 8.5 – *(a) The preoperative radiograph in this patient with pain after a THR was suspiciously normal.*

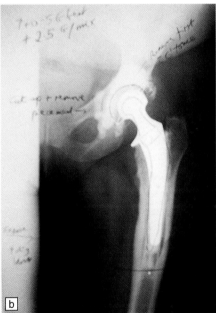

(b) Later, however the diagnosis of deep infection became clear. The handwritten notes on the X-ray are details from the pre-vision planning.

a deep infection was suspected on the basis of the complete presentation and tests; this impression was increased considerably by the patient subsequently reporting temporary worsening of the symptoms with the transient appearance of a lump.

Perioperative details of the THR

Depending on the circumstances of the case, it may be possible to establish whether the hip was originally replaced in a laminar-flow, ultra-clean-air operating theatre. If carried out in ultra-clean air (unfortunately, the type of clothing other than body exhaust suits worn by the operating team will hardly ever be known), infection seeded at the time of operation is less likely. Fortunately, the use of such operating theatres is steadily increasing. There is, however, one caveat: if it is seen from the operation notes, deduced from the scar, or otherwise known that the hip was inserted with the patient in a lateral position (i.e. usually through a posterior approach), the possibility of a deep infection may actually be increased if the operating team did not wear either exhaust suits or hoods and suits of appropriate material (e.g. Rotecno or Fabric 450). The patient shown in Figure 8.5 had pain after a THR carried out in this way. She appeared initially to be in group 1A(ii), because the preoperative hip radiograph (Fig. 8.5a) had shown minimal osteoarthritis, but soon

afterwards endosteal lysis appeared near the tip of the stem (Fig. 8.5b) and the diagnosis became clear. Investigation in this case showed a *Staphylococcus epidermidis* infection.

Statistically speaking, urethral instrumentation at the time of the THR (usually as a result of a failure to resolve urinary difficulties thoroughly in elderly men before surgery), psoriasis, and diabetes are also associated with an increase in infection rate. In balancing the evidence, the existence of such factors tends towards a feeling that infection may be present. A history of early post-operative, but perhaps seemingly insignificant, wound problems with a note, for example, that the patient had required dressings by the district nurse for a few weeks after leaving hospital, should be taken into account. Finally, the patient will often report that the hip 'was never right'.

Examination

Unless a definite wound problem, such as a sinus or sinuses, is present, examination is unlikely to be very helpful. The patient will almost certainly walk with a limp and be in some discomfort. An abnormal range of motion in the hip may, however, equally result from severe preoperative stiffness or an abnormality in the way that the hip was inserted rather than from any later supervening problems. Occasionally, patients with a gross mechanical problem in the hip, who report intermittent symptoms, may walk easily with a normal gait. Radiographs (see below) in such cases always show, however, what may be quite a marked abnormality and subsequent revision shows severe loosening. In such patients, there are alternative positions that one component (particularly the femoral) can take up, one being stable under load and the other less stable and producing pain. Such a possibility needs to be considered, because otherwise these patients are kept going for longer than is necessary with an unsatisfactory THR. These cases are usually aseptic.

Commonly, the range of movement of a hip may seem to be good because the examination has been carried out largely passively. A repeat of the examination carried out actively will show a diminished range of motion with discomfort. Active straight leg raising is also a very good test. The ability to straight leg raise actively requires a high load on the hip. Nevertheless, none of these findings is likely to be useful in determining whether or not infection is present.

Radiography

Plain radiographs are seldom diagnostic and some reported studies have suggested that they are of little use in distinguishing between aseptic and infective loosening. In practice, however, much useful information can be gleaned when taken together with the facts of the case already assembled.

If available, the complete radiograph series from the time of the original THR is extremely useful. Great

efforts should be made to obtain these. One can then work out what the hip was like before replacement, the nature and the quality of the replacement, what serial changes there may have been since then, and the speed of any such changes. From the point of view of distinction between aseptic and septic loosening, bearing in mind a number of the statements already made, we may analyse the radiographs from the following points of view.

The type of components inserted

This may of course already be known; alternatively it remains largely unknown even after inspection of the radiographs (the Hamburg Endo Klinik's PUO or 'prosthesis of unknown origin'). The type of prosthesis inserted is very important in the diagnosis as described above, quite apart from technical considerations relating to any planned later revision.

Technical competence

The technical competence of the way in which these components were inserted, in terms of both the positioning of the components and (if cemented) the cementation of each component. If only a moderately well-inserted but good type of implant, or a poor type of implant that is apparently very well inserted, comes loose early, then this raises the index of suspicion about infection being present.

Radiolucent lines

The width, distribution, and most particularly the changes in radiolucent lines are compared between serial radiographs.

In the acetabulum, a thin radiolucent line in Charnley zone 3 is more common than it should be, even when THR is relatively well performed. This results simply from the cortical nature of the acetabular floor, in combination with the fact that the margin of the bone–cement junction in this region is immediately adjacent to the teardrop, quite deeply placed, and, therefore, relatively inaccessible. In the absence of special measures, such as grafting, sufficient cement impaction in this region for complete elimination of radiolucencies can be difficult to achieve. Similarly, a short, thin radiolucency in zone 1 is quite common even with the use of flanged cups; this area of the acetabulum is often sclerotic. In the femur, insignificant radiolucencies are often also seen in Gruen zone 7, when the trochanter has not been osteotomized for the THR. Much greater significance should be ascribed to increasing distribution of these radiolucencies around the interface, especially in combination with increases in their width.

Localized endosteal lysis

Such areas of lysis may be seen in both mechanical and infective loosening. When seen in a case of mechanical loosening of the stem, the mechanism is believed to result from a defect in the cement mantle around the stem, which derives from the time of the THR. Particulate debris from the hip then works its way down between the stem and the cement (where there is frequently a very small gap, even if it does not appear radiologically), escapes through the defect in the cement mantle, and reaches the endosteal surface. Fluid pressure is almost certainly also required, and the effect will be worsened by any abrasion of the cement that may occur adjacent to the stem, producing an increase in the quantity of particles. In these circumstances, an area of lysis at some point around the stem will appear in a case that has functioned extremely well and in which infection has not been considered likely. If the radiographs suggest that there may be a defect of the mantle or an apparently very thin mantle near to the area of lysis, this fits with the rest of the picture and adds weight to the concept of mechanical loosening.

If the endosteal lysis is caused by sepsis (Fig. 8.6), the cement mantle may not show any such defect. Other features suggestive of infection, shown by the patient's clinical course, are present. Lysis in these cases can show as a very localized thumb print. More than one such area strongly suggests infection. The remainder of the interface may well be virtually perfect and the appearances may suggest that the implant had otherwise been well fixed. Localized lysis in relation to an implant of poor design, now known to produce large quantities of debris, particularly titanium (Fig. 8.7), is easy to explain on aseptic grounds alone. Similar appearances with a better designed implant, probably well fixed, would point towards infection.

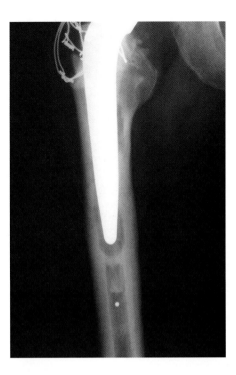

Figure 8.6 – *Endosteal lysis resulting from deep infection.*

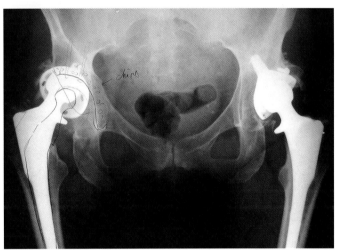

Figure 8.7 – *The X-rays also show the pre-operative planning. Gross acetabular lysis with migration caused by titanium debris.*

Periosteal reaction

In a case with early pain after THR, a periosteal reaction with new bone formation is diagnostic of a deep infection (Fig. 8.3b). An 'onion skin' effect may be seen. In such cases, there is also rarefaction and the appearances are those of osteomyelitis. Such cases are unusual, but when this appearance is seen the diagnosis is certain.

Cloacae

This is another sign of osteomyelitis, but in this case it is chronic. Often, cloacae are simply seen when inspecting the radiograph of a patient with a discharging sinus in

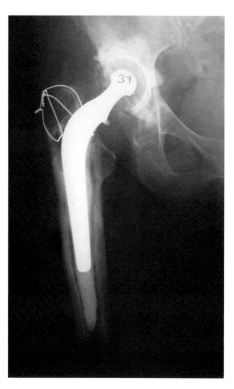

Figure 8.8 – *Apart from the thick complete femoral lucency, the gross enlargement of the wire entry hole is strongly suggestive of infection.*

through which a wire enters the upper femur (Fig. 8.8) or elsewhere (Fig. 8.9). A cloaca may be very small and difficult to see, as a result of the presence of normal cortex in front of and behind it. Figure 8.10 shows an example of this.

Cortical thickening

A dense, rather uniform, cortical thickening around the inferior part of the stem is quite often seen on well-functioning THRs, the implication clearly being that proximal load transference is taking place only to a minor degree. Such thickening is present only if the hip has at some point been functioning well; if this appearance is present in association with other radiological signs of loosening, it favours a mechanical problem.

Component migration, particularly femoral component subsidence

By themselves, migration and subsidence are clearly not directly diagnostic of either aseptic or septic loosening. Components tend to move if the loading to which they are subjected is consistently greater than the strength of the fixation. However, a crude assessment of the loading will have already been made from knowledge of the type of patient, and the solidity of the fixation by inspection,

whom a diagnosis of infection has already been made. If seen on careful inspection of a patient with a painful hip, but a healed wound, this favours infection. The cloacae may be seen as an enlargement of a hole

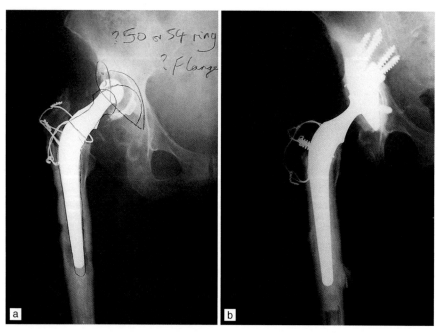

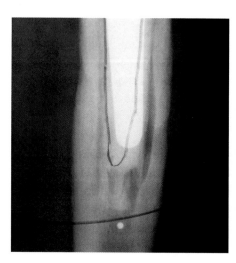

Figure 8.10 – *Easily missed femoral cloaca just lateral to the tip of the stem.*

Figure 8.9 – *(a) Multiple cloacae in the femur caused by deep infection, as well as severe acetabular migration. (b) The cloacae were not large enough to be detectable from within the femur and a 'cementogram' has been produced by femoral pressurization. Appearances at 10 years from one-stage exchange.*

particularly of the early postoperative radiographs; as a result of this analysis, it may not be surprising that a given component has migrated on straightforward mechanical grounds. Figure 8.11(a) shows an early post-operative radiograph of an extremely large and heavy man aged 50. From the radiograph it is seen that femoral component cementation is somewhat deficient. The marked subsidence seen in Figure 8.11(b) is therefore simple to explain on mechanical grounds alone. Similarly, it is not necessary to adduce the presence of infection to explain migration, even if severe, of many

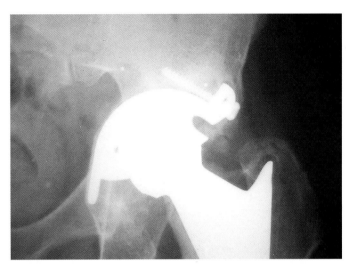

Figure 8.12 – *Gross socket migration that was easily explainable on mechanical grounds alone in this early, smooth, cementless implant.*

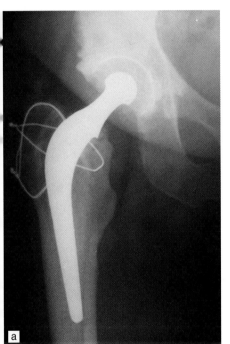

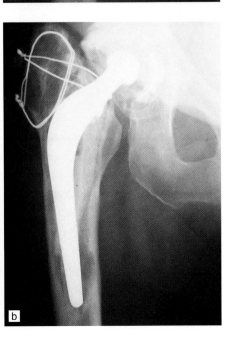

Figure 8.11 – *(a) Early post-operative radiograph of an extremely large and heavy man, aged 50. (b) Gross subsidence seen in this case was easy to explain on mechanical grounds alone (see text).*

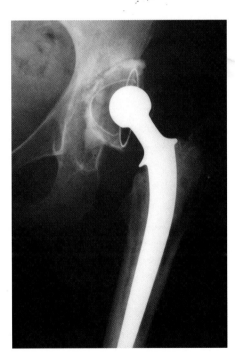

Figure 8.13 – *Severe, early socket migration resulting from infection in an otherwise mechanically adequate case.*

cementless components of early design (Fig. 8.12). As a corollary, rapid early migration in a patient in whom the loading may be expected to be low makes the presence of infection likely. An example is shown in Figure 8.13.

All patients (see below) are of course tested for the presence of infection before revision, but, on the basis of the clinical examination and plain radiographs, it should be possible in most cases to have a very good idea of whether the failure of the hip can be explained on biomechanical grounds alone, or whether it is necessary to consider that something else (i.e. infection) must be present to explain the situation. As with the rest of the analysis of the unsatisfactory THR, the radiograph as a whole must be looked at to try to interpret it in functional terms, together with the remaining facts of the case. Often, the diagnosis is clear even though the results of special tests have not yet been examined. A thick, complete, radiolucent line that has developed rapidly is highly suggestive of infection; in a THR present for many years, very similar appearances may well arise from aseptic mechanical fixation failure only.

Special tests

Further evidence about whether or not infection is present can be obtained from these. Complete reliance should not, however, be placed on any of them. As with the rest of the evidence, each is only a guide.

Erythrocyte sedimentation rate

This test is very non-specific. It is often said that 30 represents a cut-off between aseptic and septic loosening. This statement is much too definite, but nevertheless a very low erythrocyte sedimentation rate (ESR) (i.e. < 10) favours mechanical causes only. Very high ESRs (e.g. ≥ 70) tend to confirm infection in which other strongly suggestive factors are present. Statistical data in relation to loosening and the plasma viscosity test, carried out by some laboratories in place of the ESR, are unfortunately not available.

C-reactive protein

Although still rather non-specific, this appears to be a considerably better test than the ESR. This is partly because C-reactive protein (CRP) is normally present in trace amounts only, and does not have quite such a wide spectrum of normality as the ESR. Persistent elevation of CRP in otherwise healthy people is uncommon. After THR, CRP concentrations reach 200–400mg/l within 48 hours, returning to normal in about 3 weeks. A CRP of more than 20mg/l suggests infection. CRP, however, can rise for short periods even with trivial unrelated illnesses, and stronger evidence of infection is therefore obtained by repeating the test [1].

Scans

Technetium

A 'cold' scan strongly suggests that there is nothing wrong with the hip itself and is very helpful in relation

to patients in groups 1A(i) and (ii), although again some increase in such patients, perhaps around the greater trochanter, is quite common. It is important for the scan to be reported on in both its blood (diffusion) and its static (bone) phases. A scan that is 'hot' on its bone phase only is in favour of mechanical loosening, but, if 'hot' on both diffusion and bone phases, this favours infection. The diffusion phase can, however, be 'hot' when other causes of severe lysis (associated with increased vascularity) are present – notably lysis by particulate debris. As with all other tests, therefore, the scan result must not be taken in isolation.

Gallium

Originally it was thought that sequential technetium/gallium scanning would be very useful for diagnosing infection, the concept being that the gallium scan would be positive only in the presence of infection. In fact the gallium scan usually simply reflects the diffusion phase of the technetium scan, and serves as confirmatory evidence of the correctness of that scan only.

Labelled white cell scans

These are established as a method of localizing occult acute infections and initial experience with indium (indium oxime) was promising. It looked as if this could be improved on by labelling with ^{99m}Tc-HMPAO (hexamethylpropylene-amineoxime), which allows improved resolution and also scanning on the same day as removal of cells from the patient for labelling. The initial enthusiastic reports were, however, mainly based on earlier, and probably more acute, joint replacement infections, and later reports, attempting to identify the types of low-grade chronic infections that are the source of confusion, show these tests not to be any more effective than sequential technetium/gallium scanning [2].

Scanning, as well as an ESR and CRP estimation, should be carried out routinely in every patient who is to have a revision. Whether, however, a technetium scan, reporting on both the diffusion and bone phases, sequential technetium/gallium, or labelled WBC scan (In- or ^{99m}Tc-HMPAO) is carried out legitimately depends just as much on the facilities and experience of the available laboratory as on the independently assessed value of the scans themselves.

Aspiration/biopsy

Consistently good results cannot be obtained in revision surgery for deep infection, unless every attempt is made to identify the responsible organism preoperatively. It is true that many are still sensitive to gentamicin, the antibiotic most commonly used, but nevertheless organisms resistant to gentamicin are now common (notably coagulase-negative staphylococci) and this tendency is unfortunately very likely to increase. Some form of preoperative aspiration or biopsy is therefore mandatory in any patient in whom sepsis is suspected. Ideally, all patients should have at least an aspiration before revision. This may not, however, be logistically possible and an acceptable alternative is simply to omit this test in those cases in which a careful analysis of all the evidence makes it overwhelmingly likely that loosening is purely mechanical.

The hip may be aspirated under local anaesthesia, or a tissue specimen can be taken under general anaesthesia. A slightly higher accuracy is probably obtained using the latter, but the accurate and consistent conduct of the test is at least as important. Much the best thing is if the test is performed by the surgeon who is to do the revision. A perfect aseptic ritual in a suitable environment, with transfer of the specimen into appropriate media and properly organized transport to a designated bacteriologist, is essential. If the procedure is poorly delegated, or carried out on an ad hoc basis, then the numbers of false positives and false negatives will rise and the test may

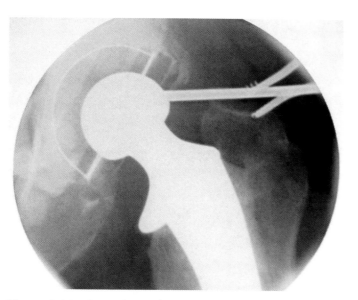

Figure 8.14 – *Image intensifier appearance during core biopsy using a Craig biopsy apparatus. A small self-retaining retractor shows the stab wound in the skin.*

well become meaningless. The author's practice is to use Craig biopsy instruments under general anaesthesia in an ultra-clean-air operating room. An image intensifier is useful (Fig. 8.14), but not essential. If it is not to be used, the surface position of the hip anteriorly is located (2.5 cm lateral to and just distal to the midpoint of the inguinal ligament) and a 1.5-cm long incision is made in the skin and held open with a very small (e.g. Alm's) retractor. The serrated biopsy instrument with its internal trochar is inserted and, when in the neighbourhood of the hip, the trochar is removed and the instrument screwed through the pseudocapsule; it should be felt to touch the neck of the prosthesis.

As the hip is to be revised anyway, scratching of this component is unimportant. A core can then be withdrawn in almost all cases. It is sometimes necessary to apply suction with a syringe to keep this within the end of the instrument. The author's practice is to put the core into a bottle of fluid intended for anaerobic culture and to swill the instruments out in a second bottle intended for aerobic culture. The incision is then closed with one stitch. If an image intensifier is available, then the precise position for the skin incision is less important and a slightly more lateral position is convenient. The approach of the instruments to the hip can then be seen and the trochar removed quite easily at a suitably early moment. If the trochar is left within the instrument until it actually enters the hip, the effect may be that a perforation is made in the pseudocapsule without actually cutting out a core of tissue. Failure may result.

Clearly, a second insertion of the same instruments is possible, but there is an increased risk of contamination and a false-positive result. If a sinus is present, specimens can also be taken from this and put into a second set of bottles, but very little reliability can be placed on the result because a sinus is open to direct external contamination, and correct labelling of the separate specimens is vital. The request card needs to indicate that the specimens are for the special attention of the particular bacteriologist involved in the work. In the laboratory used by the author, brain–heart infusion broth is the preferred medium. Incubation is carried out for a minimum of 5 days with subculture aerobically and anaerobically to non-selective blood agar. Anaerobic culture plates are then monitored for a minimum of 5 days, prolonged incubation for 10 days, with the use of special media or chocolate agar sometimes being appropriate. Isolates of coagulase-negative staphylococci have

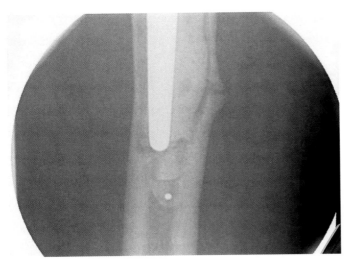

Figure 8.15 – *The sudden onset of severe pain in this THR was difficult to explain, until the small crack was noticed in the lateral femoral cortex during screening at biopsy.*

to be fully identified to species levels, and multiple isolates need to be checked by susceptibility tests because mixed infections often occur. A full 'antibiogram' is essential and sophisticated laboratory methods are required, and must be made available, to achieve this.

In certain cases an image intensifier is essential. This applies, for example, if a Girdlestone pseudarthrosis is present because there is nothing to hit with the instruments; where very severe, component migration is present and the standard hip landmarks become unreliable. If an image intensifier has been used, then it is sensible to screen the remainder of the hip with the leg in different positions. Sometimes surprising information can be obtained from this – for example, a small crack in the cortex visible only in a certain plane and responsible for hitherto undiagnosed pain (Fig. 8.15). Unexpectedly severe thinning of the cortex may also be seen in certain areas, which is helpful in the planning of a subsequent revision. Rarely, a separate biopsy of an area of lysis in the femoral shaft may be appropriate. Depending on the strength of the femur in the neighbourhood of the region to be biopsied, a more formal drilling technique may be required or a minimalist open biopsy with a small fenestration of the cortex. In almost all cases, however, infection sufficient to produce distal lysis is also present in the hip itself.

Group 1E: fracture of the stem

This diagnosis is surprisingly easy to miss. The history is

of a patient (usually a strong active male) who has had a THR for osteoarthritis with an excellent result. Some years later (depending on the type of implant) pain suddenly appears. A relative loss of function usually occurs and this may rapidly get worse and the leg shorten; on the other hand, the symptoms may improve and become quite slight.

Physical examination

The physical examination may show shortening with obvious diminution of active movement, but the findings may be minimal.

Radiography

Stem fractures usually occur at the same place for a given type of implant – for example, fractures of the Charnley stem (now rare) occur about one-third of the way down, whereas some stems fracture more distally. Fractures of the original Madreporique stem occurred through a casting port in the stem. The fracture is usually obvious, but it is most important to note that sometimes it is practically invisible and can be missed. Occasionally, patients are seen who for one reason or another have had a correct diagnosis made of a fracture of the stem, but rather minor symptoms, and who have not come to a revision. The radiographs may then show a grossly varus position of the upper stem fragment, with massive cortical thickening sufficient laterally to hold it in place. The author has also seen a case of a patient who had had a total knee replacement beneath a THR. Pain relief did not occur and the cause of the pain was later shown to be a pre-existing fracture of the stem. The radiograph, at least in the case of an implant with a 22.5-mm head, may well also show acetabular wear consistent with prior good function; sometimes this is associated with a degree of scalloping or lysis in the upper part of the femur as a result of the particulate wear debris, probably reducing the torsional support of the upper part of the implant and being one factor responsible for the fracture.

Special tests

An ESR, CRP, and scan(s) should still be done. The results should simply confirm the absence of infection, although there is likely to be activity in the upper femur. If the acetabular scan is quiet, then this is reassuring if, on exploration, it is felt that the acetabulum can be left in situ.

Modular implants

Modularity has produced a large number of possible ways in which mechanical failure of implants can occur. All these give rise to pain and some loss of function, but usually close inspection of the radiographs makes the diagnosis obvious. This applies particularly to insert failure in metal-backed polyethylene sockets; in these, close inspection shows a lack of concentricity between the centre of the femoral head and the centre of the external surface of the acetabular component. Cementless implants with fixation augmented by screws usually fail leaving the screws intact, a process that is often worsened, if not initiated, by fretting between the implant and the screw; nevertheless broken screws are sometimes seen. The breakage of the screws is, however, secondary to loss of fixation and not a primary event, and it is therefore unlikely to be heralded by sudden pain as in the classic stem fracture.

Group 1F: problems associated with trochanteric fixation

Pain apparently derived from a THR is all too commonly attributed to trochanteric wires (or other fixation – see below), which may have been used for reattachment of the greater trochanter when osteotomized at the primary operation. Such an attribution is frequently false and may lead to unnecessary surgery, perhaps producing a complication of its own. Leaving aside patients whose main problem is instability, which is discussed later, patients with pain are often seen for whom the general practitioner has requested a radiograph. The radiograph then shows the presence of broken trochanteric wires and at once a connection is made between the wires and the pain.

Careful evaluation is needed, particularly as the patient will have been told the results of the radiograph and so may well have become convinced that the problem is the wires.

Wires may be:

■ broken, with a mass of scattered fragments and the trochanter separated

■ broken, but without fragmentation and the trochanter widely separated

■ broken, and with the trochanter not united, but hardly if at all elevated

■ broken, but with sound trochanteric union with or without some loss of position

■ intact, with or without some loss of position.

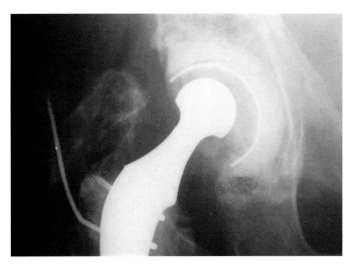

Figure 8.16 – *Multiple small cable fragments. The Dall-Miles grip itself had already been removed in an attempt to relieve symptoms.*

Similar variations apply to other types of device such as the Dall-Miles cable grip, the difference with this device being, however, that multiple, very small cable fragments may be present (Fig. 8.16).

Pain may quite possibly be genuinely a wire problem in the first category, but a connection becomes less and less likely the further down the list one goes and it is extremely unlikely that the pain is in any way related to the wires in the last category. Patients in the first two categories may complain of a limp, especially on starting to walk, but this is not helpful in relation to whether or not the pain is coming from the wires.

The question of why a patient with gross trochanteric separation can have completely normal function is of great interest, as discussed by Ling and O'Connor [3]. Biomechanical models and computer simulations have all too frequently modelled the hip with the body-weight torque countered only by gluteal abduction. Were this to be the case, patients with wide trochanteric separation would have completely absent abduction and inevitably a very severe limp. In fact (although this is not yet widely recognized), a major abduction source is produced by the iliotibial band attached to the tibia distally, and pulled on at the upper end by the tensor fascia lata and gluteus maximus muscles. Calculations, for example, show that, if this were not the case, the femur would bend when the patient stood on one leg. The same principle probably accounts for the excellent function seen after a number of approaches to the hip, in which abductor detachment is used, some of these not necessarily healing soundly. It is in no way surprising, therefore, that wide trochanteric separation can be symptomless as far as function is concerned. With regard to pain, exploration often shows a very smooth area at the area of the non-union beneath the fascia lata. As well as maintaining a 'doubting Thomas' attitude to broken wires as a cause of pain, it is also necessary to evaluate thoroughly the patient who may turn out to be in group 1A(i) or (ii), or may in fact have early aseptic loosening.

If the patient's symptoms seem to justify it (e.g. wire removal is seriously being considered), a technetium scan should certainly be done and this should reinforce the view that the problem is related to the trochanter only. Local infiltration into the wires may be helpful. Regrettably, as the patient knows exactly where the injection has been placed, a misleading non-specific improvement in the symptoms may be seen.

The patient shown in Figure 8.17 was referred with pain. This was initially attributed to loosening based on a very thin periacetabular radiolucency. Further reflection, however, suggested that this was insufficient and attention was focused on the wires. A local infiltration appeared to be confirmatory. The wires were therefore removed and the following day the patient said that she was hugely better. Unfortunately she also said that symptoms in many other parts of the body had been relieved. Later she returned to the outpatient clinic with completely unchanged symptoms.

A cavalier approach to wire removal should be condemned. Patients are referred to revision centres where the outer parts of intact wires have been removed

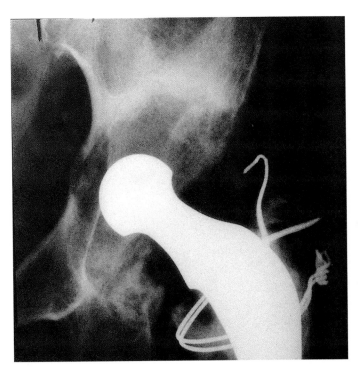

Figure 8.18 – *Radiographic appearance at referral of a young woman in whom the socket had already been removed. The poorly indicated partial excision of trochanteric wires made subsequent reconstruction much more difficult.*

without change in the symptoms; later these are found to be from some more sinister cause that needs full revision. If a trochanteric osteotomy is to be used in this revision, the removal of the external parts of the wires, as shown in Figure 8.18, will make what might have been a perfectly satisfactory trochanteric osteotomy remarkably difficult. Removal of loose and easily accessible parts of broken wires may certainly be justified at times, but there is very unlikely ever to be a case for removal of intact wires with a healed greater trochanter.

Bulkier fixation devices may sometimes be responsible for the symptoms even though correctly inserted and with sound union, but caution is still recommended.

A rare, but genuine, cause of obscure trochanteric symptoms after osteotomy is the result of an exostosis that sometimes forms laterally at the healed osteotomy site at or just below the vastus ridge, which may become several centimetres long. An example is shown in Figure 8.19. Before referral back to the author, who had replaced the patient's hip originally, part of the wires had been removed. A more thoughtful assessment would at least have questioned this diagnosis, which resulted in entirely unnecessary and ineffective surgery. The patient's symptom was of clicking, presumably

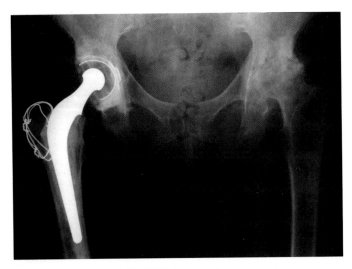

Figure 8.17 – *A painful THR incorrectly ascribed to trochanteric wiring (see text).*

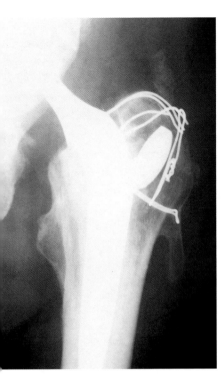

Figure 8.19 – *Exostosis producing minor trochanteric symptoms in an otherwise soundly healed trochanter.*

caused by the tip of the exostosis rubbing the scar on the underside of the fascia lata.

Group 1G: other cryptic source of pain

When THR was in its infancy, the pain relief after cemented replacements was so striking that it was assumed that pain should be completely absent in a cemented THR. With the later, very widespread use of cementless implants, pain was soon found to be a significant problem, at least in the early postoperative period. Careful studies of its incidence in comparison with cemented THRs showed that pain is by no means infrequently present after a cemented THR. Very close questioning of patients who are extremely pleased with their operations quite commonly shows, for example, some anterior discomfort or hesitancy for a few seconds after sitting for some time. Occasionally this symptom is sufficient for a patient to report it spontaneously and to require reassurance. The cause is obscure. It may result from the fact that the iliacus muscle and the psoas tendon, which before surgery ran over the smooth anterior surface of the hip and femoral head, perhaps with an intervening bursa, run postoperatively over a defect, because at least the upper section of the neck has been excised. Whether this is one reason why hip resurfacing procedures may show such excellent clinical results is unknown; certainly the underlying surface over which these powerful muscles run is bound to be very much more normal.

Patients are sometimes referred whose problems appear genuine, but in whom the only abnormality found is a relatively lateral position of the socket. Such a symptom may be associated with incipient mechanical loosening of the socket, although scans may be normal. The lateral position is bound to produce some increase in hip loading (the antithesis of the medialization of the socket originally proposed by Charnley), but the precise connection between any such overload and pain is uncertain. Such patients should, however, be kept under review and not reassured and discharged.

There are also other rare causes such as pelvic stress fractures. If the patient appears genuine, all other causes of pain have been eliminated so that the hip remains a probable culprit, and plain radiographs are completely normal, computed tomography (CT) or magnetic resonance imaging (MRI) should be considered although the presence of implants unfortunately interferes with the former.

The above completes the list of situations in which the patient's main complaint is of pain.

Other presenting complaints

Group 4: stiff or immobile hip

The patient in this group has great difficulty in getting about and in simple tasks of daily living. This symptom is unusual, but specific. It may be associated with pain, but this is not the primary presentation. The history is that the patient, of either sex and any age, has had an apparently straightforward replacement, and that the hip has not moved properly ever since. Physiotherapy may have been prescribed, but without effect. Later radiographs are then found to show marked heterotopic ossification. Occasionally, there may be some apparent predisposing factor such as early reoperation: for example, early conversion of failed subcapital fracture fixation to an endoprosthesis (Figure 8.20).

The following questions from the assessment should be answered from the assessment:
- Can the patient be helped by removing the blocks to motion by themselves?
- If so, when should this be done?
- Does the patient require not only removal of blocks to motion, but a complete revision?
- Should the patient be left alone?

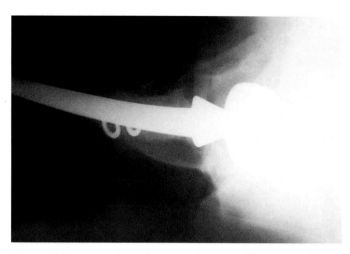

Figure 8.20 – *Large complete anterior strut of heterotopic bone.*

Clinical

Clinically the patient is well, but the hip is immobile. It is rather likely that the leg is in a somewhat unsatisfactory position, such as marked external rotation, because otherwise the symptoms from the stiffness are less likely to have been sufficient for the patient to be referred.

Radiography

In a favourable case (i.e. one in which operation might be considered – see below), well-localized areas of heterotopic ossification are seen, together with a perfectly satisfactory implant in a good position. Not infrequently, however, the replacement itself may be not beyond criticism, the implication being that more than the usual amount of surgical trauma may have taken place, perhaps increasing the likelihood of heterotopic ossification. Thus, for example, large cement fragments are sometimes seen within the joint (see Fig. 12.20).

The radiographs need to be very carefully scrutinized to see whether there is any evidence of loosening.

After inspection of the plain radiographs (and perhaps an ultrasonogram), it should be possible provisionally to decide that the patient may be someone who will benefit from removal of the blocks to motion or someone who will need a full revision. Further tests are therefore directed towards making this decision, and include an ESR, alkaline phosphatase test, and a technetium scan.

The technetium scan helps to confirm that the main implants are well fixed. Assuming that this is the case, and that the THR is sufficiently well positioned for reasonable function to be expected if the blocks to motion are removed, the special tests are required to

decide when to do this. If carried out too early, a recurrence of ossification is likely despite appropriate treatment (see Chapter 12). In theory it is best to await normality of the alkaline phosphatase and quiescence of the technetium scan. Complete quiescence is rather unlikely unless an absolutely clearly defined and solid bar of bone is present that blocks all motion entirely. Often there is a pseudarthrosis somewhere within the bar, allowing a very small amount of (painful) movement, and the area of this pseudarthrosis may remain 'hot'. Serial scans are helpful. It is unlikely that surgery will be sensible in less than 2 years from the time of the replacement. Operative treatment requires further investigation by CT scanning to delineate exactly where the bars are, as discussed in Chapter 12.

Group 5: dislocation

Here the diagnosis is obvious and the question is what to do about it.

The management of early postoperative dislocation in THR is dealt with in Chapter 5. A dislocation at more than 3–4 months after THR needs more careful assessment. Although conservative management is, at least initially, almost always likely to be appropriate, it is certainly necessary to tell the patient that further surgery may be required and to make some provisional plans.

Radiography

This is discussed in greater detail in the section on 'Revision for recurrent dislocation' in Chapter 12. Factors that suggest that conservative treatment may not be effective are severe malposition of the socket (open if an anterior dislocation and closed if a posterior dislocation) and trochanteric non-union with wide separation if a trochanteric osteotomy has been used. In a posterior dislocation, the lateral radiograph may suggest inadequate anteversion of either the socket or the stem.

History

The method of conservative treatment depends on whether the dislocation is anterior or posterior – a decision that may be obvious, but can be confusing. The history is usually helpful. If the dislocation arose when the patient was in a sitting position, it has to be posterior. This is usually confirmed by inspection of the dislocated radiograph in which the lesser trochanter should hardly be visible. Sometimes the patient appears to state that the hip dislocated when in an almost extended position, suggesting that the dislocation had been anterior, but this is not always confirmed by the radiograph (marked prominence of the lesser trochanter indicates external rotation). As it is vital to know which of the two has occurred, the manipulation under anaesthesia (MUA) has to be conducted in a thoughtful manner, deliberately seeking this information. After reduction of the dislocation, the hip should be screened in extension; gradually increasing external rotation, 'levering out' should be watched for, and the same done in flexion and internal rotation, although only an imperfect view with the image intensifier can be obtained. The hip should not be re-dislocated because this increases the soft tissue trauma, conceivably worsens the potential instability, and may also scratch the head.

Whenever possible, a surgeon should try to reduce his or her own dislocation. Dislocation is always an embarrassment and delegation is very tempting. However, absent or misleading information about the anterior or posterior nature of the dislocation may be the result, with more serious consequences later.

If it is felt that the dislocation is posterior, the best treatment is to immobilize the hip in a solid hip spica. This is uncomfortable and extremely awkward for the patient, but is much more likely to be effective because the torn posterior tissues will be allowed to heal in as short a position as possible. A much more acceptable, but unfortunately also less effective, substitute is a brace with a block to flexion of perhaps 45°. The effect of the brace-on-hip motion needs to be inspected carefully. Figures on the hinges of the brace often bear very little relation to the actual position of flexion of the hip, because of the looseness of the waist band part of the device. If the dislocation has occurred at more than 2 months postoperatively, the brace needs to be kept on for quite a prolonged period, e.g. 3–4 months. A shorter period is almost certainly doomed to failure.

If the dislocation is anterior (unusual), it is necessary for the hip to be prevented from externally rotating in the extended position, and a complex brace is required with hip and knee hinges. No limitation needs to be given to hip flexion, this part of the device simply ensuring that the thigh section is fixed in a rotational sense. The knee hinges have to be so arranged that, whenever the patient flexes his or her knee, the thigh is bound to rotate internally. The device will probably need to extend down to the heel, with an ankle hinge and a heel cup to keep it up in the necessary position. Decisions are also needed on whether the brace should be made non-removable (e.g. Scotch Cast) or removable (e.g. plastic or leather). Clearly, the former can be worn only for a short period, and a comfortable brace made of one of the latter may be sufficiently acceptable to the patient to be worn for a long enough period to stabilize the hip.

Recurrent dislocation

There is no fixed boundary between early and isolated dislocations in which conservative treatment is likely to work and recurrent dislocations requiring either long-term bracing or surgery, but any hip that dislocates at all beyond a year to 18 months after THR, or more than two to three times in the early postoperative period, almost certainly falls into the latter group. The only effective treatment for recurrent dislocation is reoperation (see Chapter 12). Long-term bracing on the lines indicated above may be tried for patients who have become medically unfit or who are particularly averse to further surgery. Patients who have become medically unfit may also, however, have major difficulties with any form of brace. If so, it is best to leave the hip dislocated and continue with mobilization. This may gradually produce a result that, in the circumstances, is acceptable, the patient being able to get about in a limited way. The hip will effectively become a Girdlestone, although peculiar noises may be produced on certain movements. Occasionally patients are seen who have come to this result unknowingly, having had a dislocation that has never been detected. If it is unacceptable to leave the hip in a dislocated position in a patient who is too unfit for a full revision, a form of Girdlestone will be slightly better in which the femoral component alone is removed, leaving the socket and all the cement in situ. An imaginary line can then be drawn and the patient's treatment considered finished. Such a situation is also the unfortunate occasional outcome of failed revision surgery for recurrent dislocation.

Less common symptoms

Group 6: clunking

The patient does not entirely trust the hip and can make it produce internal knocking feelings or audible clunking. This is a 'forme fruste' of recurrent dislocation. Sometimes the hip can be made clinically to telescope

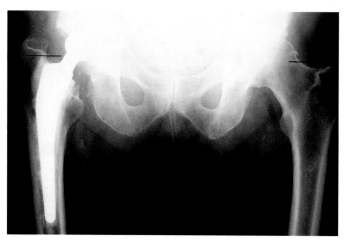

Figure 8.21 – *Patient with a clunking sensation, in this case after revision. The hip is seen not to be out to length.*

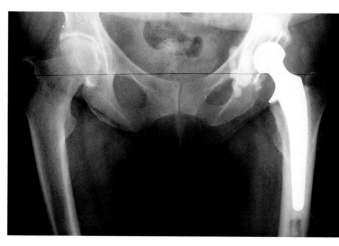

Figure 8.22 – *Lengthening: the hips were originally identical. Note that the femoral neck was somewhat varus.*

by traction on the leg with the patient awake, the head going back into the socket with a quite easily audible knocking sound when the traction is released. AP and lateral radiographs show what initially looks to be entirely normal appearances, but careful inspection of the radiograph series will show that the hip is not out to length (Fig. 8.21). Management is then simply a question of whether the symptoms are bad enough to merit revision.

Group 7: wrong leg length

Patients are often unhappy if the leg has been made too long (Fig. 8.22). The complaint needs to be handled rather carefully because almost certainly nothing can be done about it. It may be that the lengthening is some-thing that the patient has developed a fixation about along with general dissatisfaction with his or her management. Such patients are sometimes in group 1A(i) and the lengthening is then doubly unfortunate. The patient's treatment may, however, have been perfectly satisfactory and he or she may simply state that

the leg feels long. Both hips may have been arthritic and short preoperatively, and the THR has simply brought the affected leg out to length; this is something that patients should always be warned about preoperatively. However, quite frequently, it is seen from the pre-operative radiographs that the femoral neck was markedly varus (often associated with protrusio-type osteoarthritis). The lengthening has then been produced by a failure to accommodate this fact by distal position-ing of the stem. This is discussed in Section II. The radio-graphs may also show that the stem has not been sunk deeply enough into a narrow femoral canal, the head/neck junction of the stem being clearly above the cut surface of the neck; or it may be that too large a cementless stem, whose level cannot be adjusted, has been used.

Patients do also complain that the leg is short, but this seems much less noticeable to patients than lengthening, unless caused by gross femoral sub-sidence, when it is associated with other symptoms of loosening.

References

1. Sanzen L, Carlsson AS. The diagnostic value of C-reactive protein in infected total hip arthroplasties. *J Bone Joint Surg* 1989; 71B: 638–41.

2. Glithero PR, Grigoris P, Harding LK *et al*. White cell scans and infected joint replacements. Failure to detect chronic infection. *J Bone Joint Surg* 1993; 75B: 371–4.

3. Ling RSM, O'Connor JJ, Lu TU *et al*. Muscular activity and the biomechanics of the hip. Review article. *Hip International* 1996; 6: 91–105.

CHAPTER 9

Preoperative planning and notes on surgical approaches

M. D. Northmore-Ball

Planning

Planning is strongly recommended in all hip surgery. In revision surgery, it is vital. It is extraordinary how often this step is completely omitted or, at least, seriously skimped; a brief waving of an acetate sheet in front of the radiograph when the patient is being anaesthetized greatly reduces the likelihood of a successful outcome. It is appreciated that this book will be read in several countries and, in a number, these remarks are in no way necessary, but the point still needs to be stressed.

Planning is not just a matter of drawing with a wax pencil on a radiograph. It is a question of going through the entire operation in one's head, preferably in association with one's assistant. Many points may arise, such as the necessity to check that a certain instrument will be available in the operating room or a need to indicate its requirement on the operating room list or schedule. The drawing of the position of the intended implants on to the radiograph is simply part of this process. It needs to be done at leisure and, in the case of revision surgery, in ample time to put any arrangements that seem to be necessary into effect. Planning also needs to include appropriate decisions on non-surgical measures, such as the antibiotics to be included in the cement and to be given systemically in a case believed to be septic (see Chapter 12) or drugs to be given to counteract heterotopic ossification (see Chapter 12). The remainder of this section relates to radiographs. The following radiographs are required:

- Anteroposterior (AP) radiograph of the pelvis to show both hips.
- AP radiograph of the affected hip, including the whole of the femoral component and the whole of the distal cement, if cement is present.

- A lateral radiograph of the affected hip, centred on the hip.
- A cross-table lateral radiograph of the affected hip, centred on the tip of the femoral component (Fig. 9.1).

Occasionally, other plain films are needed – for example, when the distal femoral cement plug is so long (Fig. 9.2) that it extends off the end of the ordinary AP film of the hip. The lateral radiograph centred on the tip of the stem is not a conventional film, and will almost certainly initially require a special one-to-one discussion with the radiographer. However, it is a perfectly straightforward radiograph to produce. In association with the AP radiographs, it gives essential information about the direction of the axis of the stem (and, therefore, of the void left in the cement after stem removal) and the exact shape of the distal cement plug, if present (the latter, of course, frequently includes some form of restrictor).

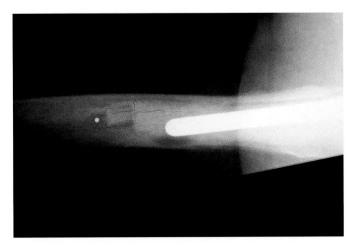

Figure 9.1 – *Cross-table lateral radiograph showing relationship between direction of stem axis and distal medullary canal.*

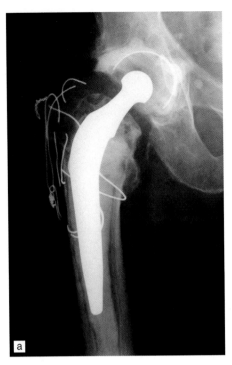

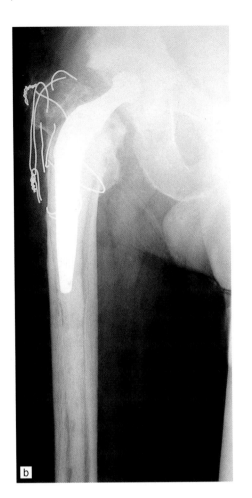

Figure 9.2 – *Extent of distal cement. In (a) this extends off the radiograph. (b) The immense length of distal cement down the femur, requiring special planning measures.*

In most cases, plain radiographs taken more than a very short time before revision (2 weeks, say) should not be accepted. A longer period may be safe in the case of a patient whose symptoms have not significantly deteriorated since the radiographs were taken and who has aseptic loosening with good underlying bone, but, if the symptoms seem to have worsened or the femoral cortex is thin, then absolutely up-to-date information is mandatory. Sometimes a combination of older and up-to-date films is acceptable, a new small AP film simply indicating that no change has occurred since the radiographs used for planning.

Planning then relates to the approach and component removal, and to reconstruction.

The approach and component removal

The trochanter (if applicable)

If a trochanteric osteotomy has been done, then any remaining wires (or other fixation device) need to be removed. As far as possible, the position of the wires, and particularly of their knots or twists,

should be determined. If a trochanteric osteotomy is proposed for the revision, the lateral position of this should be determined in relation to the loops and this can be marked before complete wire removal. This is best estimated initially at the planning stage; this is particularly important if the trochanter has united in a proximal position when the standard landmarks are not available at surgery. Careful reflection is needed at this stage if the trochanter has separated with a very wide gap or is small or fragmented. Should we attempt to reattach it? Should we use a component with a larger head (see Chapter 12)? Should we tell the patient that the hip might need to be immobilized in a spica afterwards? Sometimes, a very unusual form of fixation device is present, such as various forms of staple or clamp. Often research reveals (if carried out in time) its precise nature and shows how best to remove it; this may allow a suitable device to be obtained. A neat removal may then result without fragmentation and with a much greater subsequent likelihood of good abductor function.

The socket

Proper thinking at this stage means that many of the procedures described in Chapter 10 become entirely predictable. With cemented sockets that have not previously been revised, perusal simply shows that no special measures are likely to be necessary. It may, for example, be seen that removal is likely to be extremely easy. However, the socket may be deep, having been placed at the depth of a protrusio-type osteoarthritis; this may be associated with a very thin or absent acetabular floor. This gives a warning that it may not be safe to put curved chisels down behind the socket. Commonly, with hips originally replaced using the Charnley type of central pilot hole, there is leakage of cement medially. Although in a case that is definitely aseptic it may be perfectly safe to leave the plug, this is not desirable and the aim should always be to remove all vestige of previous implants. Therefore, the size and the shape of this plug need to be carefully assessed.

Sometimes, a medial cement mass can be very large (revision is more often required in hips that have not been all that well done!) and, if such a hip is additionally infected, the removal of this mass may by itself require careful thought, which should always be done at this planning stage. Sometimes, it is obvious that there must have been a substantial perforation in the floor; this is seen particularly in THRs carried out for failed treatment of subcapital fractures in elderly people, in which the acetabulum is porotic and has never been previously arthritic. Another difficult situation arises where infection is present, but only the femoral component has become loose. A very much higher chance of success in revision accrues if the whole of the acetabular cement is also removed. Pelvic cement protrusions may not, in cases where the socket is not loose, be covered in the thick membrane that is seen in the presence of loosening. Hasty, unplanned attempts during the operation to remove these plugs are dangerous. Occasionally, a computed tomography (CT) scan is necessary to see whether the medial protrusion has come through the floor or through some other perforation, or whether it is part of a leakage that has come through the cotyloid notch and/or is associated with damage in the teardrop region. In summary, it should be possible to know the shape and size of the plug and whether any special measures will be necessary for its removal at the planning stage. The subject is discussed further later (see Chapter 10).

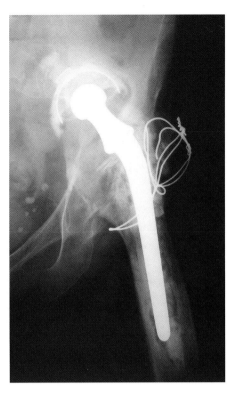

Figure 9.3 – *Case where extreme medial socket migration necessitated its removal via a medial approach.*

Rarely, it is noticed that the socket has migrated medially to a major extent, which may indicate the need for a completely different surgical approach for socket removal (Fig. 9.3); very occasionally it may also be necessary to re-schedule the revision for a time when a vascular surgeon is available.

Some of the above also relates to cementless sockets. The main function of the component removal step of planning, however, in these cases is to try to determine the nature of the original component, so that an appropriate insertion/extraction device can be obtained. Sometimes, the type is obvious; sometimes, considerable research is necessary, and this should have been carried out some weeks previously. If it is known at what hospital and at what period a cementless THR was inserted, then, in association with the radiograph, its precise type can often be accurately identified. An appropriate commercial representative can then usually be located to supply the instruments.

If broken screws are found, however tempting it is to leave this *in situ*, a much more certain and radiologically pleasing result accrues if they are removed. For this it is necessary to have something such as the AO/ASIF Broken Screw Removal Kit available. If the hip is ever revised again, the surgeon will be pleased that this trouble was taken.

The stem

With loose cemented stems, the main input from this phase of planning is into the method of removal of the more distal femoral cement and, particularly, the distal plug. The centrality or otherwise of the tip of the stem, the direction of its axis, and the presence of any severe cortical thinning in this region all determine the safety or otherwise of using the position of the tip of the stem for locating a drill. The AP and side-to-side location of the upper part of the distal cement plug, and any radiolucencies that may or may not be present around it, its position in relation to the femoral isthmus, and, if below the isthmus, its diameter in relation to the isthmus above, and its length all need to be worked out accurately and appropriate plans made for its removal. Occasionally, large leakages of cement are seen outside the femur (formerly relatively common in replacements done through limited anterolateral approaches, but more often seen now in failed previous revisions), and their size and position need to be accurately worked out. It may be necessary to measure the distance down from the top of the trochanter using the enlarged scale on one of the templates.

If there is a cementless stem, the above remarks about instrumentation apply and, indeed, this is of more significance on the femoral than on the acetabular side. If the femoral component does not appear loose (but has to be changed), an exact plan needs to be made for the necessary work on the femur, to allow for its removal in the event that it cannot be knocked out with the extraction device. A device such as the Anspach high-speed burr, with long, thin flexible cutters, needs to be requested. In the absence of such a high-speed burr, unless the cementless stem appears loose, the patient should almost certainly be referred elsewhere.

In the case of a fractured stem, the centrality of the distal fragment within the canal, its size, and whether there appears to be a complete mantle of cement around it (which is likely, because stem fractures occur only when the distal section is soundly fixed) need to be examined in terms of the type of fractured stem extraction kit to be used (see Chapter 10).

Reconstruction

This can be given only in general terms because the precise details depend on the type of implant to be used. Examples are shown in Figures 9.4 and 9.5, 10.3, 11.3, and 12.5.

In this phase, the following need to be determined:

- The sizes of the components to be inserted
- The positions in which these components need to be inserted
- How the components are to be supported in that position.

The first step is to draw a horizontal line across the pelvis using any convenient landmarks still present, such as the distal edges of the ischial tuberosities or the teardrops, and compare the positions of the lesser trochanters in relation to this line. The lengthening

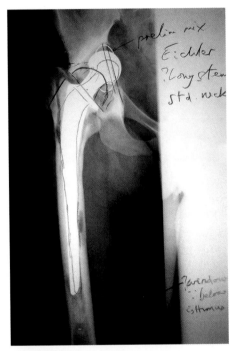

Figure 9.4 – *Drawing of reconstruction on pre-revision radiograph. The patient had had a failed prior revision of the stem only for a deep infection. It was clear that an Eichler ring would be needed to take the load on the rim of the socket. The position of a preliminary mix of cement to block the acetabular floor is shown. Fenestration of the femur was not, in fact, required.*

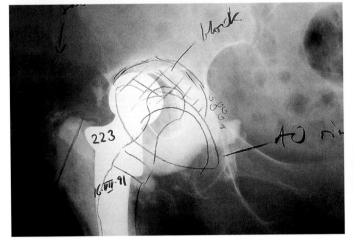

Figure 9.5 – *Drawing of reconstruction in an aseptic hip with severe acetabular destruction. The positions for a trochanteric osteotomy, a block graft, chips, a ring, and the stem are seen.*

required can then be estimated. If the position of the femoral head is to be normalized by placing its centre on a level with the tip of the greater trochanter, an appropriate position for the socket in a proximal/distal sense can be determined and marked, with suitable compromises if necessary.

Acetabular sizing

Planning diagrams are sometimes seen with very large semicircles drawn on an AP radiograph. Such drawings are, however, not sensible. The AP dimension of the residual socket is much more important. A rough assessment of this can be made (on the assumption that both hips were originally similar) by measuring the diameter of the opposite femoral head on the ordinary AP radiograph with the scale on the template, plus four thicknesses of articular cartilage, and allowing for some bone loss. Occasionally, if the original operation note is available and is a detailed one, the size of the final reamer or the previous socket will be known.

Femoral sizing

Having positioned the centre of the femoral head, as noted above, the size, neck length, and insertion depth of the femoral component should be determinable with some precision with a good set of templates (Figs 9.4, 9.5).

The radiograph then needs to be scrutinized very carefully for acetabular and femoral defects, and their positions, shapes, and sizes determined. If significant defects are present, the reconstructional method to be used, or a choice of no more than two very specific methods, needs to be decided on. The question of which is best in a given case is discussed in Chapter 11; two of the main determinants (i.e. the patient's age and whether infection is present or not) are already known before the planning stage, but the degree of bone loss is, of course, critical. This should be carefully thought about at this stage. A decision must be made about whether the implantation is done purely using cement, cement augmented by rings and screws, or so-called hybrid fixation with a cementless acetabulum, and/or using block or morselized grafting. Clearly, a number of these reconstructional techniques may be legitimate (the author's present thinking is given in Chapter 11), but, whichever method is selected, the precise methods and likely hazards in this particular case need to be gone through at this planning stage. If, for example, the acetabulum has a large floor defect (see Fig. 9.4), the method of

blocking the floor needs to be decided on and can be drawn in. If a ring is to be used, then it is possible (using home-made templates from previous revisions – see Fig. 9.5) to draw this in also. Every attempt should be made to bring the socket down to near the original level, and a provisional plan can be made about whether a block graft is needed.

If the necessity for such a graft is likely, then the operating room staff need to be warned that a solid osteoarthritic head rather than a weaker one is needed from the bone bank. In the femur, it is worth measuring the distances of defects from the tip of the trochanter so that they can be quite readily exposed through a small split in the vasti. If large, a plan can be made about how they are to be blocked. Clearly, a number of defects will be found during the operation itself, but a thorough search now for acetabular and femoral perforations pays significant dividends. This applies particularly if purely cemented fixation is to be used.

Planning in second or later revisions

The above remarks mainly apply to a first revision, which is intended as the main thrust of the revision section in this book. The same remarks still apply to second and later revisions, but additional questions may arise which can be sorted out at this planning stage. If the upper femur is badly destroyed, for example, it is necessary to make a preliminary decision about which of the reconstructional methods described in Chapter 12 should be used. If it is intended to bivalve the upper femur, the level of the femoral osteotomy must be accurately planned and marked. If the hip is a Girdlestone, then a CT scan (Fig. 9.6) is particularly helpful in delineating defects (see Chapter 12). In gross medial socket displacement, occasionally angiography may have a place.

In a number of cases with extremely severe anatomical distortion and bone loss, the drawing in of new components becomes too unrealistic to be useful. In the case shown in Figure 9.7, reconstruction was greatly facilitated by making a model from CT scans (Fig. 9.8) as described for acetabular osteotomy in Chapter 2.

Notes on surgical approaches

It is essential to have proper development of an

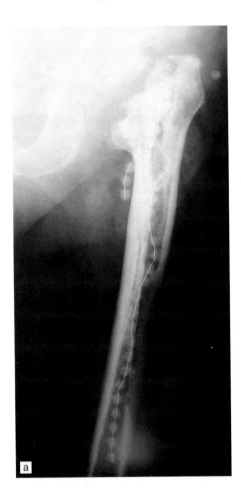

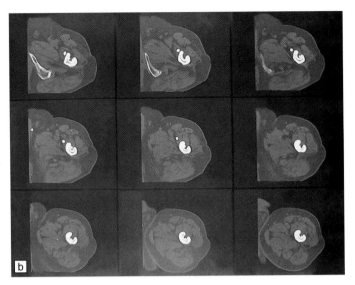

Figure 9.6 – *(a) The AP pre-revision radiograph shows a Girdlestone with chains of beads and what looks like a large lateral cortical defect in the femoral diaphysis. (b) CT scanning of the femur showed that there was, in fact, a very long gutter extending all the way up to the neck, necessitating a special component.*

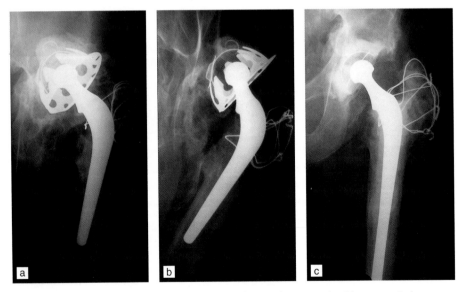

Figure 9.7 – *(a, b) In this failed hip in which a replacement had been carried out after a fracture dislocation, the socket largely having been placed in the false acetabulum, it was unclear whether there was any useful acetabular roof, and (c) how the hip could be reconstructed.*

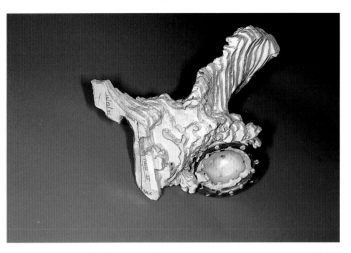

Figure 9.8 – *Planning for the reconstruction was made possible by a model made from CT scans carried out after a first stage, converting the hip into a Girdlestone. Adequate CT scans would not have been possible with the implants in situ. For clarity, the actual removed socket and ring have been placed in the false acetabulum in the model. This is the same case as Fig.9.7.*

appropriate surgical approach giving unrestricted access to the acetabulum and the best possible direct view down the femoral canal. In practice, this means, in the author's view, using either a transtrochanteric or a posterior approach. A large number of other possibilities have been and still are being described, many of which seek to produce adequate access by a transgluteal technique. The advocates of these techniques would agree that a trochanteric osteotomy would certainly improve the access, but they would argue that this advantage is completely offset by uncertainty of trochanteric reattachment. Although this argument does have a certain validity, trochanteric reattachment should not be a major problem if an appropriate technique is used, and transgluteal approaches have the following disadvantages. The substantial gluteal/vastus flap anteriorly significantly detracts from acetabular access and gives problems particularly if it is necessary to reach anterolaterally in the neighbourhood of the lateral wall of the ilium; second, any residual attachment posteriorly of the femur to the pelvis by the intact posterior section of gluteus medius prevents the femur from coming fully out from the wound. This makes a direct view down the femoral canal much more difficult. This disadvantage is not present in the original MacFarland–Osbourne approach and recent variants, such as the Omega, but the problem produced by the anterior flap is the same, if not slightly worse. Nevertheless, a variant of this approach is described in the section on upper femoral bypass.

The transtrochanteric approach also has the significant advantage that the hip is dislocated by pure adduction rather than by torsion as in the posterior approach (and in some transgluteal approaches, depending on the way in which they are done), and this significantly reduces the chance of fracture of a fragile femur, as originally noted by Charnley.

Various details of the transtrochanteric approach as applied to revision surgery are discussed below.

The transtrochanteric approach

Patient positioning

A transtrochanteric approach can, of course, be carried out with the patient either supine or in the lateral position. The former is probably the more widely practised and is described. The principal advantages are that, with ready access to both anterosuperior iliac spines, pelvic orientation is easily determined and acetabular component orientation is, therefore, facilitated; second, the equality or otherwise of leg lengths can easily be checked intraoperatively, with opposite medial malleolus being easily palpable through the drapes and the leg flat down on the table; no special pins or markers within the wound are needed. The advantages of the lateral position are that, particularly in a fat patient, the wound edges may gape more easily, helping access, and the assistant (more significant in a teaching situation) on the opposite side of the patient from the surgeon has a good view, in marked contrast to the supine position where this assistant (or 'leg-holder') is unable to see the acetabulum.

A supine patient needs to be placed so that the lateral surface of the greater trochanter is at least on a level with the edge of the operating table. The patent's thorax also needs to be to the side of the table with the ipsilateral arm up and across the body. If the patient is placed more lateral than this, onlookers will think that he or she is in a dangerous position, but should be reassured that the patient is, in fact, lying on the ischial tuberosity which is well medial; furthermore, during draping, the patient always moves to some degree medially. A rather too lateral position initially is, therefore, in order. It is also necessary to make sure that any non-sterile coverings on the table are flat and thin. Operating department assistants are inclined to tuck these under the buttock, which produces a lump in an undesirable position.

A sandbag is often favoured and, in some circumstances, can prove helpful; it is seldom, if ever, truly necessary, however, provided that the above details are adhered to. Sandbags also have significant disadvantages: they have to be placed rather exactly because, if put under the buttock rather than more medially and proximally, the access is impaired rather than improved. It is also possible for patients to slide gradually sideways off sandbags intraoperatively. If, for some reason, it is elected to use a sandbag, it is best to add a side support on the opposite side of the pelvis so that this gradual medial migration can be avoided.

Draping

With the patient supine, it is vitally important that the buttock be lifted off the operating table by internal rotation of the slightly flexed hip, the knee being bent so that, after skin preparation, the posterior drape (or posterior limb of a split sheet) can be placed well medially. The transverse drape delineating the cephalad end of the prepared area also needs to be a hand's breadth proximal to the anterosuperior iliac spine and its posterior end tucked in well medially. Subsequent drapes need to maintain the exposure of this area. Although apparently obvious, it is surprising how often, if a wound is prepared and draped by an assistant before attempting to start the case, the vital proximal and posterior skin area is obscured, and the scene is immediately set for skimping of the proximal part of the exposure with most unsatisfactory implications. The author likes to feel that the drapes have been so placed that, in principle, a posterior approach could be made to the hip with the patient in this supine position.

Certain cases present particular difficulties in draping – for example, patients who have a pseudarthrosis where internally rotating the leg will not lift the buttock up, and patients whose hips are severely adducted and stiff (sometimes in association with an arthrodesis on the opposite side), in which groin access will be very difficult. In both cases, commonsense measures have to be carried out and accurate placing of the drapes is the start of all the predictable problems to be overcome to achieve a successful result.

In certain cases, the distal thigh may need to be exposed and it is then frequently better to be able also to see the knee. If a sinus is present, it is the author's practice to carry out exactly the same draping as usual and largely ignore it. It is sensible, however, to squeeze out as much of the discharge as possible before application of the plastic wound covering (Op-Site) or this will not stick.

The approach itself

A trochanteric osteotomy by itself in no way guarantees good access. An extensive soft tissue dissection has first to be done and then, when the trochanter is osteotomized, the view rapidly develops. The author has on occasion seen a very cramped and unsatisfactory access achieved using a transtrochanteric approach, even by surgeons of considerable experience, by making an osteotomy too early and relying on this, together with strong retraction, to produce the required view. The situation is analogous to the anterior cruciate ligament in the knee. If, in an otherwise intact knee specimen, the anterior cruciate ligament is divided, virtually no abnormal movement takes place. Instability appears only when other soft tissue laxity is present, as demonstrated by E.L. Trickey. The following description should, therefore, be considered as a complex soft tissue dissection building up to a trochanteric osteotomy after which the access is almost complete.

Skin and fascial incisions

It is best to mark the position of the greater trochanter on the skin. Its position is often quite easy to determine (the palm of one's hand is best), but in severely distorted cases (e.g. in severe shortening, severe external rotation, or where the trochanter has proximally migrated) it may well be quite difficult. It is, of course, in these cases that a correctly placed skin and fascial incision is so important. A straight longitudinal incision is marked, curving backwards at the upper end. The longitudinal limb is best placed just anterior in relation to the shaft of the femur, although its position is not particularly critical. If too anterior, the size of the posterior flap, particularly in a large patient, produces problems. If too posterior, particularly at the upper end, trochanteric wiring at the end is more difficult if one of the twists of the cruciate system (as described later) is placed in the classic position medial to the leading edge of glutei. The upper end of the longitudinal limb, where it starts to curve backwards, needs to be a full four-fingers' breadth above the tip of the greater trochanter, and must go posteriorly to a level well posterior to the back of the trochanter. It is better to err towards making the change to a posterior direction too proximal because, at worst, this will simply make slight difficulties in closure of the wound at the end, as a result of thinness of the fascia lata in this region. If this point is too distal, serious cramping of the approach results.

Parts of previous incisions can be used, but their position is, unfortunately, often unsuitable; this may sometimes be obvious, and a clue to the failure of the original THR. Fortunately, unlike in the knee, it is almost always safe to ignore previous incisions, skin necrosis between the scars resulting very seldom, provided only that none of the incisions is in any way recent. If revision has to be done in the presence of a recent scar and its position is less than ideal, it needs to be extended into the line of the normal incision described above, even though this makes a very odd shaped incision. In such cases, the fascial, as opposed to the skin, incision can still usually be made on the ordinary line. A sinus is usually present in a sufficiently suitable place for its mouth to be excised in continuity with the main incision. A probe can be placed in it and the fascia lata cleared immediately around the point where the sinus passes through it. The fascia can then be divided around it in continuity with the main fascial incision, as with the skin. In these cases, the sinus can be excised virtually to its complete depth in one piece (Fig. 9.9). If the sinus opening is more distant from the wound, its mouth can still be excised, but deeper débridement of the track needs to be carried out in a more ad hoc fashion as granulation tissue is discovered. More distant sinuses (unusual) may need to be left alone entirely. There need, however, be no concern about this because, provided that the focus of the infection in the hip itself is properly dealt with, healing still results. It is, in fact, probably safe to completely ignore the presence of the sinus in the soft tissue dissection, even when this appears near to the wound, but this seems an unnecessary compromise of the technique.

Often, as soon as the skin and fat are incised, tissue that at first looks like the fascia lata is seen, but on closer inspection it is in fact vastus lateralis, there being an overlying deficiency in the fascia lata. It is probable in these circumstances that closure of the wound at the end of the original THR has been skimped. If this point is not appreciated, then immediate major problems in identification of the deeper layers result. The whole of the fascia lata needs to be identified before it is incised. The margins of defects can almost always be palpated and quite accurately defined. The fascia is then divided between the defects. A marker suture at the point where the longitudinal section of the fascial incision goes backwards is helpful in closure.

In a primary THR, the fascia can be stripped with blunt dissection of the leading edge of the glutei and the initial incision (self-retaining fascia lata) retractor immediately inserted and opened, making the wound into a diamond shape. In a revision, several quite taxing steps may be needed before this retractor can be inserted.

Posterior dissection of the fascia lata

Finger dissection can be used posteriorly and distally to feel round to the linea aspera. The fascia may be extremely thick over the greater trochanter. If wires are present, they may appear, surrounded by a bursa, indicating that the full depth has been reached. When the flap is taken backwards off the trochanter, and particularly if the hip has significantly shortened so that gluteus medius is lax, it is all too easy to cut deeply into gluteus medius rather than simply taking the fascia off with gluteus maximus. If the hip is strongly adducted at this point, then medius straightens out and the correct plane is easier to define (Fig. 9.10). Careful sharp dissection at the back of medius is necessary, particularly if a posterior approach has been used before. As the flap is taken backwards, the tendon of gluteus maximus, which is very frequently still present, can be seen as an important landmark. The posterior dissection is complete when it is possible to get the flat of one's hand in behind the greater trochanter (i.e. as with a primary case) with flesh of medius easily visible running proximally and some way deeply.

Anterior dissection of the fascia lata

If a posterior approach has been used before, the anterior dissection is almost the same as that for primary surgery.

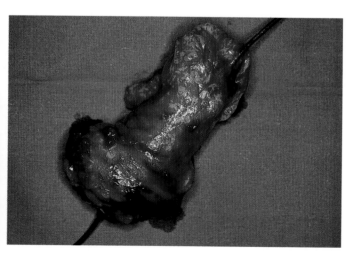

Figure 9.9 – *Sinus excised en bloc at a one-stage exchange as part of the surgical approach.*

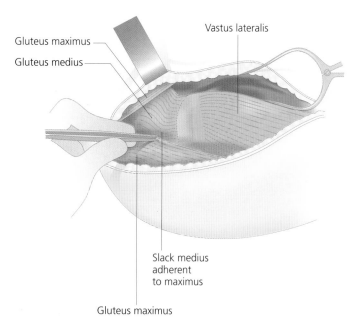

Figure 9.10 – *If the hip is very short, the abductors may be slack and very easily damaged at dissection. Correct identification posteriorly of the plane between maximus and medius is much easier if the hip is strongly adducted, straightening out medius. Adduction may also facilitate definition of medius anteriorly, especially if the trochanter is un-united or in a very proximal position (see text).*

In most cases, however, variable amounts of sharp dissection are needed. The space deep to the fascia lata in front of the vasti needs to be identified distally and running proximally with finger dissection (almost always virgin terrain at a sufficient depth). With sharp dissection, the fascia lata can be taken off vastus lateralis, taking great care not to enter muscle. The dissection comes up to the vastus lateralis ridge and the place where the leading edge of gluteus medius ought, in theory, to be. It is very helpful in the dissection at this stage to have some knowledge of what type of anterior or anterolateral approach has been used. In a previously well carried out McKee approach, it may still be possible to find flesh of gluteus medius in the normal position by sharp dissection and, with a thumb under fascia lata and the region of tensor, sharp dissection can be continued along the front of medius under direct vision so that the fascia comes forward widely quite quickly.

Usually, however, damage to the front of medius has occurred, sometimes quite badly. The correct procedure in these cases is the sharp dissection of tissue beneath the fascia lata on the correct line, and then usually more proximally and anteriorly living muscle fibres are found.

If dissection is proceeded with along the front of the trochanter, looking for the leading edge of medius, major destruction of the residual abductors occurs. If a transgluteal approach has been used, not infrequently the leading edge of medius is normal, but in a more proximal position than usual. Once the leading edge of medius has been identified, however, the fascia strips off it quite readily. If a trochanteric osteotomy has been used and union has resulted without loss of position, there is no great problem in establishing the soft tissue abductor anatomy. If, however, the trochanter has migrated proximally before union, or is un-united or malpositioned, a very careful and thoughtful search is required. Once again, if the hip is strongly adducted, a more normal position of medius is found. It tends to come out from underneath the fascia lata and its attached gluteus maximus and, by sharp dissection lateral to medius and distal to its leading edge, a satisfactory quantity of healthy looking muscle can often be found. Unless this step is carried out at this early stage, there is very little chance of sound trochanteric reattachment at the end. The specific subject of the treatment of trochanteric non-union is discussed in Chapter 12.

With completion of the above steps, the fascia lata edges should come very easily and widely apart, exposing a large area of healthy looking gluteus medius. If a self-retaining retractor is being used, this can then be inserted.

Deeper dissection
The temptation to dissect from an anterolateral direction and try to find the neck of the prosthesis by ad hoc soft tissue excision, as the next step, is not recommended. The correct step should be to clear the (pseudo)capsule and, in so doing, the iliacus should be clearly visible. There is unfortunately no anterior landmark equivalent to the posterior landmark of the tendon of gluteus maximus, but the author always feels that a major step has been accomplished anteriorly when the flesh of iliacus, which has a quite distinctive appearance and direction, is found. A Homan retractor can then be put beneath it over the front of the acetabulum (Fig. 9.11). When this retractor is lifted up, the psoas tendon is often seen and the Homan retractor may need to be re-positioned. Safe sharp dissection, albeit with some bleeding from small vessels between iliacus and the (pseudo)capsule, can then be done until a wide area of (pseudo)capsule is seen. It is frequently possible to put a curved instrument (such as a Moynihan) extracapsularly

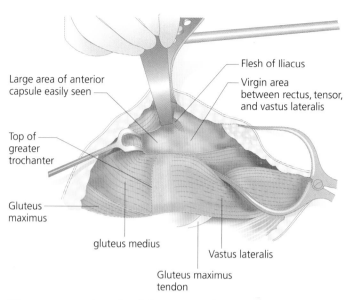

Large area of anterior capsule easily seen

Top of greater trochanter

Gluteus maximus

gluteus medius

Gluteus maximus tendon

Flesh of Iliacus

Virgin area between rectus, tensor, and vastus lateralis

Vastus lateralis

Figure 9.11 – *Completed dissection before anterior capsulectomy, wire removal (if needed) and trochanteric osteotomy. A large area of anterior (pseudo)capsule is seen. Iliacus has been clearly identified and is held forwards by a Homan retractor. The abductors have been completely mobilized anteriorly and posteriorly.*

and inferomedially from front to back, and to feel this with the middle finger of the opposite hand from posteriorly.

If the greater trochanter needs to be distalized, it may also be sensible to dissect in an extracapsular plane deep to glutei. The position of the lateral side of the ilium can also be defined. When this has all been done, a bold and deep cut can be made right through the (pseudo)capsule and two large pieces of it excised from inferomedially and superolaterally. Quite a wide view of the components can usually be achieved immediately. Not only is there then a feeling that the exposure has almost been completed, but there is the knowledge that the deeper planes have been identified clearly. If attempts are made to carry out a further capsulectomy at a later stage, when the plane between iliacus and the (pseudo)capsule has not been properly identified, there will be concerns about major vascular damage anteriorly.

Removal of wire/trochanteric fixation devices

Wires

If the operation has been properly planned, incision and partial removal of tissues on the outer side of the greater trochanter soon reveal the essential twists. In the great majority of cases, it is possible to remove all or almost all of the wires. This greatly facilitates trochanteric

osteotomy, and time should be spent on wire removal. Once the direction of the wires associated with each twist is identified, an appropriate cut can be made and that wire withdrawn. If the wire is not first properly identified, even after being cut, it cannot be extracted and there is then a danger that attempts to remove it forcibly will cause damage to the trochanter. It is also possible to cause wires to 'cheese-wire' completely through the trochanter. It may sometimes be necessary to identify wires anterior to the top of the femur deep to gluteus medius. This applies, for example, to the spring wire system. Sometimes, also, when wires are twisted or knotted lateral to the trochanter, but known not to be passing through drill holes in the trochanter, they can be divided and easily pulled away from the trochanter at the back and brought sufficiently forwards for a saw to be inserted, even if it is not possible to remove them bodily.

Other devices

A reference has already been made to this under 'Planning'. Most devices should be completely removable. Much care is, however, required with larger devices. For example, the Dall-Miles cable grip device needs some cautious removal of bone from around its spikes; forcible removal leads to a major fracture of the probably porotic lateral trochanteric cortex. It is often not possible with this device also to pull the cables completely out because they become firmly integrated. Nevertheless, they can be got out of the way sufficiently to allow a normal trochanteric osteotomy.

The trochanteric osteotomy

A chevron osteotomy with a saw (Fig. 9.12) is strongly recommended. The midpoint of the trochanter from front to back (bearing in mind that the trochanter is a somewhat posterior structure) is marked laterally and the leg put into neutral rotation. It is convenient temporarily to place a blunt instrument, such as a Moynihan, through the hip intracapsularly from front to back to delineate the deep end of the osteotomy. The anterior cut is first made using an oscillating saw. The direction of the cut should be at about 40–45° to the axis of the shaft of the femur, viewed frontally. Occasionally, there may be an indication for a shallower angle, but a 40–45° cut gives a good solid trochanteric piece, greatly helping later reattachment.

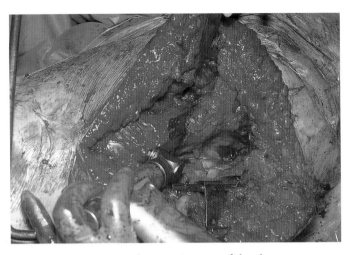

Figure 9.12 – *Cutting the posterior part of the chevron osteotomy. The anterior cut has already been made and a spare saw blade has been put in it to show its position exactly and guide the posterior cut.*

A saw blade is then placed in the anterior limb of the cut and the leg is internally rotated. A Homan retractor should be placed behind the trochanter to guard the sciatic nerve should the saw slip; then the posterior half of the osteotomy is made at an angle of between 110° and 140° to the anterior cut, the main concern being that the posterior end of the top of the trochanter (so often very medial and something that should be deliberately searched for) is included. It is important to make sure that both cuts are absolutely complete before attempting to move the trochanter or else a fracture results. Remaining soft tissue attachments in front and behind can then be divided and a laminar spreader inserted deeply. The trochanter can be quite easily mobilized a long way proximally. This method leaves nice flat surfaces, enabling much more satisfactory reattachment and advancement if required – applicable particularly to revision (see below).

Technique in the presence of a previous trochanteric non-union

The precise position of the non-union can be found by inserting a needle or the tip of a cutting diathermy. It may be obvious, but in cases of a short fibrous non-union it may not be, as a result of the very small amount of abnormal movement. The non-union is then entered and a laminar spreader can be inserted. This facilitates the dissection greatly. If it has been intended from the planning to try to achieve bony union at the end of the revision, the trochanter should be mobilized at this early stage. Failure to do so simply means that mobilization is skimped at the end of the procedure when the surgeon is tired. Persisting non-union then results. The trochanter is held (e.g. with the trochanteric holder), traction applied, and the pseudocapsule removed from deep to glutei. It may be necessary to take the muscle off the underlying ilium to some degree with an elevator. Mobilization in special cases of a high non-union where reattachment is particularly important, as in the case of revision for recurrent dislocation, is considered in Chapter 12.

Dislocation

It is again tempting to place a hook around the neck of the prosthesis and dislocate the hip at this stage. In many cases, this is perfectly satisfactory, but sometimes force is needed and something breaks – for example, weak bone in the region of the lesser trochanter. It is much better to bring the hip gradually into a dislocated position and divide pseudocapsular attachments close to the upper femur in a progressive fashion. A Moynihan can be put extracapsularly (easy, because this plane was identified much earlier) and the remaining medial and inferomedial capsule divided. The hip is then, in almost all cases, easy to dislocate and can be extracted from the wound. Some special situations naturally arise and these are discussed in Chapter 12.

CHAPTER 10

Removal of failed prostheses

M. D. Northmore-Ball

General remarks – one or both components?

In the great majority of cases of failed prostheses, it is best to change both components. Changing only one appears simpler, but it can very easily lead to the need for further revision with change of both components very quickly afterwards. In the case of a proven deep infection, it is essential to change both, even if one may appear to be securely fixed still. The reasons for this are discussed further in the appropriate section. In aseptic loosening, with a definitely loose symptomatic stem, the socket may appear well fixed even on fairly careful intra-operative examination, but frequently on removal it is found to be sitting on a thick soft tissue membrane. This membrane may then grow bacteria (i.e. the hip was, in fact, infected); alternatively, its fixation may have appeared to be sufficient in the presence of a poorly functioning stem, but, with revision of the stem with increased loading, acetabular fixation might fail. If there is a temptation to leave a correctly positioned stem *in situ*, the head should be inspected extremely carefully, especially if significant acetabular wear is present. The author has seen at least one experienced surgeon leave a stem with a very doubtful head in place when changing a socket for loosening and wear. Assuming that wear products were a factor in the loosening, such a policy would represent short termism at it worst. There is also the danger that instability will result, because the position of the second component cannot be changed after insertion of the first. To place a component deliberately in an abnormal position (e.g. to retrovert a socket to cope with an apparently abnormal anteverted stem) is simply to dig an even deeper hole for the surgeon and patient.

There are, of course, exceptions. In the case of a fractured stem, only the stem may be changed. This is because both components must have been functioning extremely well in order to produce sufficient fatigue to fracture the stem. The change of one component only may also occasionally be appropriate in mechanical loosening. This would apply if there was some extremely obvious problem on one side with remarkable normality on the other. The situation is sometimes seen with hybrid systems or some of the earlier ill-fated designs of cementless total hip replacements (THRs). Nevertheless, the much safer plan, although requiring more operating time, is to change both components.

Practical details

The following assumes that the trochanter has now been removed, the hip dislocated, and the prosthetic head and neck and the upper end of the femur properly exposed.

The author's sequence in aseptic loosening is to remove the stem, change the socket, and remove the femoral cement (if present).

Component/cement removal should be considered as a necessary 'chore' preceding the much more challenging reinsertion of new components as perfectly as possible to produce good long-term function. The reconstructional phase of the operation (see Chapter 11) is greatly facilitated if every care is taken to avoid the occurrence of any damage whatsoever during component removal. One hears it said that at a certain stage 'it' broke. This is usually nonsense. Most fractures occur because insufficient care is being taken with the fragile structures seen in failed THRs.

Stem removal

The complete upper end of the stem and any collar must be cleared of overhanging soft tissue, bone, and cement, if present, so that there no overhang. A burr is often best.

Chisels have to be used extremely carefully or marginal fractures will occur immediately, especially if there are thick blocks of cement. It is all too easy to knock off one complete section of the trochanteric bed if the trochanter has been osteotomized.

With monoblock stems, it is much better to use an extractor with a slap hammer (Fig. 10.1). This is much more satisfactory than hitting the femoral head with a hammer or the collar with a punch. With an extractor, the direction of the pull can be adjusted exactly and any load, from an extremely gentle tap to quite a heavy impact, can be delivered. Old banana-shaped stems come

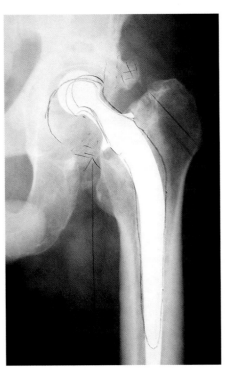

Figure 10.3 – *Stem with a long curve at the upper end, more difficult to extract (in this case Stanmore).*

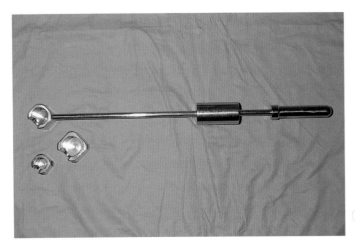

Figure 10.1 – *One variety of universal extractor for monoblock stems. The different ends accommodate different sizes of head.*

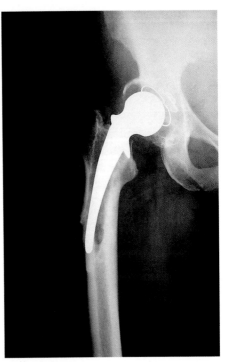

Figure 10.2 – *Banana-shaped stem which easily comes out of its cement bed (in this case McKee–Arden).*

out very easily (sometimes falling out as the hip is dislocated) (Fig. 10.2). The shape of other stems must, however, be carefully inspected. Charnley stems require removal of about 2.5–3 cm of cement from superolaterally. If forcibly knocked out, although the stem will gradually allow itself to go into varus as the distal stem becomes disimpacted from the cement, a fracture is likely superolaterally. Stems of a shape such as the Stanmore (Fig. 10.3) are more difficult. Once again, these are straight distally, but the upper curvature goes down a greater distance and clearance is needed a considerably longer way down the femur on the outer side. A drill or burr is needed, kept close to the prosthesis.

In all cases, if the stem comes some way and jams, it should be knocked back in and the cause of the obstruction remedied.

Modular stems
An extraction instrument designed to lock on to the trunnion is essential (Fig. 10.4).

Cementless stems
Some form of extractor must be arranged that has an extremely secure hold on the stem and allows very hard hammer blows in the axis of the shaft of the femur. This is through one of the devices already described or a specialized device, as referred to under 'Planning' in

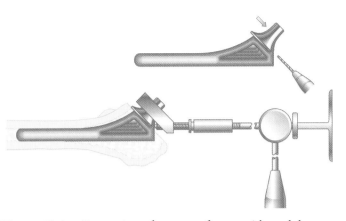

Figure 10.4 – *One variety of extractor for use with modular stems. A high-speed burr and appropriate bits may be necessary.*

Chapter 9. Time should be spent on getting this apparatus very well secured and in good alignment. Unless the stem quite readily comes out, the device should be removed and attention directed to releasing the stem from at least the upper femur. A high-speed burr, such as the Anspach, is essential if the procedure is to be undertaken reliably. Using a very thin end and side cutting bit (the Silver 2), a space can be developed around the stem. A narrow saw is occasionally possible, depending on the shape of the collar, if present. Once 2–3 cm have been cleared anteriorly, posteriorly, and laterally, firmer blows can be safely put on the extraction device. If the stem is still securely fixed, progressively longer fine flexible bits (the Micro Revision MR8 in its three lengths) can be used, which can be advanced further and further down the stem. There may be space to use very thin osteotomes with extreme caution. With care and patience, it should be possible to remove virtually all stems in this way.

If, however, there is still failure, the following procedure is best. The femoral cortex over the part of the stem that is still firmly fixed (judged from the pre-operative radiograph and the point down to which the stem has been freed) is exposed and the position of a window, which may or may not be required, is marked and its corners drilled. A small longitudinal cut is then made between two of the holes only, taking the cut right through to the stem. An old and rather thick osteotome is inserted into this saw cut and banged in. There is then usually a 'click', with the femur expanding just sufficiently to free the stem; this can be extracted. Provided that care is taken and the drill holes are sufficiently distal, the femur will not split above the

proximal of the two drill holes, and subsequent reconstruction will not be greatly compromised.

Occasionally, a fenestrated stem such as an Austin Moore or early type Ring can be difficult to extract as a result of solid fibrous tissue or bone growing through the fenestrations. It is most important to recognize this because firm hammering on the head simply produces a fracture. The bony bridge can be very carefully transected with a saw. In principle, it would be very much better to expose any such bridge through a carefully placed femoral fenestration, and then to divide it under direct vision, rather than risk a fracture. Such holes can be later blocked during reconstruction (see Chapter 11).

In the special case of polymer stems, and notably the RM-Isoelastic stem, these are usually completely loose, although occasionally they can be solidly fixed. Attempts to grasp the polymer trunnion are unlikely to be successful. The best procedure is to remove piecemeal the plastic in the upper section of the femur, revealing the metal core. The metal core can then be grasped. In the case of the Isoelastic stem, the core is perforated, and a wire or cable can be threaded through one of these holes and hitched to the end of an intramedullary nail-extraction device. It is likely that the stem, together with the remainder of the implant, can be removed. If not, further plastic should be removed, in which case the core may come out from the centre of the stem (Fig. 10.5). Although this seems a perplexing situation, it is in fact quite a straightforward one, because the plastic stem with its central hole becomes analogous to a long distal femoral cement plug. Its removal is, therefore, exactly on the lines of removal of these plugs described below.

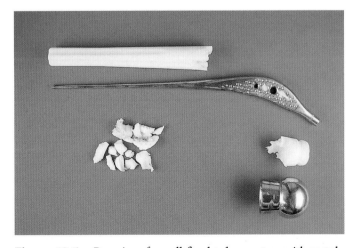

Figure 10.5 – *Remains of a well-fixed polymer stem with metal core (RM-Isoelastic) after piecemeal removal. The metal core came out initially, leaving the polymer behind.*

Acetabular component removal

Hasty attempts at removal of the socket may well produce acetabular fractures. These will not be major, but an acetabulum that is completely free from fractures is much simpler to reconstruct. The reconstructional phase of the revision should be borne in mind continuously during the component removal phase.

It is safest to expose the entire bony acetabular periphery around the socket and to insert any preferred retraction system next. More than one insertion of a retractor (e.g. a Homan) is necessary in any position because, initially, it is difficult to tell the bony margin from the edge of the socket. Posteriorly, the bony margin should be felt and a pointed Homan retractor inserted in a vertical fashion (assuming that the patient is supine), bringing it horizontal to make absolutely certain that the sciatic nerve (which cannot always be felt) is pushed safely posteriorly. This retractor can then be banged into the ischium. Inferiorly, the true acetabular floor in the neighbourhood of the teardrop can often be found at this early stage; the retractor is inserted. Anteriorly, a Homan may need to be inserted two or three times, progressively defining the anterior rim. Having inserted these retractors, the socket/cement (if present)/bone region can be carefully examined circumferentially. Overhanging bone and cement can easily be removed with chisels.

All-plastic cemented sockets

These can be drilled and the appropriate tap (Fig. 10.6) inserted. It is vital that the drill be sharp so that the plastic is easily drilled. Pressure on the drill could, of course, be highly dangerous. The acetabulum can then be manipulated, at least to a limited degree, and the slap hammer used to extract it. Often, obvious minor obstructions are seen part way through removal and these can be easily relieved with chisels to avoid any fractures.

A device that is probably slightly better is shown in Figure 10.7: this allows for more certain manipulation of the socket. Force, however, must not be used.

Usually, much of the cement comes out with the socket. The residual cement then has to be removed. It is safe to use chisels only if that particular bit of cement is backed by solid bone; if not, a fracture or perforation results. Instead, it can be drilled and the Wroblewski drill and tap (Fig. 10.8) used.

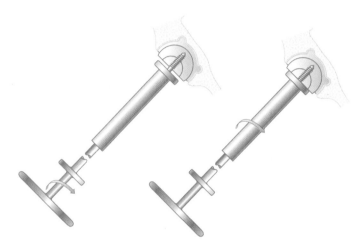

Figure 10.7 – *Moreland acetabular extractor: the socket can be manipulated without the threaded part losing its hold.*

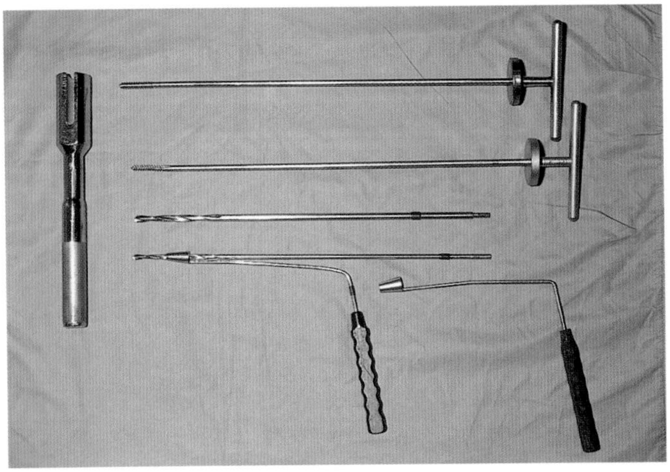

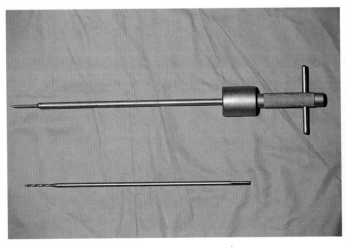

Figure 10.6 – *Set of Waldemar Link drills, drill guides, taps, and slap hammer.*

Figure 10.8 – *Wroblewski drill and tap, with sliding hammer.*

Cement in keyholes and plugs

Cement in keyholes can be either carefully picked out with a chisel or removed with the drill and tap. Removal of small medial plugs can also be done with the drill and tap. The removal method for larger plugs has been discussed under 'Planning' in Chapter 9. The requirements are:

- to hold the plug in some way
- to have a sufficient hole in the floor of the acetabulum for extraction.

Parts of the plug can usually be grasped with a Kocher's forceps and membrane teased from the sides with a blunt instrument, such as a ring-handled spike. It is best if the plug can eventually be turned almost completely round, because then one can be absolutely sure that, if knocked out, no damage will accrue. Sometimes, in a large plug, a drill and tap can be used, but the drill should go only a short way into the plug. If the hole in the floor of the socket is smaller than the plug (quite common), it is much better to enlarge this in a controlled fashion with a spinal instrument, such as a Kerrison's rongeur (i.e. as if it were a vertebral lamina). A large central hole of known size. with a relatively solid rim (which can be easily blocked up later) through which the plug can easily be withdrawn, is hugely better than somewhat frantic scrabblings, loss of hold on the plug, and repeated semi-blind and medial insertion of grasping instruments.

Sets of cement chisels usually include one with a long curve intended for use in the acetabulum (Fig. 10.9). This chisel should be used only very cautiously. The method given above is better. Attempts to loosen a socket with it, particularly in cases with a medial position or rather thin medial cement, are potentially dangerous. Serious bleeding can result. Occasionally, the acetabulum can be levered out with a large broad instrument, such as a Watson-Jones gouge, inserted between the bone and cement from superiorly. This can be quick and easy but, nevertheless, is not recommended unless the socket is manifestly loose and the ilium very solid. In other cases, damage that is irritating or worse to the ilium in the vital weight-bearing zone will result.

If the socket needs to be changed, but is barely loose, the cement is thick, and the bone very osteoporotic and/ or thin (for example, the revision of a cemented socket inserted for a subcapital fracture), unacceptable force may be required to knock a socket out with the slap hammer. In these cases, cement should be removed using a combination of high-speed burr and narrow chisels, with deliberate controlled sacrifice of some bone, and any large ischial or iliac plugs are transected with a chisel. The component can then be removed and the remaining cement taken out in a controlled fashion without problem. If it is felt that insufficient access to cement can be obtained in this way (e.g. the remaining anterior and posterior walls are already extremely thin), it may be safer to transect the socket and remove it piecemeal from the cement bed. A drill of about 6 mm can be used in cruciform fashion and the holes joined together with a very sharp, thin osteotome. It may be necessary to remove a wire marker from the plastic at some point. The sectors then need to be grasped with a strong instrument, such as sequestrum forceps, because the plastic can be surprisingly resistant to removal. The author has not found the process greatly facilitated by the use of high-speed burrs. Once the plastic (or perhaps only one sector) is out, unimpaired access to the underlying cement can then be achieved. This should be removed cautiously in small pieces.

The achievement of an empty acetabulum, which has been seriously eroded, but has no further surgical damage, is demanding but very satisfactory.

Sockets with extreme medial or superomedial migration can virtually always be removed in standard fashion from laterally, although the margin of the acetabulum may well need to be enlarged (analogous to the enlargement of the floor of the acetabulum for removal of large plugs), and drilling of the plastic will be neither necessary nor desirable. Only in extreme cases (perhaps 1% of revisions) is it necessary to perform a medial approach. To do this, a separate incision is made over the anterior

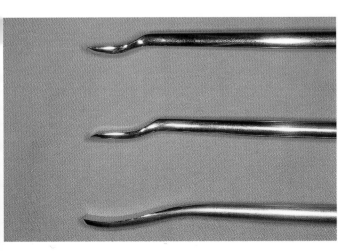

Figure 10.9 – *Negative-cut (top), positive-cut (middle), and acetabular (bottom) cement chisels.*

third of the iliac crest. As this situation will have been anticipated from the planning, the initial skin incision should have been made somewhat more posteriorly than usual to allow for a wide skin bridge between the two incisions. Iliacus is then taken off from medially. This limited medial approach, however, only just reaches to the lip of the true pelvis, and the socket is not reached as easily as might be anticipated. Figure 9.3 shows the case of a socket removed in this way.

Cementless sockets

Unless very loose, these sockets can often present quite serious difficulties. If there is a plastic liner inside a cementless metal-back, it will certainly be necessary to remove this first. A neat solution is to drill a small hole in the plastic and insert a screw. By turning the screw, the plastic can then be jacked out of the metal-back.

Many cementless sockets requiring removal are threaded. They may be sufficiently loose to cause symptoms but, unfortunately, not sufficiently loose to allow easy removal (as occasionally seen with an Austin Moore in the femur). The two possible methods for extracting the socket are (1) rocking and (2) unscrewing it.

Rocking

Bone can be cautiously removed using a drill or narrow burr from superiorly, and this space can then be developed anteriorly and posteriorly using the narrowest instruments possible. It is assumed that the inferomedial region has been thoroughly cleared. Using blows with a punch, the acetabulum can then gradually be rocked on an anteroposterior axis. By knocking it back into its original position and repeating this manoeuvre and cautiously removing further anterior and posterior bone, it will eventually come out.

Unscrewing

Hopefully, a suitable insertion/extraction instrument has been made available. However, the best efforts sometimes fail and the available instrument may not fit. In this case, rotation has to be applied to the socket with a punch directed tangentially, or some form of grasping forceps applied superiorly after removal of some bone from the ilium. It is usually found that minor rotation of a few degrees can be achieved, but that the component then becomes completely jammed once again. Bone removal, as described earlier under 'Rocking', should

then be carried out; it may be possible to employ some of the discontinuities between the threads of the socket to insert instruments. Sometimes the socket eventually spins, but with stripped threads, and is still difficult to extract. With patience, it can be rocked out. With all-ceramic sockets, exactly the same applies, but a sharp centre punch should be available because it may be possible deliberately to break the socket up, as described by Neider.

If, by any unfortunate chance, it is necessary to remove a socket cemented on to a screw-fixed reinforcement ring, a sharp instrument, such as a Kirschner wire, is needed to remove the cement from the screwdriver holes. A special ASIF chisel with a very narrow blade is also available, and, if the hexagonal socket in the screw head becomes damaged, there is also a special left-handed extraction screw that can be driven into it.

After removal of the contents of the acetabulum, it needs to be thoroughly débrided. Specimens should be sent for bacteriology and histology in all cases.

In cases thought to be infected, but in which a one-stage exchange is intended (see Chapter 12), an antiseptic swab should be placed in the acetabulum. In aseptic cases, the acetabulum can be reconstructed before femoral clearance, as noted above.

Femoral clearance/cement removal

Lesser trochanter upwards

A little cement will probably have been removed already before taking out the stem. The remaining cement in this region is very easily visible and on the face of it very easy to remove. However, it is all too easy to produce marginal fractures, or fractures of quite significant pieces of the upper femur, greatly complicating later reconstruction. The thickness and strength of cement in any given spot have, therefore, to be compared with the solidity of the bone behind it. Chisels, a burr, or ultrasound can be used, or combinations of these. Usually, chisels alone are sufficient, provided that they are used very carefully.

First of all, the bone–cement junction has to be carefully defined circumferentially. Frequently, it is found (particularly if a limited anterolateral approach has originally been used) that there is exposed cement directly underneath the muscle anteriorly for 1 or 2 cm. Elsewhere, bony erosion may have caused cement to be denuded. Such cement can be removed as a first step with chisels in a coronal plane relative to the axis of the femur, directed towards the centre of the canal. An edge running longitudinally (i.e. parallel to the femoral axis) should then be selected and cement split a few millimetres away from this. If cement is split longitudinally elsewhere, a split in the upper femur almost certainly results. Narrow or thin remaining pieces of cement running longitudinally (which are now weak in comparison with the underlying bone) can then be cautiously chipped away with a chisel running between the cement and the bone. When no cement is left around the whole of the mouth for 1 or 2 cm, the danger of producing marginal fractures is less and chisels can be used slightly more freely. Often there is very thick cement posteriorly, somewhat below the level of the lesser trochanter. This may be very difficult to split and cement somewhat distal to it can be thinned right down; this section can then be removed bodily, as it is only weakly attached to the rest of the cement column. A drill and tap can be useful.

If the upper cement is solid and thick and the bone porotic, and particularly where the femoral component may not be loose (e.g. in a case of endoprosthesis revision after subcapital fracture), it is necessary to thin the cement down or remove it completely in this region using a high-speed burr. A drawback is the amount of cement debris produced. The at-risk upper 2–3 cm of femur will, however, have been safely cleared and chisels can then be used more distally. This situation is also a very good indication for ultrasound, if available; slots can be made and the cement thinned right down without applying any load to the weak underlying bone. The use of ultrasound is considered in detail in a separate section at the end of this chapter.

Fragments of wire are often encountered. They are often responsible for difficulty in splitting cement and, if some wire is seen, it is best to hold it with an instrument inside the cement column and twist it out from within.

Lesser trochanter to tip of stem

A properly functioning light source is essential. Sometimes, systems are in use with broken cables within the fibre light, giving poor illumination. This is quite unacceptable. A battery-operated flexible light is also insufficient. A revision type of sucker with an internal filter is essential because ordinary suckers block almost immediately. A syringe is adequate for irrigation, although a specialized lavage system is very much better.

Depending on the anatomy of the column, which will have been clearly worked out from inspection at the planning stage of the anteroposterior (AP) and lateral radiographs, chisels can be used to go a variable way down this section. A combination of longitudinal splitting and cautious use of positive-cut chisels (Fig. 10.9) is required. If the cement is somewhat loose and the femur relatively solid, this is quite straightforward.

If the radiographs show that the tip of the stem is relatively central within the canal in an AP as well as a side-to-side sense (perhaps one revision in ten), and the femur is also quite strong, Wroblewski drills (Fig. 10.10) can be used. The smallest one is put all the way down the track and its depth measured from the scale on the drill against a suitable bony landmark in the trochanteric region. Progressively larger drills are then used, which cut into the cement initially just near the tip, but gradually further up the track. Cement shavings should be washed out between insertions of the drills. The diameter of the femur in the region of the plug should have been estimated from the radiographs and progressively larger drills used until this dimension is reached. Increasing care is required with the larger drills because not only is a greater torque transmitted to the femur as a result of the larger diameter of the drill, but a longer column of cement is also being cut into. With sufficient care, however, the cement column can be cut across at the level of the tip of the stem. The achievement of this can be verified by direct inspection with the light source. Chisels can be used in a very satisfactory

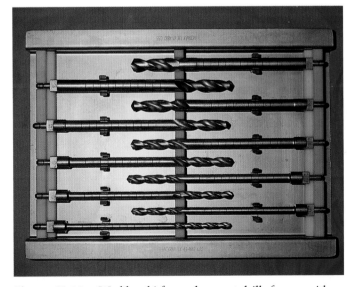

Figure 10.10 – *Wroblewski femoral cement drills for use with a low-offset hand brace.*

fashion to remove long sections of cement from the walls of the femur down to this level.

Burrs have to be used only with great caution in this region, because of the at-best limited view, which rapidly becomes obscured with cement debris, although ultrasound can be very effective. It should, however, always be possible to removal all the cement down to the level of the distal plug using the other methods already listed (but sometimes, particularly with very eccentric stems, also requiring the Charnley revision jig, or a similar instrument – see next section).

The distal plug

In virtually every case, it is possible to remove the plug without fenestrating the femur. If adequate equipment is not available for plug removal, such that fenestration is liable to be routinely required, then revision should not be carried out and the patient should be transferred. Windowing of the femur should be required only rarely, and then only with very distal cement below the isthmus. Removal of the plug should not be attempted until all the cement down to it has been removed completely. If longitudinal cement is still attached to the plug for some distance above it, it will not be possible to remove it.

A positive-cut chisel, or a chisel with a 15° angle (Fig. 10.11), is next used circumferentially round the top of the plug.

If the plug is short and weakly held, and its upper surface is relatively flat or has a suitably positioned depression from the cast of the tip of the stem, it can be

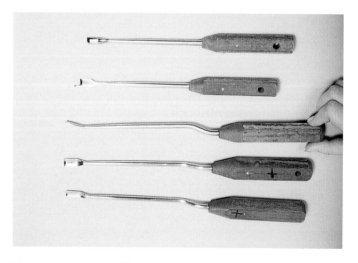

Figure 10.11 – *Set of femoral cement chisels. The 15° angle chisel is in the middle. Above this is the splitter. All but one has a hole for a Tommy bar should it become jammed.*

drilled into under direct vision with a Wroblewski drill (see Fig. 10.8) and the tap inserted; it may well be possible to remove the complete plug in one go.

If this tap strips its threads and comes out as a result of greater adherence of the plug, then the Waldemar Link drills (see Fig. 10.6) can be used. Provided that no major erosions (unfortunately quite common) are present immediately proximal to the plug, the centring cone can be used. The larger size of this system produces a better hold in the plug and it can probably then be extracted. Sometimes, on first inserting the tap, the plug remains immovable. The tap can, however, be progressively unscrewed and sometimes the upper part of the plug can be extracted. Frequently, however, the effect of this is simply that the upper parts of the thread strip.

If the upper part of the plug has an oblique surface or is very off-centre, and there are substantial erosions in the femur just proximal to it so that the conical drill centring device cannot be used, it may be possible to flatten it with a flat-ended burr or mill, and then drill under direct vision but a safer system is to use a drill guide located on the outside of the femur. At least three such devices are available: the Charnley revision jig (Fig. 10.12), the Eftekhar jig, and the Vidalain jig [1,2]. These devices are very safe and insufficiently used. The only drawback is that they require either a separate distal incision or an extension of the approach, together with splitting of the vasti. The distance over which the muscle has to be split with the Charnley revision jig is, however, very short. Two ring-handled spikes can be inserted through the muscle and spread apart at an appropriate level.

Starting with the smaller sizes, progressively larger distal elements of the jig can be offered up to the femur until one fits exactly. The jig is then assembled and the phosphor bronze bush inserted at the upper end, going down into the upper part of the femoral shaft. The position of this bush is then checked under direct vision. Allowance needs to be made for the anterior curvature of the femur. The trephine is then inserted on a power drill (Fig. 10.13). Minimal pressure is first used so that the trephine cuts into the desired part of the cement (which may have an acutely sloping surface); when it is felt no longer to be having any tendency to wander, firmer pressure is used. The trephine is extracted at intervals and the cement that has found its way into the central hole is removed with the special instrument. This is very easy. In most cases, it is possible to drill all the way through the distal plug.

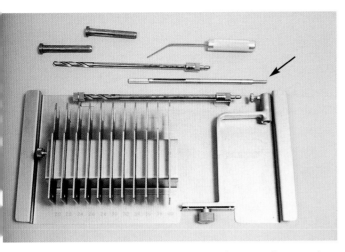

Figure 10.12 – *Charnley-type revision jig for centralizing either hand drills or a power trephine (arrowed) in the femur. The trephine has a central hole to accommodate some of the removed cement, and the instrument at top right is for removal of this cement through the slot seen in the trephine.*

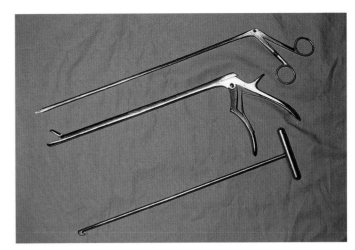

Figure 10.14 – *Long fine (top) and larger (middle) cement-grasping forceps and, at bottom, a reverse cutting hook.*

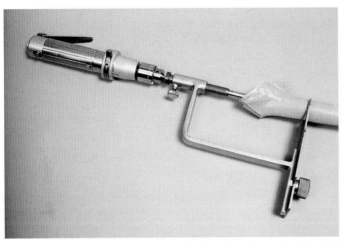

Figure 10.13 – *Revision jig assembled to show the principles. In use, it would be put more distally in the femur down to the full depth of the phosphor bronze bush. The drill is accurately centralized within the medullary canal.*

The jig can be dismantled and a tap inserted into the track, when it may be possible to extract the plug. If not, chisels can be used because there is now a central hole. A reverse cutting hook (Fig. 10.14) can be put down through the hole and knocked back up. Thought is, however, required because the view at this depth is very limited, and it is possible to get hooks jammed deep to slightly loosened cement plugs. At some point in this stage, elements of any plastic plug will be found and it should be possible to remove this completely. The plug can be grasped with fine, long, cement forceps (Fig. 10.14), moved around in the distal femur until clearly free, and

then withdrawn. If the plug is loose, but there are difficulties in withdrawing it, adherent wall cement is probably present. This can be removed with the 15° angled chisel (attacking it from proximally) and the reverse cutting hook (attacking it from distally). When all the cement has been cleared, it is possible to bring the hook back up along all sections of the femoral cortex without running into any obstructions.

Cement can usually be removed in the above way even if significantly distal to the isthmus (see Figs 9.2b and 9.4). Care must be taken, however, that the isthmus is wide enough to allow the plug to come back up. If not, the isthmus needs to be enlarged with reamers. A case in which a fenestration was planned and used is shown in Figure 10.15.

Ultrasound also has a significant place in the removal of distal plugs, particularly if the device is such that it can be sunk into the plug and rotated with the subsequent application of a slap hammer. This becomes the equivalent of drilling and tapping a plug without the requirement of any centring device.

Special situations

Often (particularly after a previous revision), as previously noted under 'Planning' in Chapter 9, there are femoral perforations. It is very helpful to locate these through splits in the vasti so that the cement can be removed from them directly. Occasionally (particularly in ill-executed anterolateral approaches), very large posterior extrusions of cement are found, which can be quite easily removed under direct vision. Often, in such cases,

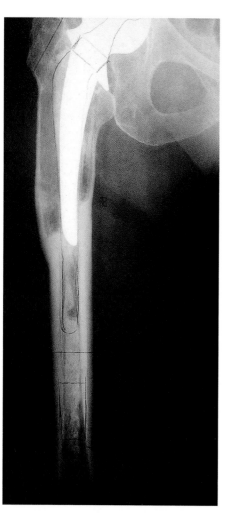

Figure 10.15 – *A case in which femoral fenestration was decided on at the planning stage (bottom two lines). The planned position for the tip of the stem is seen to be well proximal to the window. The middle line is the position of a Kirschner wire planned to prevent migration of the plug if necessary.*

much of the cement is outside the canal. With cement extrusions elsewhere, greater care is needed to avoid significant damage to vessels in the vasti.

Rarely, the whole of the femoral cement is loose in one extremely large chunk and the femur much enlarged around it, whereas the extreme upper end of the femur is still narrow. In these circumstances, the upper femur cannot be sufficiently enlarged and it is necessary to break the cement up in some way while still loose and deep within the femur. It may be possible to hold it with a drill and tap, while at the same time reducing it in size with chisels.

Stem fracture

Cement needs to be carefully removed down to the level of the fracture, although this is unlikely to be difficult. The procedure then depends on the special apparatus that is available. If apparatus is not available, the case should have been referred. Available devices include those that go round the stem and grasp it (the Zimmer stem extraction kit) and those that drill into it (principally the

Anspach and Midas Rex systems). For several years, the author used the specially made Phoenix system which simply allowed a hole to be drilled, using special hardened drills, into the distal fragment, followed by the insertion of special taps. This system (one never made commercially) worked well, but was, however, unsatisfactory with the modern, harder, stem materials. The Zimmer stem extraction kit is quite simple to use, but may give an insufficient hold with fractured stems of certain dimensions. This system drills a cylindrical slot in the cement around the distal stem fragment and grasps it by a collet system. The Anspach and Midas Rex systems can be used for stems of any material and any dimension. Dry bone practice is, however, essential before being put into practice. Both are designed to drill a hole into the fragment, which is then undercut. In the Anspach system, a rod with an attachable slap hammer has a small piece of malleable metal fixed to the end of it, which is impacted into the undercut. If correctly fashioned, there is sufficient hold on the fragment to extract it. The Midas Rex system drills an undercut of a different shape.

If irretrievable failure of the apparatus occurs, such that the hole in the fragment is stripped and no other adequate surface is available, the correct procedure is to drill a hole about 6 mm in diameter obliquely upwards and inwards through the cortex of the femur and the cement, so that the inner end is near the top of the distal fragment. Cement in the hole is cleared and a sharp chisel with the flat of its bevel pointing distally is put up against the side of the distal fragment at the distal end of the hole, and hit sharply. If all has been done correctly, the fragment shifts a few millimetres proximally and the chisel can be reinserted. This system can chiefly be applied to older types of stem of softer material when the fragment comes out with a number of transverse marks, but by using special carbide punches the same principle can be used with stems of newer and/or harder material. The method is hugely preferable to making a long very distal window that allows a punch to be put against the distal end of the stem. Such a window inevitably compromises reconstruction, whereas a small proximal hole can easily be blocked with a finger and bypassed with a stem of normal length.

As a final step, as with the acetabulum, all membranes need to be cleared. This is sometimes surprisingly difficult if the membrane is particularly adherent. A neat system is to hold it with grasping forceps and then use a cement chisel in the fashion of a periosteal elevator. Not infrequently, very large pieces of membrane can then be extracted, these sometimes (although only in the case of gross loosening) coming out in the shape of a large complete fingerstall. The distal membrane needs to be extracted with a hook.

Ultrasound (B. Bradnock)

Ultrasound is the term used for a high-frequency vibration (above 16 kHz) which travels through air, liquid, or solid media as pressure and displacement waves. In a bounded system, standing waves may be established, which produce a much greater concentration of acoustic energy and scope for rapid local heating at absorption sites. The first known experiments in the removal of bone cement using ultrasound were made at the EndoKlinik in Hamburg in the early 1970s. Bone cement is remarkable in that it can maintain a temperature gradient of 200°C over a distance of 1 mm. This means that, if molten cement can be removed rapidly, the residual cement hardly increases in temperature, thus minimizing damage to adjacent bone. In the initial studies in Hamburg, however, it was found difficult to remove the molten cement.

Over the last few years, several ultrasonic systems have been developed to assist the surgeon in revision arthroplasty. These systems are similar but not identical; the differences are discussed in detail later.

One of the major benefits of ultrasonic cement removal is that it is now possible for the probe to be de-tuned electronically when it comes into contact with bone. All commercially available systems have this technology, but the sensitivity of the de-tuning varies. Animal studies carried out by the author using a computerized system developed by Orthosonics (OSCAR – Fig. 10.16)) have demonstrated that, when the tip of the probe is in contact with the endosteal bone surface for a period of 10 s, cell death to a depth of only 50 µm occurs. This contrasts with cell death to a depth of 50 µm, which occurs when bone cement thicker than 9 mm is applied to the endosteal surface. Using this system, it is possible for the bone to be recognized and the probe to de-tune when bone is paper thin as a result of the fact that the system is computerized, unlike some other ultrasonic cement-removal systems.

It was mentioned earlier that inserting osteotomes into a ring of cement causes expansion of the ring, and thus increases the risk of fracture of the surrounding bone. This risk can be averted by using ultrasonic cement-removal techniques to remove cement in longitudinal grooves linked together by internal circumferential grooves.

Thus, with a combination of ultrasonic instrumentation and normal hand instruments, it is possible to remove segments of cement by folding the segments inwards, breaking along the lines where the grooves have been made through the cement mantle, so avoiding undue stress on the attenuated cortical bone.

This is the author's preferred option for removing cement proximally in the upper third of the cement mantle. More distally, it is possible to use ultrasonic

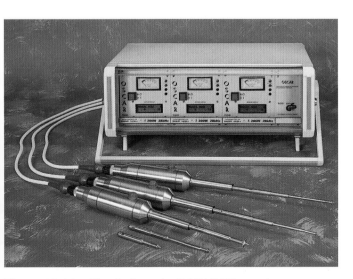

Figure 10.16 – *The Orthosonics OSCAR Ultrasonic cement removal apparatus.*

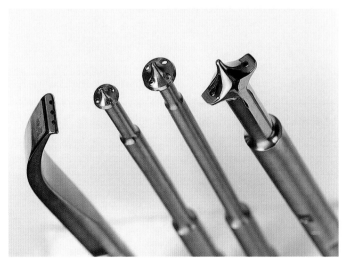

Figure 10.17 – *Ultrasonic wave guides with groover, piercer, and back scraper tips.*

equipment that is reverse cutting such as a back scraper (Fig. 10.17); this is used in a retrograde manner to remove cement from the endosteal surface down to the plug. Before attempting to remove the plug, it is necessary to remove the cement from the proximal femur down to the level of the plug. This allows the plug to be approached without the ultrasonic wave guide being compressed by bone or residual cement, which would cause the ultrasonic energy reaching the tip of the wave guide to be reduced and compromise the instrument's function.

It should also be noted that, in many instances, it is necessary to remove bone from the greater trochanter (if this has not been osteotomized), to allow straight access down the femur and to avoid bony impingement of the wave guide. Removal of the plug can be done by embedding an ultrasonic tip into the solid cement plug and applying a slap hammer. This works only if the proximal cement plug is wider than the distal cement plug, i.e. proximal to the isthmus. It is not always clear from radiographs whether or not it is possible to remove cement in this manner; in the author's experience it is preferable to embed an ultrasonic probe into the cement and try to pull it out by hand or apply gentle hammer blows to the slap hammer.

With a computerized ultrasound system, the frequency of the wave guide can be changed, depending on its impedance. The impedance of the wave guide changes quite considerably when it is embedded firmly into cement. With other systems, the wave guide is energized using a standard ultrasonic generator and, when the impedance of the wave guide changes as a result of the device becoming embedded in cement, it may not be possible for the ultrasonic generator to re-energize the wave guide; thus, it is possible for the probes to become stuck in cement.

An alternative to using a slap hammer to remove the plug is to use a piercer (see Fig. 10.17). This is a round, cone-shaped wave guide with multiple holes. The cement liquefies at the tip of this wave guide, flows through these holes, and becomes solid when outside the area of focused ultrasonic energy. After inserting the wave guide through approximately 1 cm of cement, it should be withdrawn and the cement wiped off using a damp swab.

The process can then be repeated after irrigating the femoral cavity to reduce thermal injury to the surrounding bone. When inserting the wave guide into the plug of cement, it is sometimes possible to detect thin

laminations of bone within the cement itself. These laminations are produced when blood is mixed with the cement, and over the years this layer of blood calcifies. This thin layer of bony tissue is sufficient to stop progress of a sensitive computerized ultrasonic system and, under these circumstances, it is necessary to scratch away the bone using an end-cutting, T-handled, Charnley reamer or other similar instrument. A wave guide with a gentle curve can also be of benefit because, when the wave guide tip touches bone, a new course can be made through the cement simply by rotating the handset through 90°, allowing further progress through the cement plug.

The secret in cement removal is to apply very little pressure to the handset, thus allowing the wave guide room to oscillate within the cement. If excessive pressure is applied to the handset, the wave guide vibration is dampened and the heating process of the cement reduced dramatically. When removing the distal cement plug, a polythene cement restrictor is often encountered. The polythene cement restrictor absorbs ultrasonic energy more than polymethylmethacrylate (PMMA) and thus a slight resistance is felt during the cement-removal process. On these occasions, it is necessary to wait a few seconds to allow the perforated wave guide to heat up the polythene and then make progress through the restrictor. As a consequence of this, the polythene that is heated up gets hotter than bone cement and it is necessary to irrigate the femur regularly during removal of cement and the cement plug. Once the plug is pierced, it is possible to remove the residual cement with a retrograde cutting device, such as the back scraper or some form of intramedullary hook. Alternatively, purely mechanical methods can be used, as already described.

Another method of cement removal in cases where the cement–bone interface is very poor is to remove cement from one side of the femur (usually from the side where the cement is thickest), to go through the cement plug eccentrically on the side that has had cement removed, and thus convert the cement cylinder into a C shape. When the cement is C shaped, there is some 'give' in it and it is usually possible to remove it as a single fragment.

It is possible to customize wave guides and this can be of benefit in patients with severe bowing of the femur. It is obviously preferable in such patients to remove the cement in small steps using a piercer rather than a slap hammer technique; with the latter it is possible to pull the broken fragment of cement and the wave guide itself through the thin femoral cortex.

Ultrasonic cement removal produces fumes. These fumes have been analysed in great detail. The only recognizable substance that is harmful is benzene, but, interestingly, the level of benzene that is encountered during cement removal is less than the level detected at fuel pumps when cars are being filled up with petrol.

References

1. Vidalain JP. The mechanical cement extractor: an original device for cement extraction in total hip arthroplasty revision. *Hip Int* 1996; 6: 155–158.
2. Eftekhar NS. Rechannelization guides. *Total Hip Arthroplasty,* Vol II. St. Louis: Mosley, 1993; 1221–5.

CHAPTER 11

Reconstructional techniques

M. D. Northmore-Ball

A large number of fundamentally different types of reconstruction are in current use. Proponents of any one type achieve very good results, in their own practices, with that particular technique and, as a result, its indications tend to be extended, with the consequence that it is suggested that most revisions should be done in that particular way. In fact, it is not difficult to match different types of revision case with the major different reconstructional techniques available, so that most have an assigned place.

The types of revision statistically most likely to be needed are for aseptic loosening of a total hip replacement (THR) in middle-aged or elderly people, and revision of an endoprosthesis initially inserted for a subcapital fracture in elderly people. Although, on occasion, some additional technique may be preferable, the great majority of such cases can, in the author's view, be perfectly adequately reconstructed using cement alone, provided that careful attention is paid to a large number of details. These are described in this chapter. In cases, chiefly aseptic, with severe acetabular or femoral bone destruction, restoration of the skeleton by bone grafting may very well be desirable if the patient is young and fit enough for possible further revision in the future. Whether or not bone grafting is done should be considered quite independently of what type of fixation is to be used. Grafting is for skeletal augmentation; the use of cement for fixation is a separate question. In the past, these two topics were confused. Bone grafting was formally considered to be the prerogative of those who exclusively used cementless fixation and those who employed cement were considered to be averse to it. This is of course quite wrong and a combination of cement and grafts often can be excellent, both in the acetabulum and in the femur. The indication for grafting, however, is that the clock needs to be put back, if possible, as far as

the patient's skeleton is concerned. Such a consideration is much less relevant in elderly people.

The rest of this chapter largely relates to the common types of case noted above. The indications for more special techniques are considered in Chapter 12.

Cemented fixation

In primary surgery, a micro-interlocking of cement into the trabecular system can be achieved throughout the femoral interface and over any desired percentage of the acetabular interface (see Chapter 5). In a revision, the bed available initially for fixation is usually almost entirely sclerotic, and the area that can be made suitable for micro-interlock is always small. The early advocates of low-viscosity cement used it because it could enhance micro-interlock, as a result of the greater ease of squeezing it into the intertrabecular spaces, and this effect was enhanced by deliberate attempts to pressurize the cement.

Clearly, even with reduced viscosity and pressurization, cement cannot be driven into a sclerotic surface and it is almost certainly for this reason that many have reported poor results using cemented fixation in revisions. It is the author's view, however, that very good and long-lasting results can be achieved: in a personal consecutive series of 150 hip revisions, one-third having had at least one (maximum four) previous revisions, and one-third having proven deep infection, a 95% clinical and (on exclusion of hips treated with a cementless stem) a 90% radiographic survivorship at 10 years was seen [1]. The secret of success with cement in revision surgery is to assume that a micro-interlock is extremely unlikely, except over small areas, such as keying holes (discussed later) and the lesser trochanter, secure fixation being achieved by firm impaction of standard viscosity cement into the large and, fortunately, irregularly shaped acetabular and femoral cavities.

An essential part of the technique is to ensure that the cavities are closed; if not and perforations (pre-existing, deliberate, or accidental) are detected, these must be properly exposed and blocked so that the cavity, despite its hard surface, can have standard viscosity cement jammed sufficiently firmly to produce good, long-lasting fixation. Pressurizing techniques are essential. Many tend, unfortunately, to associate pressurization only with micro-interlock. This is quite untrue. The same techniques are applicable in revision, even though micro-interlock is not expected. Lavage and drying are important, but difficult to quantify, and may be of less over-riding importance than firm impaction/pressurization. In primary surgery, the object is to clean out the inter-trabecular spaces. In revision, this can be done only in an extremely limited way, but it seems overwhelmingly likely that, the cleaner and drier the sclerotic surfaces are, the better the fixation will be.

Acetabular reconstruction

Removal of all vestiges of membrane is vital. After using a curette, a sharp, high-speed burr is convenient. Areas of membrane can easily be left in less accessible areas (e.g. under an overhanging lip anterosuperiorly or in a pre-existing pubic keying hole). All must be removed. Setting aside any worry about infection, there is no way that cement can have any fixative value unless it is on a soft-tissue-free surface.

The next step is to establish the standard landmarks. As the hip has failed, it may be found that the teardrop and, not infrequently, the true floor itself were never located at the initial operation. In some ways, this is fortunate because it may well produce some measure of virgin terrain and reamable bone. Sometimes, a great deal of dissection and removal of membrane are needed to reach this area. The lateral wall of the ilium must then be unequivocally seen.

The intention should be to try to place the centre of the socket as closely as possible to the original anatomical position. A high position should be accepted only if a much more complex reconstruction (e.g. with rings or grafts) were required in a patient not suitable for this extra work. The term 'high hip centre' is often used; such a description should, however, really be regarded only as representing acceptance of the difficulty of achieving an anatomical centre of rotation, rather than representing a

special principle in itself. Techniques for distalizing the socket are discussed later.

Cement pressurization is achieved by two completely separate mechanisms: first, a cement pressurizer and, second, the cup itself. If, therefore, a trimmable flanged cup is used, the next step should be to do the necessary minimal reaming and to trim the cup so that it can work as a pressurizer. It is likely that reaming is mainly needed on the lateral margins of the acetabulum only, although sometimes, if the acetabulum has been malpositioned, deepening may be possible. It is assumed that cheese-grater reamers are used. The acetabulum is likely to present as a rather large hole with an overhanging outer rim, so that it is larger from front to back on the inside than at the mouth. This is undesirable, and it is best to correct as far as possible, even at the expense of a degree of over-reaming laterally. The reamers should be taken down somewhat distally also in the region of the teardrop in order to make as good a seating as possible for the pressurizer (see below). The socket flange is then trimmed to the best fit, with the realization that this will be rather poor.

Cups in the DePuy–Charnley systems may have a reverse curve for the flange (the Ogee) in the region of the ischium but, if the cup does not have this feature, the flange can easily be bent appropriately outwards in the same way. Radial splits may be appropriate in the flange, especially anterosuperiorly, because it is important to make use of as much of the available fixation surface as possible. The socket is trimmed to allow about 10° of anteversion. Some monoblock revision stems with longer necks have a more valgus neck–stem angle than the equivalent primary components; if one of these should be needed, the cup would also need to be slightly 'closed'.

Small adjustments of the flange, together with repeated applications of reamers, are required until the best position and fit are obtained.

With unflanged cups, it is particularly important to preserve the residual superolateral lip, as far as possible. An eroded lip gives a very large uncovered area of cement with an unflanged cup and makes adequate cementation difficult. The reamers are chiefly used to determine the size of the socket. The maximum socket diameter that can be accommodated will be about 4 mm smaller than the reamer that fits the acetabulum from front to back, but a socket of this size often tends to be protuberant superolaterally. If the reamers are orientated in the same direction as its socket, the appropriate size (usually much smaller) to give almost complete coverage superolaterally can be determined easily. Such a reconstruction, however, tends to give a 'high hip centre'. This has a bearing on the femoral reconstruction and should have been considered in the planning.

Preparation for cementation

The best gross overall shape for the acetabulum has now been achieved, and the precise positioning and fit of the socket in it determined. It is necessary to give the cement the best possible chance of a secure fix. The previous keying holes are available. If the pubis or ischium lacks a hole, one should be made. In the pubis, it is safest to make a small initial hole with a curette or a small drill, feeling with the opposite hand for the pubic symphysis to help with the direction. The small hole in the sclerotic acetabular surface can then be enlarged, and often a blunt instrument, such as an acetabular pusher, can be impacted to give quite a large hole. The closed nature of the cavity should be checked with a small instrument. If a large drill is used initially, it is all too easy to make a perforation into the pelvis. If an ischial hole has to be made, it is a good plan to feel exactly under any residual posterior osteophyte for the lateral margin of the ischium. In the absence of normal anatomy, it is again quite easy to make this hole in the wrong position and perforate through posteriorly or medially. An unrecognized posterior hole could obviously be disastrous.

In the ilium, if not already present, a large keying hole can be made, somewhat medially and posteriorly, towards the sacroiliac joint. If too anterior, this again perforates medially. A large number of other small holes, or indentations, can then be made with a burr in the sclerotic surfaces. In the principal iliac load-bearing area, the orientation of the bone–cement surface should be considered in relation to the applied load. If the socket has migrated superiorly and the roof is therefore proximal, there may be a large superolateral sclerotic surface deep to the outer wall of the ilium in a very unfavourable direction (Fig. 11.1). This surface may act as little more than a cement restrictor, but sometimes it can be made to take the load by fashioning indentations in it in the shape of steps.

Perforations

Plans must be made for the blockage of any acetabular perforations, either pre-existing, deliberately made at the

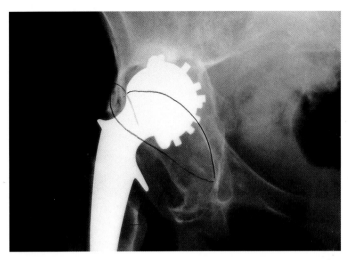

Figure 11.1 – *Severely eroded acetabulum: old-type metal/metal McKee in a very old patient reconstructed with cement only (the reinforcement ring drawn on the plan was not used). The lateral side of the inner surface of the acetabulum superiorly is in a very unfavourable direction for taking any load, and chiefly acts as a cement (or graft) restrictor.*

time – for example, of medial plug removal – or made accidentally later. In the types of case now under discussion, none of these is likely to be large. It is important, however, that they are all blocked in a thoroughly reliable fashion. Ill-placed, poorly fixed, or weak pieces of mesh can all too easily lose position during the application of cement or intrude into the pelvis during pressurization (Fig. 11.2). Proprietary mesh

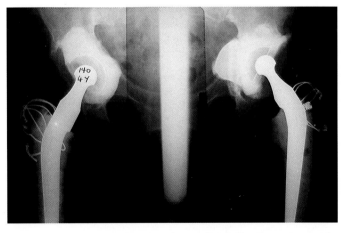

Figure 11.2 – *Composite AP pelvic radiograph of a patient with bilateral revisions and large bilateral medial floor defects, both films being at about 4 years. The defect on the left (right hip) was blocked with a firm preliminary mix of fast-setting cement. The defect on the right (left hip) was blocked with wire mesh only, which was too weak and displaced medially during pressurization. Note the large resulting lucency in zone 3 on the left.*

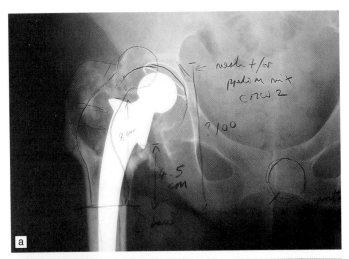

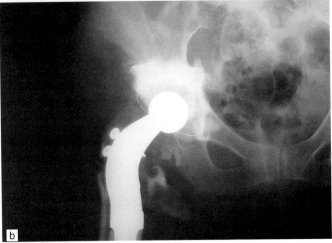

Figure 11.3 – *Planning X-ray of an elderly patient with gross failure of a Howse total hip replacement (a) before and (b) after revision to a AO tumour resection prosthesis. The superomedial acetabular defect was blocked with a proprietary mesh cement restrictor, fixed firmly enough to resist cement impaction. Mesh was also needed in this case posterosuperiorly.*

cement restrictors of the type sometimes still used to block a central pilot hole in primary surgery can be useful (Fig. 11.3 and see Fig. 11.8), but their hold is usually less secure in the sclerotic bone of the revision situation. It is often convenient to trim the edges of these restrictors and impact them with a pusher so that they are just below the surface. A simple, adaptable, and very reliable method is to use a small quantity of fast-setting (e.g. CMW2) cement as a preliminary mix (Fig. 11.4). More than one perforation, if present, can be blocked simultaneously. Combinations of mesh and cement, and grafts, are considered later. Clearly, it is not sensible to waste a large quantity of allograft simply in order to produce a small piece of femoral head to block a small perforation.

Pressurization

It would be wrong to embark on revision surgery in the absence of an effective pressurization tool. The author currently uses the Exeter balloon pressurizer (Fig. 11.5) and also a version (DePuy) of the CMW pressurizer with a 45° angle (Fig. 11.6) and [5].

Pressurizers can be placed in one of two positions. The first, and traditional, method is to place them against the mouth of the acetabulum. This unfortunately requires blocking of the cotyloid notch. This may be quite easy in a primary case, but is more difficult in a revision case and certainly requires a preliminary mix of fast-setting cement. Even then the seal may not be entirely trustworthy. The second position, favoured by

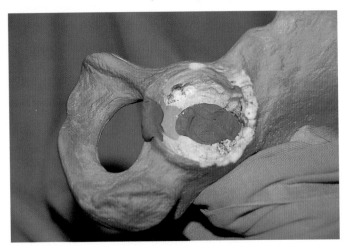

Figure 11.4 – *Laboratory model to show blockage of a central defect (and in this case also the cotyloid notch) with a small quantity of fast-setting cement.*

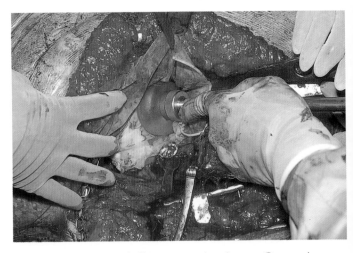

Figure 11.5 – *Exeter balloon pressurizer in use. Cement is gradually oozing out from posterosuperiorly, indicating a persistent positive pressure within the socket.*

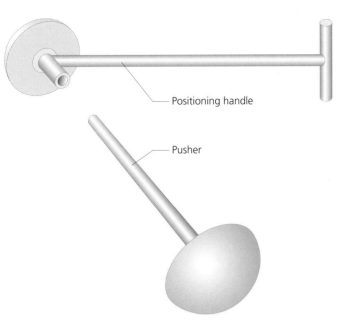

Figure 11.6 – *The angled acetabular pressurizer.*

the author (Fig. 11.7), is to disregard the area of the acetabulum distal to the teardrop and make the seal with the pressurizer against the floor of the acetabulum in that region. The cotyloid notch does not then need to

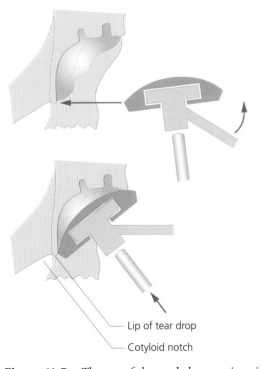

Figure 11.7 – *The use of the angled pressurizer, in which its rim abuts distally against the acetabular floor adjacent to the teardrop rather than against the acetabular rim; this principle overcomes the problem of cement leakage through the large acetabular wall defect represented by the cotyloid notch.*

be blocked. This is usually the best option in revision surgery. If the Exeter device is used, it is important to check that the annular balloon is properly filled without air bubbles so that it can expand adequately to seal around the enlarged socket properly. If the straight or angled CMW instrument is used, a head size is selected about 0.5–1 cm larger than the anteroposterior dimension of the acetabulum, as judged by reamers.

The angled CMW instrument is simple to use but, if the acetabulum is extremely irregular, the Exeter device may be preferable. Whichever device is used, it is extremely important to do a trial insertion of it into the empty acetabulum. The way it sits and its fit can then be judged. It is one thing to use a pressurizer, but, unfortunately, quite another to achieve pressurization, as can be quite easily demonstrated.

Cementation

Everything is now set up and the final rituals of a rotary brush followed by pulsed lavage and drying can be done. After drying, small swabs soaked in hydrogen peroxide may be inserted into the keying holes and pressure applied. It is important to make sure that, when the swabs are withdrawn, any mesh which may have been used to block a perforation is not dislodged. The swabs are then removed and the socket filled with cement and pushed digitally into the keying holes. The pressurizer and the socket are effectively a very crude piston in a cylinder. The travel of the 'piston' is extremely limited and it is vital, therefore, that the 'cylinder' is completely filled with cement initially. The pressurizer is then inserted and, on the assumption that it has been decided to use it in the second of the two methods given above, its inferomedial edge is pressed firmly against the region of the teardrop, while the remainder of the device (expanded in the case of the balloon pressurizer) is then brought up against the remainder of the cement, sealing against the insides of the anterior and posterior walls and against the supero-lateral lip. The Exeter pressurizer needs to be covered in a piece of glove rubber and it may be necessary also to put some sort of detaching agent on to the surface of the head of the DePuy device. Cement should then be seen gradually to leak out superolaterally. The instrument can be removed (by sliding it off the cement superolaterally in the case of the angled pressurizer) and reapplied if necessary. The author also puts cement under the flange of flanged cups before insertion to reduce the dead space, although the effect of this is unquantifiable.

The time for which cementation should be maintained is determined by how good the fit of the socket is into the acetabulum. If a flanged cup is being used and a very good rim seal has been achieved, the pressurizer can be removed relatively early (say, at 3 min) and the socket inserted. If, however, there are large gaps around it or, alternatively, if an unflanged socket is being used, the socket itself will only achieve very little, if any, pressurization and the pressurizer should be left on for a considerably longer period. With standard viscosity cement at ordinary operating room temperature, however, it is unlikely that it will be safe to leave it in place until more than about 4.5 min from the start of mixing, desirable though this might be.

Socket orientation

This has already been referred to. It is vital, however, that the socket is put exactly into the previously rehearsed position. The feel of the socket going in is quite different from at the trial insertion and, in addition, there is some obscuring of the periphery by extruded cement; it is all too easy for the socket to be cemented in in a position slightly different from the one intended. It is most important, therefore, to clear cement quickly from some easily visible part of the periphery, such as superolaterally, to make sure that the rehearsed position has been exactly achieved. The best position depends, to some degree, on the components used, but has been referred to above. If the socket is to be put in a somewhat closed position, it is particularly important to antevert it. Failure to do this results in the femoral neck hitting the rim of the socket in flexion and, although the horizontal position of the socket has a subjectively stable appearance when seen on an antero-posterior (AP) radiograph, impingement in flexion will occur with the strong likelihood of a posterior dislocation.

The final step is to remove any residual overhanging bone, particularly anteriorly; a deliberate search needs to be made for anything likely to cause impingement.

Use of reinforcement rings

Purely cemented fixation, as described above, has a very wide application. In certain badly destroyed acetabula, however, it may be inadequate, particularly in the following circumstances:

- It is clear that, after making a seriously or multiply perforated acetabulum into a closed cavity, very little host bone will be available for fixation (i.e. direct cement–host bone contact)

- The shape of the remaining acetabular rim makes the fit of any pressurizer too poor
- There is such severe superior resorption that without the use of some special method the socket will be too proximal. In these circumstances reconstruction may be supplemented by screw-fixed rings without necessarily having any recourse to a bone bank.

The first indication is found most commonly in severe protrusio, with an acetabular floor deficient over a large area such that the acetabulum is simply a cylinder with no bottom (see Fig. 9.4). The second two indications are often found together in severe erosion of the acetabular roof (Fig. 11.8, and see Fig. 8.9). The latter is the more common situation. The reconstructional steps are then: reamers are used cautiously, partly as sizers, and an AO roof reinforcement ring 4 mm smaller than the last reamer is chosen. It is made to sit in the acetabulum in a stable position; it will almost certainly be quite proximal, and there will be some gaps superolaterally.

Having decided on its position, a plan can be made about blockage of acetabular defects. Although the socket is now being fixed largely by screws (i.e. largely cementless), cement leakage must still be prevented. Defects may be blocked before or after ring insertion, depending on their size and position. Sometimes, the ring needs to be screwed in place with one screw, removed, mesh and a small

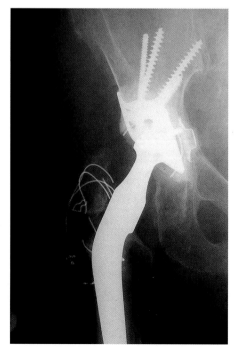

Figure 11.8 – *Eleven-year postoperative radiograph after a one-stage exchange for deep infection, the acetabulum being reconstructed using an AO hook ring as a result of severe proximal acetabular migration.*

preliminary mix inserted over a defect, and then the ring screwed back before the cement sets. This can be extremely effective. It is essential to screw the supero-medial screws up tight first. A position for the ring in which tightening of this screw produces a tendency to rock, particularly into a more open position, should not be accepted. Very occasionally, a superolateral screw whose head sits underneath the ring may be appro-priate – for example, in a one-stage exchange for infection in which the area is not filled by grafts (see Chapter 12).

Combinations of cortical and fully threaded cancellous screws may be used. It is not necessary to use a cancellous screw if the cortical screw gets a very firm hold (as it frequently does) in the sclerotic acetabular surface. Once one solid medial screw has been inserted, others can be put in, to a total of four or five. It may be best not to tighten superolateral screws maximally for fear of rocking the ring, but the others should be tightened maximally. Effectively, a partly screw-fixed, metal neoacetabulum has now been constructed which is continent and ready for contained cement. A socket is also quite easily cemented into the ring. Keying holes in the pubis and ischium are usually still available, or can be made. A gun may be required because it is most important to make sure that any spaces under the ring are thoroughly filled with cement, the effect of which is to lock together the screws and prevent any possible fretting between the screw heads and the ring. If a flanged socket is used, the roof to which the flange has to reach is now formed by the ring, and a much closer anatomical position can be achieved. There is then also no inhibition about putting the socket in in absolutely the desired position from the point of view of stability. Without the ring, there is a danger of being guided by the deficient rim and malpositioning the socket, with a risk of later instability.

In the first situation (Fig. 11.9a), where the acetabulum has no floor, the load has to be transferred on to the rim of the acetabulum and an Eichler ring is usually best. It may be possible to fix this with screws (Fig. 11.9b), although this may well not be possible. The sequence is as follows: the acetabulum is sized with reamers, and the rim is trimmed and flattened with hand tools and a burr (and the special Eichler reamers if available). A stable position for the Eichler ring on the

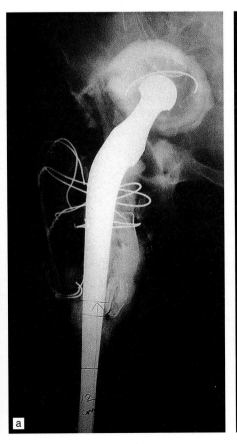
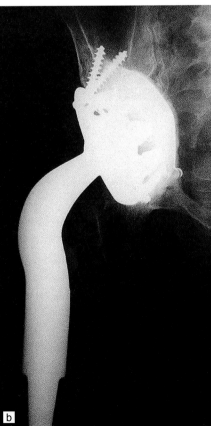

Figure 11.9 – *(a) Pre-revision radiograph of a previously multiply revised infected hip with complete medial dislocation of the socket. The anterior acetabular wall was also incomplete in this case. (b) Post-revision radiograph. In the reconstruction, a floor was made using wire mesh and a preliminary mix of cement and load was taken through an Eichler ring screw fixed on to the residual acetabular rim.*

177

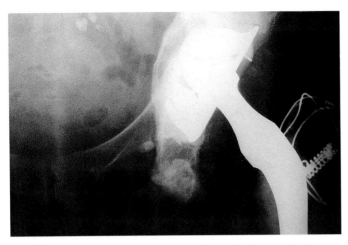

Figure 11.10 – *Late post-revision radiograph of a similar, but less severe and aseptic, case to that shown in Figures 11.10 and 11.11; the floor defect was blocked by a large corticocancellous graft from the inner table of the ilium.*

outside of the acetabulum should then be achieved, accepting the fact that it will be in a somewhat vertical position, inappropriate for the socket itself. A plan now needs to be made for blockage of the floor. In aseptic cases, a large corticocancellous graft from the inner table of the ilium can be taken (Fig. 11.10) and fashioned to fit the floor defect. The walls of the cylindrical acetabulum around the edges of this graft need to be fashioned with a burr, so that a preliminary mix of cement can be put around the margins of the graft to seal it, and probably over the graft itself unless it is quite strong. If the ring is being screwed into position, this can be done and the socket inserted. If the ring is not being screwed in, it is safest to cement it in next without the acetabular component, using a pusher or pressurizer to keep the inner side of the ring free from cement. The socket is then cemented in to this space as a further step. With very careful rehearsal, it is possible to put the ring in place and cement the socket into it in one procedure, but there is severe danger that either the ring will rock, weakening the fix greatly, or, worse still, the socket will not be inserted in the correct orientation. In septic cases (Fig. 11.9b), the same procedure can be done, but with a large piece of stiff wire mesh in the place of the graft.

Insertion of the stem

To make a trial stem sit in approximately the right position, it is almost certainly necessary to remove bone from the back of the lateral part of the upper femur in the region of the residual trochanteric bed, or the inside of the greater trochanter if not osteotomized. It is essential to have a 'straight shot' down the femur. If the femur has been walled across distal to the implant (pedestal formation in a cementless stem or its equivalent in a cemented stem), it is best to perforate through this and reach into the distal medullary canal. Successful entry is accompanied by marrow coming up the femur. Provided that the remainder of the cement has been removed in a logical fashion, so that the exact orientation of the femoral canal is known, there should be no difficulty in doing this. A drill is occasionally necessary. It should be possible now to place a long straight instrument down the femur through the isthmus, determining the position of the upper end within the femur.

A trial reduction is required. One of two unsatisfactory techniques is often used. These are, first, to use a very fat stem which jams within the femur and, second, to hold the trial stem in position in the expanded femur with small swabs. Neither of these works at all well. The principle of using a large stem within the femur is a bad one because it is bound to imply an incomplete cement mantle, and attempts to hold a smaller stem with swabs are very hit and miss. The bony landmarks at the top of the femur in a revision are poor, and it is all too easy to cement the stem in the wrong position. If it is put in too far and the system is modular all may be well, but most varieties of modularity (the Waldemar Link Reconstruction stem is an exception) do not allow for changes of version.

There are two ways, in principle, in which this problem can be overcome: to use an oversized rasp with a head neck unit or a trial prosthesis with adjustable dimensions.

Use of over-sized rasp

When using an over-sized rasp, the handle can be detached and replaced by a head-neck unit. With care, this will usually be successful, but it relies on one of quite a small range of rasp sizes being of just the right dimensions, and on the definitive prosthesis, smaller in size than the rasp, then being cemented in with exactly the same protrusion from the femur and exactly the same orientation. Although relatively easy in a primary case, the rasp may well be supported only at limited points and significant errors in positioning the prosthesis, perhaps sufficient to cause dislocation, can come about. This problem did not arise with the straight-stem Muller system, but the duo-lock principle whereby the stem was expected to jam within the femur, leaving cement to fill the remaining space, goes against modern thinking in terms of cement mantles, as noted above.

Use of an adjustable trial prosthesis

This involves use of a trial prosthesis whose dimensions are adjustable. In this system, the trial prosthesis is inserted, a trial reduction is done, the position of the head and neck is adjusted, and the size of the prosthesis to be inserted, and a landmark on the femur, are determined so that the definitive prosthesis can be inserted exactly in this chosen position. Such a system is currently available for the Charnley and DePuy Elite systems only (although one has been specially made for the author for the Elite Plus) but, as the apparatus has, in principle, a very wide possible applicability (i.e. to many other types of stem), it seems appropriate to describe it briefly here. The only other prosthesis available with an adjustable trial, although not

relevant to the present chapter, is the AO tumour resection prosthesis, in which the trial is extensile. At the trial reduction, its length can be adjusted until stability is found and then the appropriate prosthesis selected.

The principle of the adjustable trial prosthesis and the method of using it are shown in the laboratory series in Figure 11.11. A long spigot, which has tapered wings at the upper end (Fig. 11.11a), is impacted into the shaft of the femur. Its upper end has a rod attached to it. After impaction of the spigot, the rod is in an exact line with the medullary canal (Fig. 11.11b). An adjustable head-neck unit is then slid on to this rod. Figure 11.13b shows one with a head of 22.25 mm, but heads of 28 mm and 32 mm are also available. The head-neck unit can then be locked in any position by a screw. A trial reduction is done and the position of the head neck unit can be adjusted to the desired position, in terms of soft tissue tension, leg length, and anteversion, and locked (Fig. 11.11c,d). The drill guide is then fixed on to it. This guide has a number of holes corresponding to the neck–

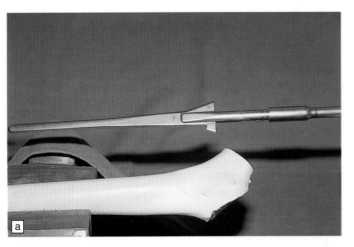
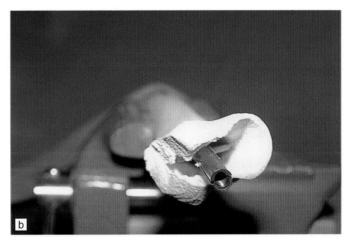
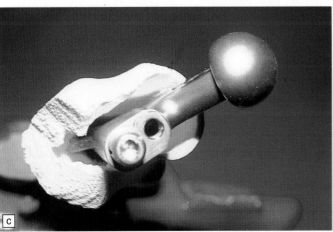
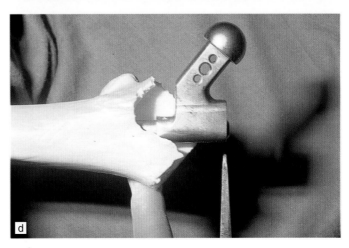

Figure 11.11 – *Steps in the use of the adjustable trial prosthesis (see text).*

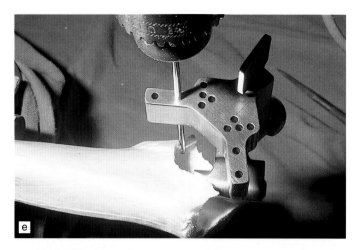

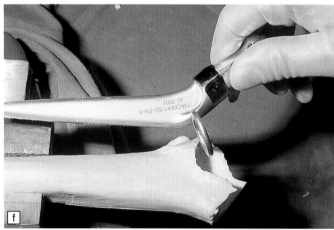

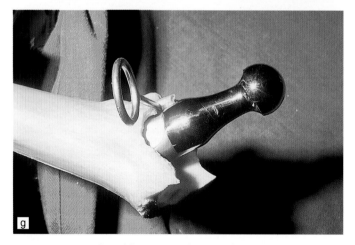

Figure 11.11 – *(cont'd) Steps in the use of the adjustable trial prosthesis (see text).*

removed from the femur, the position of the head, in terms of leg length and anteversion, will be exactly the same as the adjustable head when the chosen prosthesis is used and its neck–stem junction is put up against the pin; the stem of the prosthesis is also exactly neutral in a varus/valgus sense. In primary surgery, the femoral neck is cut-off flush with the pin, but in a revision this is not usually necessary. Finally, a soft pin, which will not scratch the prosthesis, is substituted for the hard pin (Fig. 11.11f,g) before cementation. As with all devices, the adjustable trial prosthesis has its limitations, particularly in cases of more severe than usual bone loss in the trochanteric region. It is best if a neck length of prosthesis can be selected so that the pin is held both anteriorly and posteriorly. Nevertheless, quite frequently, a hold in the posterior cortex only has to be accepted. With care, however, this is quite sufficient.

Trial reduction

Correct femoral orientation at the trial reduction, and its reproduction when the definitive stem is inserted, is crucial to stability. Whether or not an adjustable trial prosthesis is used, the femoral stem has to be sufficiently anteverted so that the front of the femoral neck does not impinge on the edge of the socket until at least 90° of flexion in some internal rotation. Too great an anteversion, however, causes impingement of the back of the neck against the posterior lip of the socket in extension, so a compromise has to be selected. With most systems, an anteversion of 10–15° is about right. Ideally, the length should be such that the tightness of the reduction is correct when the leg lengths are equalized and this can often be achieved, although it is safer to concentrate on the tightness of the reduction. This should be such that, when moderate traction is applied (telescoping) by the surgeon and his opposite thumb is on the articulation, the surfaces just perceptibly come apart. A tighter reduction is perfectly acceptable, provided that the greater trochanter, if osteotomized, then comes down to the right position. If the tightness of the reduction is such that more than moderate tension is put on the trochanter, the potential gain in terms of stability from the tightness is more than offset by potential trochanteric escape. Attempts to simplify trochanteric reattachment by allowing a deliberately slack reduction are, however, unwise.

stem junction, i.e. the re-entrance immediately below the collar, of several different sizes of prosthesis.

A hole is made in the residual femoral neck or trochanteric region by drilling through one of these holes (Fig. 11.11e) and a hard pin is put through this hole after removing the jig. When the adjustable trial prosthesis is

Length of femoral stem

Provided that all the details of cementation have been given proper attention, fixation in the upper femur should be such that a stem of standard length can often be employed. If, however, there is quite severe erosion, so that a neck more than about 1 cm longer than standard is required, it is safer to use a slightly longer stem. How much longer than usual is determined largely by the available choice of implants. The stem does not need to be much longer than the standard one; stems with the tip reaching too far below the isthmus should be avoided if possible (see below).

As with the acetabulum, the femur now has to be made into a closed cavity.

Plugging the femur

Plugging the femur in revision surgery is more difficult than in primary surgery for three reasons: first, the walls are smooth; second, the medullary canal may be large; and, third, whereas in a primary case the plug is situated in the upper femur where the diameter is narrowing down distally, in a revision the walls may be parallel sided or, if below the isthmus, widening distally. Excluding cement plugs, all the available proprietary plastic or bioabsorbable intramedullary plugs may well not be sufficiently secure so that they slip distally during the pressure rises that occur during cement injection and stem insertion. A secure plug is nevertheless essential. Distal migration impairs cement pressurization. If pressurization is maintained, despite migration, fixation may be adequate, but the long distal plug of cement will make any subsequent revision much more difficult (see Fig. 9.2b).

Fortunately, migration of plugs is not a difficult thing to prevent [3]. If, when the plug is inserted, it is felt to have a weak hold at the desired position in the femur (i.e. immediately distal to the planned position of the tip of the stem), it should be extracted. Through a small split in vastus lateralis, a Kirschner wire is driven across the medullary cavity distally, as shown in Figure 11.12a and b. A fresh plug can then be inserted and it will impact against the Kirschner wire Fig. 11.12c. After cementation, the wire is withdrawn Fig. 11.12d. It is necessary to check that the wire is central in the medullary canal. An instrument may be put down to assess this. If it is too much off-centre, a second wire can be inserted. If the plug has to be in a very distal position (see Chapter 12) some way below the isthmus in the distal femur, two wires are

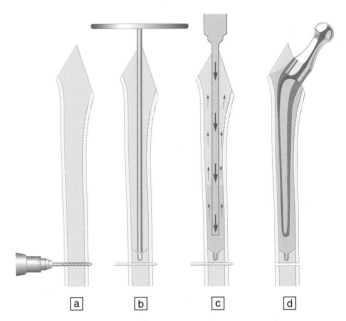

Figure 11.12 – *The transfemoral Kirschner wire technique to prevent distal migration of plastic plugs under cement pressure. In many femora, the femur can be transfixed with a Kirschner wire without first using the drill shown on the left. The procedure is particularly useful at and below the isthmus. Distally, two wires can be used if necessary.*

essential. A Steinman pin can be used percutaneously, but this has the disadvantage of producing a larger stress rising hole within the femur. An alternative is a cement plug; this, however, is much less convenient and may not be so secure. The Kirschner wire technique is free from complications and is recommended.

All holes in the femur must then be blocked, including defects diagnosed preoperatively, other smaller pre-existing defects found at prosthesis removal, a fenestration, if it was necessary to make one, and any accidental perforations. It is most important to acknowledge the last and locate them. If sufficiently big to impair cementation, it should have been possible to recognize them when made. A long curved forceps can be put down the femur and pushed out through the defect; its tip is felt and the vasti split. Small perforations can easily be blocked by the tip of an assistant's finger (Fig. 11.13). If slightly larger, a preliminary mix of fast-setting cement is convenient. A trial stem, or its equivalent, covered in glove rubber needs to be put down the femur to make quite sure that the lumen is not obstructed. If CMW2 is used, gentamicin may be added. If the defect is even larger, the pure cement technique becomes difficult to control and it is necessary to use mesh. Mesh by itself, however, is weak and it is best to seal it thoroughly and fix it with fast-setting cement

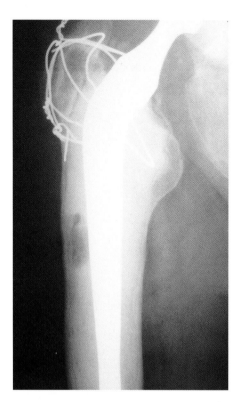

Figure 11.13 –
*Appearance
produced by
blockage of a
femoral defect by
an assistant's
fingers. In this case,
a defect was
produced in the
mantle down to the
stem itself, but this
late radiograph
shows that no
problem resulted.
The lesser
trochanter has also
been excavated to
produce anti-
rotational load
transmission.*

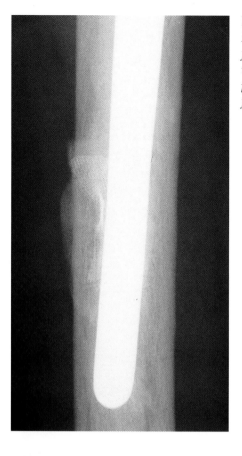

Figure 11.14 –
*Blockage of a
femoral defect
using mesh and a
preliminary mix of
fast-setting cement.*

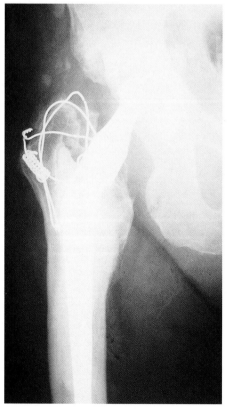

Figure 11.15 –
*Appearance 8 years
after one-stage
exchange of a
previously revised
infected hip with
several femoral
defects blocked at
operation by the
methods described.
There is a small
non-progressive
radiolucency in
Gruen zone 1 only.*

(Fig. 11.14). If the femur is being grafted endosteally (see Chapter 12), then a completely leak-proof seal is not required and the mesh can be held on with circlage wires. With pure cement fixation, however, a seal is essential or the cement, unlike graft, will ooze out, perhaps seriously, around the mesh.

A decision needs to be made about any defects in the upper femur, perhaps anteriorly running below the level of the lesser trochanter. The effective size of the defect is partly determined by how far down in the femur the stem is to be seated. Smallish defects can be excluded from cement fixation by an assistant's digit.

Slightly larger defects can, if necessary, be blocked easily with a preliminary mix of cement. Subsequent cementation is then likely to be very much easier. Figure 11.16 shows an AP radiograph of a femoral component 8 years after cementation, in which several holes had been blocked in this way.

Wires now need to be inserted. A modified cruciate system is recommended and is described below. The advantage of wiring systems is their adaptability.

Just before or after inserting the wires, the lesser trochanter should be excavated (see Fig. 11.13), as recommended by Wroblewski. The lesser trochanter is still present in the great majority of revisions and forms an excellent anti-rotational key. As it is virgin terrain, a degree of micro-interlock is also possible. A number of other indentations can be made with a burr in residual bone in the upper femur, concentrating on trying to prevent rotation. These are particularly vital if, for some reason, the lesser trochanteric keying hole is not available.

Femoral cementation

The femoral canal should be washed with pulsed lavage and dried. A catheter should then be put in the femur and a hydrogen peroxide-soaked swab is pushed down alongside it. It seems possible, however, that the hydrogen peroxide is unnecessary and that, instead, the femur should be washed and dried immediately before the insertion of cement. Sufficient cement should be available to fill the femur amply and this always implies two 40-g mixes, sometimes an extra 20-g mix, and, occasionally, another 40-g mix. No compunction should be felt about apparently wasting cement. The swab is removed from the femur and the femur filled using a gun with minimal delay. Delay at this moment causes pooling of blood in the neighbourhood of the plug. The femur should then be filled as quickly as possible.

The upper end now has to be sealed. Proprietary devices are available for this, but, particularly in the revision situation where the upper femoral edge is irregular, an adequate seal can be obtained simply by wrapping a gauze swab in glove rubber, applying a detaching agent to it if needed, and wrapping this around the nozzle. The seal is held with one hand while the other is used to work the gun (Fig. 11.16) and, at the same time, to prevent

the gun from pushing itself up out of the femur. The catheter is withdrawn, nipping it to try to prevent any blood inside it from being left in the femur.

If an unblocked femoral defect is present, a trial cementation should have been done so that the exact position of an assistant's fingers can be rehearsed. The nozzle of the gun is allowed to pump itself back out through the gauze and glove rubber seal and, with the same gauze and glove rubber, direct pressure is applied digitally. This simple method requires no special apparatus. If the femur has been very well filled, then quite a solid resistance is felt when the upper cement is pressed on. The upper cement, which is in contact with the femoral stem, is carefully dried and the stem should be insertable in one long smooth movement. No obstructions should be encountered and, if the cement has been properly impacted, considerable resistance should be felt. The holder should be removed just before the last few millimetres of seating to make absolutely certain that component orientation is correct. The component can then be pushed into its definitive position.

If an adjustable trial prosthesis is used, this is when the neck–stem angle is up against the pin, and is soon afterwards withdrawn. In other circumstances, some other local datum needs to have been selected. Assuming, as it should be, that there is a good mantle of cement all the way round the stem, it is all too easy for the stem to be pushed further into the femur, or its version changed, with potentially disastrous consequences, after full insertion and before the cement is set. An assistant can produce some gentle longitudinal pressure on the stem, sufficient to prevent it coming out, while the surgeon holds it very

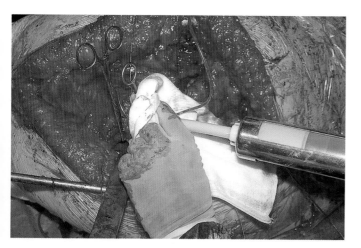

Figure 11.16 – *Femoral cementation in revision. The upper femur is obturated digitally with gauze over glove rubber; the irregularity of the upper end precludes the effective use of proprietary seals.*

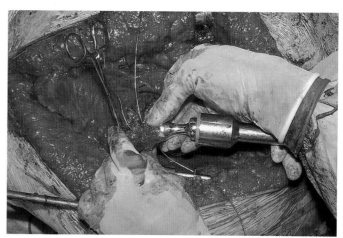

Figure 11.17 – *Maintaining digital pressure on exposed cement until curing.*

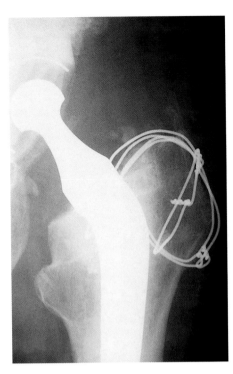

Figure 11.18 – *Appearance after cruciate wiring.*

may yet be well, although it might be necessary to guard against certain movements in the postoperative period (e.g. if the stem is slightly less anteverted than intended, the physiotherapist should be particularly warned about potential instability in flexion).

Trochanteric reattachment

The author has experience of the following: the original Charnley two-wire system; later modifications of the two-wire system; the Wroblewski spring-wire system used with a chevron osteotomy made with a Gigli saw; the Charnley three-wire cruciate technique; the Dall-Miles cable grip system; the Charnley staple clamp in association with cruciate wiring and a flat osteotomy; the Weber-type of chevron osteotomy made with a saw; and a modification of the Charnley cruciate wiring system. The last two in combination are strongly recommended. The basic wiring sequence is shown in Figure 11.19. The differences from the system described in Charnley's book *Low Friction Arthroplasty of the Hip: Theory and Practice* [4] are:

■ When the anteromedial wire is passed over the top of the trochanter (Fig. 11.19b,c), it is bent backwards as soon as it leaves the femur so that it passes posterior to the upper end of the femur at the front of the trochanteric bed. This step ensures that the wire remains truly running over the top of the trochanter rather than sliding around to the front.

■ The cruciate wiring system is done up completely (Fig. 11.19l) before tightening of the double vertical wire (Fig. 11.18m) and not the other way around.

carefully in position and, at the same time, blocks as much of the remaining exposed cement surface as possible; this should be almost invisible (Fig. 11.17) if it is being properly contained. After cementation, any blocked defect should be examined to check for cement leaks. Extruded cement can easily be removed.

The whole of the hip, and particularly the articulating surfaces of the socket and the stem, should be very carefully washed to reduce possible third body wear. It is surprising how often this step seems to be omitted.

The hip is then reduced and the appearance of the articulation should show precisely the same orientation as at the trial reduction. If it is not quite the same, all

Figure 11.19 – *(Facing page) (a) The wires have been inserted and the femoral component cemented in. Blue: double vertical wire (DVW); red: medial wire of the cruciate system; green: lateral wire of the cruciate system. (b/c) A thick awl is used to make a passage through the glutei hard up against the bone at the top of the trochanter and with a wire passer (not shown) the DVW is passed through. (d) A drill hole is made proximally and posteriorly (through two cortices), and through this is passed the postero-medial wire. (e) A fine awl is passed through the distal part of the trochanter bearing in mind that by muscle action it is now flexed. (f) The trochanter is extended (if necessary the hip is flexed at the same time) and the trochanter is harpooned onto its bed, making sure the chevron surfaces match. The insets show the trochanter anatomically reduced or advanced. (g) The DVW is tightened though not maximally. The wire tightener is left in place. The DVW is omitted from the following sequence for clarity. (h) The antero-medial wire is passed making sure that it is bent just below the anterior lip of the trochanteric bed, and passes also closely over the top of the trochanter, rather than anteriorly. This is an important step. (i) The postero-lateral wire is brought 'towards the patient's opposite shoulder (Charnley)', and the medial wires are crossed over it. (j) The medial wire is tightened up against a fine awl placed to stop the junction from migrating upwards and medially over the top of the trochanter. The fine awl is then removed; the medial wire slackens slightly. (k) The postero-lateral wire is now passed medially. (l) The lateral wire is tightened deep to the glutei. Before fully tightening, the twist in the medial wire is bent upwards and inwards. The DVW is then fully tightened and both wires are then finally tightened sequentially. (m) This shows the final position.*

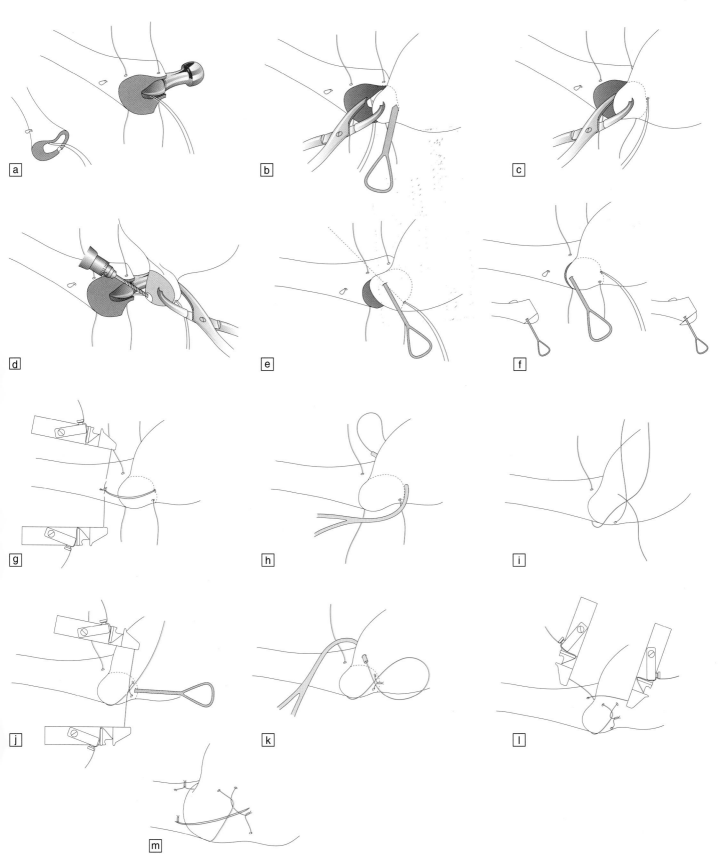

■ Before final tightening of the cruciate system (i.e. the twist in the lateral wire), the twist in the medial wire on the outside of the trochanter is bent upwards out of the way, and this twist is not then buried in the trochanter at the end of the cruciate tightening.

The final radiological appearance is seen in Figure 11.18. Although burying the wire in the trochanter, as in the traditional system, produces a very neat effect, it can very easily produce some slackening off of the cruciate compression system. Modifications to wire insertion may be needed. For example, the anterior drill hole for the medial wire may need to accommodate an anterior femoral deficiency, thus exiting the femur either much more medially or more laterally than usual. Sometimes, it is also necessary to take this wire round to the lateral side of the stem rather than medially. Occasionally, it may be found most convenient to pass the medial wire either through a drill hole in the lesser trochanter or even occasionally round the outside of the femoral cortex medially, just distal to the lesser trochanter.

In the reattachment, the trochanteric bed may be quite defective but, even then, the cruciate system can still produce sound union. In these circumstances, it is best to distalize the greater trochanter, mobilizing it if required (see Chapter 12), so that it sits well overhanging the distal end of the residual trochanteric bed. It is best then to connect up the double vertical wire (DVW) system, but not to tighten it until the cruciate wires have snugged the trochanter down in this new position. If the DVW is done up first, the trochanter is very likely to twist or tip out of the right position. An element of distal advancement is, in fact, highly desirable for union in all cases, but not to the extreme degree required when the trochanteric bed is seriously deficient.

Technique with a previous trochanteric non-union

A preliminary decision should have been made at the planning stage about whether to attempt a reattachment intended to achieve bony union (see Chapter 9). The practicability of this will have been decided on during the surgical approach, bearing in mind the lengthening of the hip with distalization of the trochanteric bed that almost certainly occurs. Suitable mobilization should, therefore, have been carried out. Further mobilization may need to be done at this stage. It is essential to mobilize the trochanter by deep dissection, so that it can be got down to the level of the trochanteric bed with only minor tension. If the trochanteric bed is quite good and the trochanter, after scarification of the non-union and flattening it with a saw, is large enough to feel that the wires will have a solid hold, a little tension, even with the leg slightly abducted, is acceptable. Significant tension so that the leg has to be markedly abducted, especially if in combination with doubtful wiring capability, is certain to result in early failure and is not worthwhile. The aim should still be to advance the trochanter slightly; this greatly increases its stability on the bed, as noted above. Dissection needs to be deep and not near to the trochanter; if the latter is done, the trochanter may be mobilized, but there will be little effective muscle still attached to it. In extreme cases, if this is carried out, the residual muscle attachment sometimes tears.

If it becomes clear (hopefully, at planning, but at least before wire insertion in the femur) that bony union is 'pie in the sky', the trochanter should be mobilized sufficiently for a strong soft tissue repair, if necessary using drill holes in the residual trochanter. In these circumstances, an abductor repair with the leg quite widely abducted may still be possible.

References

1. Izquierdo RJ, Northmore-Ball MD. Long-term results of revision hip arthroplasty. Survival analysis with special reference to the femoral component. *J Bone Joint Surg* 1994; 76B: 34–9.

2. New AMR, Northmore-Ball MD, Tanner KE, Cheah SK. *In vivo* measurement of acetabular cement pressurization using a simple new design of cement pressurizer. *J Arthroplasty* 1999; 14: 854–859.

3. Northmore-Ball MD, Narang OV, Vergroesen D. Distal femoral plug migration with cement pressurization in revision surgery and simple technique for its prevention. *J Arthroplasty* 1991; 6: 199–201.

4. Charnley J. *Low Friction Arthroplasty of the Hip. Theory and Practice*. New York: Springer-Verlag, 1979.

CHAPTER 12

Special problems in revision

M. D. Northmore-Ball

Revision for deep infection

This should be embarked upon only if (1) there is sufficient through-put of aseptic revisions for everyone concerned in the patient's treatment to be very familiar with them, and (2) an interested bacteriologist with a commitment to this type of work, together with suitable transport arrangements for specimens, is available. These matters have been referred to earlier (see Chapter 8).

One- or two-stage?

Many papers have been written on this subject, of which a selection are listed at the end of this chapter. The centre that probably has more experience of revision for infection than any other in the world is the EndoKlinik in Hamburg, where one-stage exchange is the rule and two-stage the exception, with very good results. However, numerically, there are probably more advocates of two-stage revision. Nevertheless, this is partly the result of the fact that one-stage exchange requires the addition of antibiotics of different types and often in substantial quantities to bone cement, and this procedure is not universally available. This, for example, is probably the reason for the lack of popularity of one-stage exchange in the USA.

One-stage exchange, if successful, has the following advantages. First, only one operation and one anaesthetic are required; although the operation may be a long one, it is not as long as two procedures, because the wound does not have to be closed and later reopened. Second, the patient is likely to have a considerably shorter period in bed and probably, therefore, a somewhat reduced risk of medical complications, such as venous thrombosis.

The advantages of two stages are: first, there is an opportunity to change the antibiotics in the cement at the second stage if bacteriology at the first stage gives an unexpected result. Second, if the bacteriology is correct at the first stage, there are two separate surgical and antibiotic assaults on the infection rather than only one; third, the surgeon will be fresh at the start of the reconstructional procedure in the second stage. The author has a policy of usually doing a one-stage exchange, but carrying out a two-stage exchange in the following circumstances:

- The biopsy has revealed an unusual organism or, alternatively, a common organism (notably *Staphylococcus epidermidis*), but with multiple antibiotic resistance
- The patient has diabetes or there is a particularly bad soft tissue infection, e.g. with multiple sinuses or tissue loss
- The soft tissue dissection and removal of previous implants and probably cement are very complex (particularly where previous revisions have been done)
- It is felt to be necessary to use bone grafts or an upper femoral bypass (see later), notably in a young patient, because in these circumstances no antibiotic will be present around significant parts of the implant
- Where the patient has had a previous one-stage exchange for infection that has failed, despite being carried out correctly.

Notes on operative technique in one-stage exchange

The débridement has to be very carefully carried out on the lines described Chapter 10 with removal of all foreign material, even if this is not apparently involved in the infective loosening process. Reconstruction techniques, but without using grafts, are then employed, as in Chapter 11. Antibiotics are added to the cement up to a total of 4 g in one 40-g mix (although usually not more than 3 or 3.5 g). At the present time, this is commonly gentamicin, although, unfortunately, resistance of *Staphylococcus epidermidis* to gentamicin is increasing. Others, such as a cephalosporin, a penicillin derivative, and, increasingly, vancomycin may be needed. It is best to withhold parenteral antibiotics until after the specimens have been taken so as to increase the chance of accurate bacteriology. If the antibiotics are started before the operation, there could in theory be a slightly increased chance of success, but the operative specimens might well be falsely negative. The author's practice is to keep the patient in bed for 3 weeks and to review the systemic antibiotics when the bacteriology is available, continuing with an appropriate oral antibiotic until about 6 weeks after surgery. There is, unfortunately, no reliable scientific basis on which to decide for how long antibiotics should be continued. Sound arguments can be made for a very much shorter period and there should be no concern about this if, for example, allergy occurs, so that the chosen antibiotic has to be withdrawn at a very early stage.

Notes on technique in two-stage exchange
The same minutely detailed débridement has to be done as if the components were about to be reimplanted. Unfortunately, it is common to receive patients who have nominally had the first stage of a two-stage exchange and then been referred, but in whom retained cement or other material may make a repeat first stage necessary

(Fig. 12.1). As the hip will shorten before the second stage, it is most important to mobilize the trochanter thoroughly and it is best to reattach this with rather marked distalization. The femur can, for example, be deliberately moved proximally while the trochanter is reattached. A double vertical wire works quite well, with a firm soft tissue reattachment, or a screw can be used.

Bony union is not aimed for but, when the hip is put on traction, the glutei are stretched and, at the second stage when the hip itself is once again brought out to length, the trochanter is much more likely to come down to the right position. Proprietary Septopal chains are quite inadequate and, because the cement is only acting in this case as a depot for antibiotics, there does not need to be any concern about weakening it by the addition of large quantities of antibiotics. The 4 g/40 g mix level can, therefore, be exceeded if necessary. The cement is fashioned into irregularly shaped small beads on braided wire, with a number of knots in it to prevent the beads coming off (Fig. 12.2). The beads need to be small enough to go down the femoral canal, but a neat shape is not important. An irregularly shaped bead (or a small plate) has a greater surface area than a sphere and, therefore, allows larger quantities of antibiotic to leach out. Three to five

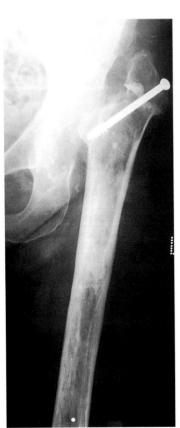

Figure 12.1 – *Appearance at referral of a patient with a deep infection who had nominally had the first stage of a planned two-stage exchange. The trochanter has been nicely fixed with a screw, but the femur still retains the plastic restrictor and some cement requiring a repeat of the first stage.*

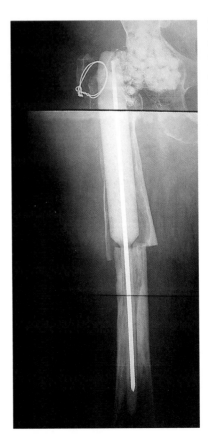

Figure 12.2 – *The appearance of 'home-made' beads. A stent was also made for the femur by allowing cement to set in a cement gun, the cement in the nozzle being stiffened with a Steinman pin followed by cutting away the plastic. The patient had already had a previous revision and the hip was discharging and growing a highly resistant organism.*

'home-made' bead chains are made. These are put down the femur and put curled up, into the acetabulum. An alternative is to make a stent by wrapping an old prosthesis in cement; a suitably shaped head can be made by using an old vitallium cup arthroplasty as a mould. This procedure may reduce shortening between the stages and may make the soft tissue dissection at the second stage easier. In addition, traction may not be needed and it may be possible to mobilize the patient, and perhaps for him or her to leave hospital. There are significant disadvantages, however: the surface area of cement from which antibiotics leach out is much less, there is the possibility of soft tissue irritation from the rather rough cement surface, dislocation may occur, and there is also the rather worrying possibility of a fracture.

Just as with the duration of systemic antibiotics, there is no uniformity about the time between stages. The effects of the depot antibiotic will have largely dissipated by 3 weeks and, with this gap, the soft tissue dissection at the second stage is quite easy, requiring finger dissection only. Excessive bleeding can, however, be a problem. At 4 weeks, bleeding is less, but the soft tissues are already beginning to heal, and at 6 weeks and beyond the dissection at the second stage is taxing. Not only have all the tissues healed, but the hip has shortened and the implant is no longer available as a landmark. Nevertheless, it is much better to accept these problems than to embark on the second stage at a time when wound healing appears uncertain. Delays may also be necessary because of the general condition of the patient.

Gross bone destruction in infected cases

In the acetabulum, bony destruction, even if very severe, can almost always be dealt with by the measures described in Chapter 11. Hips with an acetabulum that cannot be reconstructed may be salvageable without a true Girdlestone by means of a saddle prosthesis (Figs 12.3, 12.4), in which the saddle-shaped upper end is made to articulate directly with the residual acetabular roof or iliac wing; a description of the use of this implant is, however, beyond the scope of this book. If the upper femur is so destroyed that it is clearly unsuitable for any load-bearing, then a distally fixed implant is needed. It is best to preserve the upper femur (for further details, see below under 'Bypass') so as to retain muscular attachments (Fig. 12.5). This requires a two-stage procedure, as

indicated above. A one-stage exchange resecting the upper femur completely is effective (see Fig. 11.9b), but, as a result of the lack of muscular attachment to the upper femur, it is liable to be unstable.

Cases in which femoral destruction is so severe and extends so far distally that none of the femur is suitable for stem fixation require total femoral replacement, the distal prosthetic anchorage being via a total knee replacement into the tibia. This procedure, which although extremely major can be very effective, is preferably done using a push-through type of prosthesis in which the distal femur is preserved; if necessary, however, the whole

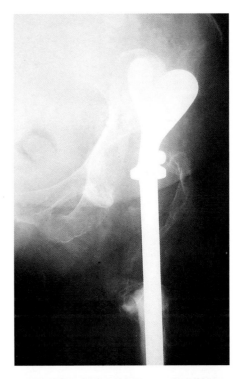

Figure 12.3 – *Radiological appearance of the Saddle prosthesis. The sclerosis around the upper end is indicative of weight-bearing on the wing of ilium.*

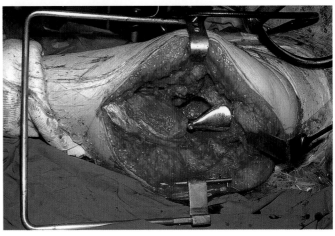

Figure 12.4 – *Intraoperative photograph of the saddle prosthesis articulating with the ilium.*

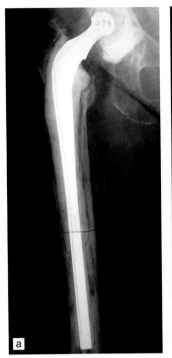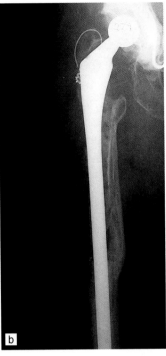

Figure 12.5 – *(a) Preoperative and (b) late postoperative film of the case shown in Figure 12.2. The upper femur was unsuitable for load-bearing with large areas of complete cortical loss. A distally fixed (Orthogenesis) implant was used, preserving the remains of the upper femur. An acetabular ring was also required.*

of the femur can be resected. Such procedures, as with the acetabulum that cannot be reconstructed, are beyond the scope of this book.

Skeletal augmentation by grafting

This is a very attractive concept in any patient young and fit enough for the possibility of further revision. It is seldom, if ever, necessary simply for fixation purposes; all hips can be treated without grafting. Access to a bone bank is required.

Notes on technique

The acetabulum

Decisions have to be made about (1) graft size, (2) whether or not cement should be used, (3) if cement is to be used, whether it is put directly on to the graft or with intervening mesh, and (4) whether a ring is to be used and, if so, of what type. It is best to adopt one single technique that has a wide applicability.

Graft size

Regarding graft size, the poor reputation of blocks in terms of late fatigue failure may well be unjustified if careful thought is given to how they are fixed and loaded at revision (Figs 12.7, 12.8). Poor long-term results are associated with heavily loaded block grafts, particularly when not supported by rings and/or which are fixed with screws that are not in the load-bearing direction and, therefore, subject to excessive repetitive bending loads. Small particle-sized grafts made with a power mill are initially much more like a fluid in mechanical terms, bearing load only if completely contained, although later incorporated. Between these two types of grafts, chips are compressed together to form a semi-solid structure, which still has the capability of complete incorporation. Combinations of the three may be used.

Cementless fixation

Cementless fixation currently seems to be working quite well in revision situations associated with morselized grafting. However, such sockets have to be hemispherical and need to fit against host bone over a substantial area. They are, therefore, liable to be large in diameter to fit the anteroposterior (AP) dimension of the acetabulum, and it is seldom possible to achieve an anatomical reconstruction.

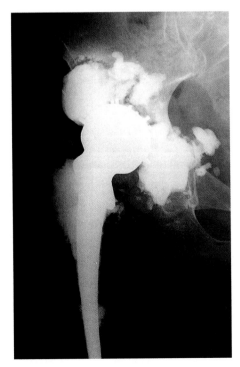

Figure 12.6 – *Bizarre appearances of a failed metal/metal McKee inserted in the early days of total hip replacement after failure of an upper femoral osteotomy. The socket had originally been severely malpositioned as well as being loose at the time of revision.*

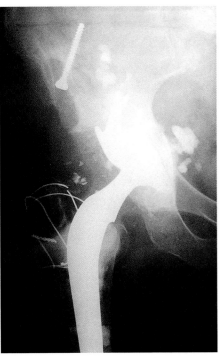

Figure 12.7 – *Twelve-year postoperative appearance. The screw indicates the upper limit of a very large block graft. The reconstruction has been stabilized using an AO roof reinforcement ring.*

and bone cutters. Part, or the second head, can be made into mush using a power-driven mill, such as the Aesculap. The overall quantities of each can be adjusted to suit the circumstances; it may be necessary to keep some bone as slightly larger blocks. Meanwhile, the teardrop region is very clearly visualized and a blunt instrument, or perhaps a finger, put down around it. The socket is gently reamed, usually inferomedially and to the rim, and a hook ring 4 mm smaller than the last reamer is offered up. Ideally, when inserted around the teardrop, its superolateral flange should come into contact with the outer edge of the residual acetabular roof. It may be necessary to bend the hook section slightly.

Direct cementation or via mesh

The distance into which the cement should interdigitate with the graft is not known at present. Clearly, if it goes too far, much of the graft never incorporates, because mesh prevents this. Nevertheless, if the graft at least has impacted small particles on its surface, the cement will fix on to these particles, producing an implant with an allograft surface, which is obviously highly desirable.

Type of ring

If bony erosion is not very severe and host bone is still available in an appropriate position, directly cementing a socket on to the graft may well work very well. If, however, the socket is much enlarged, either an extremely large cup is needed, or the cup sits entirely on graft. It is then not strictly speaking fixed (complete displacement from the graft later in the same operation has been reported) and the possibility of later migration must be increased. This potential problem is obviated if a ring is used. One technique is discussed below.

Acetabular impaction technique using the AO (Ganz) hook ring (Figs 12.8–12.11)

One, and sometimes two, femoral heads are required. While the surgeon is carrying out the earlier stages of the operation, the scrub nurse can cut these up suitably. One can be made into chips, somewhat smaller than the size of the end of a little finger, using a saw, an osteotome,

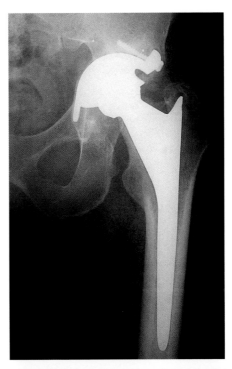

Figure 12.8 – *Failure of a cementless total hip replacement with quite severe socket migration and lysis, treated by impaction grafting.*

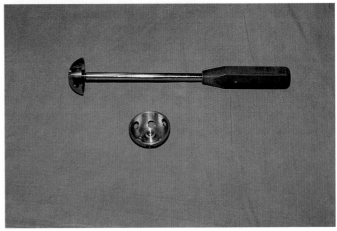

Figure 12.9 – *The author's special acetabular graft impactors.*

193

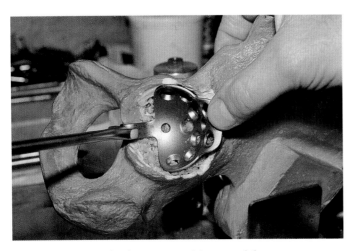

Figure 12.10 – *A hook ring in position on a laboratory specimen. The hook is being retained in position over the teardrop, in this case by the use of the special AO ring impacting punch. At surgery, the same effect may be achieved by a normal curved Homan acetabular retractor.*

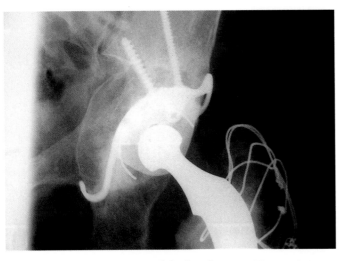

Figure 12.11 – *Appearance of the hip shown in Figure 12.8 after impaction grafting. An iliac graft was also used in this case in the distal part of the floor defect.*

Next, with the ring held in the desired position, a trial insertion of the flexi-drill is made to see which hole is most convenient to start with and to ensure that the drill will have solid bone to go into. A drill inserted through other holes may go deeply into previous fixation pits or on to a very oblique surface, and so may be difficult to drill at first. This trial of drill insertion is important and facilitates later screw fixation greatly. The ring is then removed. If there are particularly large defects or a floor defect, smallish blocks may be inserted next and the socket is partly filled with the chips which need to be solidly impacted using some instrument, as shown in

Figure 12.10. The position of the surface of the graft should have been estimated from the position of the ring at the earlier insertion. When this is appropriate, mush may also be used on the surface which tends (as in Roman road building) to hold the chips together; the ring is then reinserted. It is important to make sure that the hook is properly engaged around the teardrop and it should be deliberately held in this position with a retractor in the cotyloid notch (Fig. 12.10). Otherwise failure may result. The ring should sit in good contact with the graft at all positions and the first screw is inserted through the previously planned hole.

If a proper trial has been done and the graft has been solidly impacted, this should not be difficult. If, however, these conditions are not met, it may be almost impossible, the screw simply not finding the hole in the now invisible acetabular roof. Once one screw is inserted, the whole construct should immediately become extremely solid. Further screws are then inserted, as in Chapter 11. As the screws are progressively tightened, marrow should be seen to be squeezed out through the remaining holes in the ring, indicating firm compression of the graft (Fig. 12.11). If there is a significant rim defect, a block may need to be held in place temporarily with a Kirschner wire during ring and screw insertion. Subsequently, the wire can often be simply removed or it can be replaced with a screw.

Severe roof erosion

The precise limits of the above technique are unknown. A very large uncontained superolateral deficiency can be filled with a large piece of head as a block (Fig. 12.12). The surface of the head is thoroughly scarified and it may be necessary to ream gently on the opposing eroded surface. The head can then be somewhat reduced in size inferiorly before insertion, but in the main it needs to be shaped and reamed *in situ*. To avoid gaps deep to it, mush is placed, and the head positioned and held with two or three Kirschner wires. Definitive shaping of the inferior section of the graft is then carried out with a combination of instruments, such as the Anspach, high-speed burrs, and finally reamers. If reamers, especially large ones, are used too early, the graft, only rather feebly held by the Kirschner wires, moves. After reaming, there are then three possibilities:

■ Gaps around the head can be filled with mush and chips and impacted (although the impaction will not be as solid as in other cases) and then a screw-fixed hook ring inserted exactly as described previously.

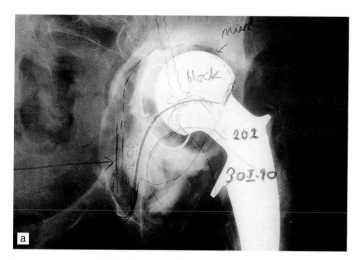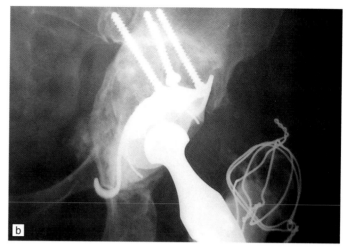

Figure 12.12 – *(a) Planning of the reconstruction in a patient with very severe superior acetabular migration. (b) The late film after reconstruction using a large superior block and impacted chips.*

The Kirschner wires need to be removed before final screw tightening or it is impossible to get them out. The lateral surface of the head is then trimmed off. In this case, the screws are in the most favourable mechanical situation (i.e. in the load-bearing axis), but the chips and mush are not so firmly impacted.

- A screw can be put in the load-bearing axis through the graft with its head buried, so that it lies underneath the ring (Fig. 12.12b). This is much easier and allows solid surrounding impaction, although the position of the screw needs to be very carefully selected or it will be in precisely the position required for one of the screws that have to run through the ring.

- Screws may be put superolateral to the ring and still be in an axis not far from the load-bearing one. This is possible only if the graft has to be a very large one. If carried out when the graft is smaller, the screws are undesirably transverse and much more likely to break later. After the ring is solidly fixed, it may be appropriate to remove some of these screws, trim excess graft, and reinsert shorter screws. This technique is also sometimes applicable to total hip replacement (THR) for old unreduced fracture dislocations (see Chapter 7).

An alternative to the AO hook ring is the Kerboull ring. The main differences from the AO ring are that the screws are inserted through the superolateral flange as with the Burch-Schneider cage, the ring is somewhat more flexible, and cement is in contact with graft over a larger area in the weight-bearing zone. With the patient in the supine rather than the lateral position, however, perfect control of the graft by the metal plate in the weight-bearing zone is advantageous, and biomechanically the construct is significantly different, because the main load-bearing part of the graft is solidly compressed by the screws in the AO hook ring, although not to such a degree with the Kerboull ring. With these provisos, however, the indications for and principles of use of these two rings are broadly similar.

The femur

There are a large number of different types of classification of femoral bone loss. The types of loss that need grafting can also be conveniently divided into three groups in a simple practical way, each requiring completely different treatment, as follows:

- The extreme upper femur is seriously eroded or may have wall deficiencies down to about 2 cm below the lesser trochanter, but the femur distal to this is solid and virtually normal, and in some circumstances not only solid and normal, but narrow as well. This situation is usually seen in gross acetabular loosening which produces major erosion by high-density polyethylene (HDP) debris, but in which the femoral component has remained solidly fixed.

- Severe lysis is present over a major part of the femur around the stem, perhaps with cortical defects, but the residual cortex still appears strong enough to be used for load transmission.

- The femur around the stem is so eroded, or so perforated, that using it for load transmission is either a doubtful proposition or impossible. Alternatively, a fracture of the femoral shaft is present either around the distal part of the stem or distal to it in association with a loose femoral component.

Accepting that there is obviously overlap between the above groups, and bearing in mind the comments at the start of Chapter 11, the three groups may be appropriately treated as follows.

Group with serious erosion of the femur

The femur is turned back into a tube by filling the defect with a block firmly held in position by screws or a small reconstruction plate (Fig. 12.13). Small gaps around its edges can be filled with chips or mush and/or an extremely small quantity of fast-setting cement. It is essential to make the repair solid. If a piece of ilium has been used, then it is almost certainly necessary to strengthen it by the use of fast-setting cement. An external protuberance of graft is quite unimportant and can be easily trimmed down after femoral component cementation, if necessary, as in the acetabulum.

Group with severe lysis (Fig. 12.14)

This is the group to be treated by impaction grafting. This technique was originally described with cementless implants and Figure 12.15 shows a case treated in this fashion in 1986, using an RM-Isoelastic stem. The concept of impaction grafting using cemented fixation was first applied to the femur by Ling and Gie as an extension of the work in the acetabulum by Sloof. The

principles of the technique are simple, the main requirements being the following:

- The femur, if not so already, is made into a sufficiently strong tube and the canal is solidly blocked distally by a firmly fixed intramedullary plug
- The graft is very firmly impacted.

If these conditions are not met, then subsidence, and perhaps early failure, are likely. Radiographs are sometimes shown purporting to represent a failure of the technique, in which it is clear that there have been significant technical deficiencies in the operation. Femoral impaction grafting, though extremely effective when carried out, is highly surgical technique-dependent, as with so many other aspects of revision. There are several as yet unanswered theoretical questions relating to graft type, size, and size variability, the effect of prophylactic anticoagulants on the blood which becomes mixed with the graft, the viscosity of the cement used and the degree to which it infiltrates the graft, and the effects on subsidence under repeated loading of tamp and stem geometry. In practice, mush made with a power mill seems to be best, and recent work certainly suggests (Smith *et al.*) that mechanical rather than pharmacological methods of deep vein thrombosis (DVT) prophylaxis should be used, if available, because the ability of the blood to clot seems be important in solidifying the impacted graft.

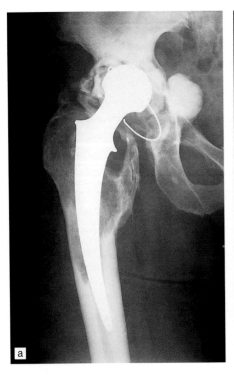 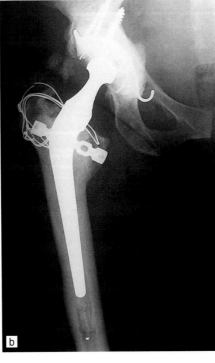

Figure 12.13 – *Appearances (a) before and (b) after revision of a 45-year-old patient with severe acetabular and upper femoral bone loss. Distally, the femur is quite solid and narrow.*

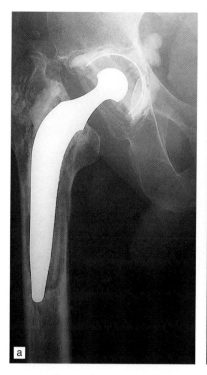
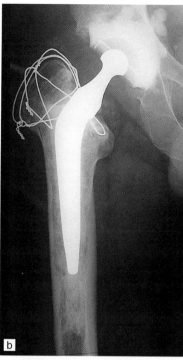

Figure 12.14 – *Appearances (a) before and (b) after revision of a 55-year-old man with severe upper femoral lysis and an incipient fracture medially below the lesser trochanter. The upper femur, though severely eroded, is still suitable for taking load and has been treated by impaction grafting using the author's instruments and a Charnley prosthesis.*

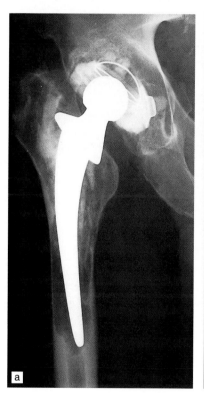
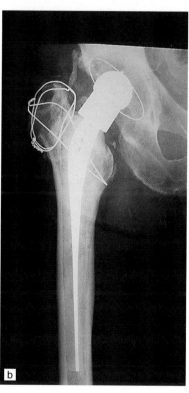

Figure 12.15 – *(a) Pre- and (b) late postoperative appearances after endosteal/ impaction grafting using the now-abandoned RM-Isoelastic prosthesis. Cortical restoration is particularly striking, but subsidence gradually occurred and endosteal lysis later reappeared distally, probably as a result of polyacetal debris.*

Regarding which system to use, the technique was originally described with impaction using over-sized Exeter trial components only, and the author has successfully used specially made double-tapered tamps, as shown in Figure 12.16. The first commercially available grafting equipment was designed for the Exeter stem, but others, such as the DePuy/Charnley/Elite/Elite Plus, the Zimmer for the CPT stem, and the Osteonics system are now available. The last has a special syringe system for filling the femur with a tube of graft, but apart from this the systems appear (at least superficially) to be similar. In all types, the diameter of the femoral canal at an

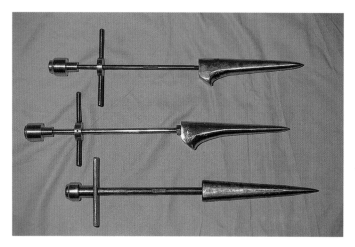

Figure 12.16 – *Very simple impaction grafting instruments (see text).*

appropriate level distal to the tip of the stem is measured and a plug inserted. If necessary, the plug can be held in place by a Kirschner wire distal to it (see Chapter 11). The femur is then filled with graft, which is impacted with cylindrical cannulated tamps up to or somewhat above the planned position of the tip of the stem and then, using a tapered tamp or tamps, the upper section is filled and impacted. A trial reduction is done with a head-neck unit attached to the top of the last tamp. Cement is mixed and immediately before its insertion the trial and guide rod is withdrawn. The cement is then pressurized and the definitive component inserted.

It is certainly best to use the impaction system that corresponds to the implant with which the surgeon is most familiar. However, although the systems appear similar, the long-term results, not currently known, may not necessarily be the same, because the geometry of the tamps, which determines the external shape of the cement mantle, shows important differences. Using trial Exeter components or the Howmedica systems, the shape of the cement mantle is tapered in both AP and lateral planes; with the DePuy system, modelled on the Charnley implant, which is of uniform AP thickness, the cement mantle is tapered only in the mediolateral sense. Clearly, this may have a significant effect on graft impaction as well as on subsidence of the cement mantle (i.e. of the allograft-coated implant) within the graft after cement curing. Hopefully, clinical and experimental work currently under way will eventually give the answers to these questions. It is also unclear whether it is strictly necessary to graft the femur down to the most distal lytic area. It may be necessary for geometrical reasons to make the

tamp/cement mantle go some way distal to the stem; if freed from the osteoclastic effects of wear debris, however, the femoral cortex is almost certain to hypertrophy with appropriate loading in the lytic area without grafting. It may also be possible to block the femur very effectively with allograft rather than a plastic plug by using the transfemoral Kirschner wire technique (see Chapter 11).

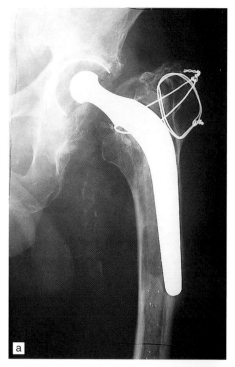

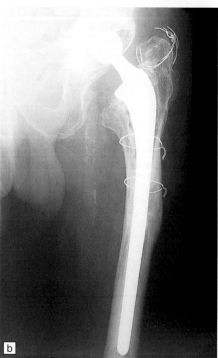

Figure 12.17 – *(a) Preoperative appearance of a hip in which the upper femur was felt to be too weakened to transmit load. The postoperative appearance is shown in Figure 12.17(b). (b) Postoperative appearance of a hip in which the upper femur was felt to be too weakened to transmit load. The hip was treated by upper femoral bypass using a distally cemented Weber stem, proximally hydroxyapatite coated, and proximal grafting.*

Relatively small defects in the femur may be blocked with wire mesh applied externally and held solidly with circlage wires, or cable fixed with crimping blocks. Circlage around the femur is not, as previously thought, a problem and there also does not need to be concern (i.e. from the point of view of bone viability) about stripping quite significant areas of the femur. The defect has to be sufficiently solidly blocked so that very firm impaction of the graft can be carried out. If this is not done, failure is inevitable. If large defects, or multiple defects, are present, it is probably safer to consider the femur as being in the last group below.

Postoperatively, a period of at least 6 weeks of minimal weight-bearing is necessary.

Group with perforation or erosion of stem

This group requires upper femoral bypass (Figs 12.17a and b). The component is fixed only distally and the residual upper femur, which is deficient and/or fragmentary and may have been bivalved, is reassembled around the upper part of the implant with or without intervening graft. Several types of stem are available. The main decisions to be made are whether the distal fixation should be with or without cement and whether or not a transfemoral approach, bivalving the upper femur, should be used. Secondary decisions concern whether the upper part of the implant should be coated with hydroxyapatite and whether or not bone graft should be used.

Distal fixation

The distal end of the stem is unfortunately in the middle or lower femur where, as noted earlier, the medullary canal is parallel-sided or becoming wider distally. This geometry could cause potential difficulty with any form of intramedullary fixation. The chief systems and their advantages and disadvantages are considered below.

Cementless stems

These stems have a taper and flutes (notably Wagner and Waldemar Link Reconstruction).

Advantages
- Simple to carry out in theory
- If failure results, extraction should be simple
- Bivalving of the upper femur may not strictly be necessary (for fuller discussion, see below).

Disadvantages
- The femoral component may not solidly impact at exactly the planned depth, and it may or may not be

possible to compensate for the position of impaction by modularity at the upper end. In this respect, the modularity in the Waldemar Link Reconstruction stem has the great advantage that it is adjustable rotationally (as with the S-ROM) as well as in length, the length adjustment also being considerably greater than in the Wagner.
- With the greatest attention to component sizing, reaming, and solidity of impaction with or without prophylactic circlage, subsidence is still a significant problem. Secondary rotational instability may also result.

Theoretically, the advantages listed above can be retained and the chief disadvantage of subsidence removed by using a locking-screw form of distal cementless fixation (e.g. Huckstep, Kent, and Cannulok hips). This principle is, however, borrowed from fracture technology where it is assumed that long-term fixation is not required. Unless carried out for a transverse femoral fracture where, for some reason, the upper end can be solidly fixed for later load transmission, there are theoretical worries about this system.

Cement

Advantages
- The great advantage of this is that the position of implantation is completely adjustable, so that the length of the thigh, tightness of reduction, and version can be set to a nicety.
- Subsidence should be less of a problem, provided that the Kirschner wire technique is used to block distal migration of the plug, which is in an expanding section of the canal; combined with the usual other measures, properly pressurized cementation can be done. Two Kirschner wires may well be necessary.

Disadvantages

It is necessary to bivalve the upper femur to get access to the upper end of the distal part of the stem for proper cementation. Although bivalving of the femur is usually given as an intrinsic part of the Wagner insertion technique, the main original reason for bivalving was to facilitate removal of the previous implant and the cement. Such a reason is, of course, no longer valid. With cemented distal fixation, the easy implant and cement extraction from bivalving should merely be considered as a bonus factor in terms of the ease of the operation. It is not advantageous in any other way.

Notes on using a distally cemented stem

A transgluteal approach can be used, provided that acetabular reconstruction is not too complicated. The femur and the vasti are split laterally from the top of the trochanter down to a planned anterior corticotomy level. An anterior capsulectomy is done and glutei split. The medial femur is then perforated with narrow osteotomes made through splits in quadriceps and the anterior section lifted forwards, as in other transgluteal techniques. The posterior part of the trochanter is usually then osteotomized. It is a good plan to leave some membrane in the femur at this stage to reduce blood loss and deal with the acetabulum next. Some reaming of the distal femur is required and a trial reduction is done, the component being clamped to the femur at the site of the osteotomy.

After accurate measurement of the insertion depth, a rotational datum made with a notch in the femur or a short Kirschner wire, and sometimes with a small cement occluder around the implant at the upper end of the distal section, is then cemented in, as described above. The test reduction should have been done with a standard head-neck unit which can later be adjusted if necessary. The upper femur is then reconstructed by circlage and the trochanter reattached. The upper femur may be extensively grafted, but the necessity for this is uncertain.

Revision for recurrent dislocation

In contrast with early dislocation, there is always, with one exception, something significantly amiss with a hip that dislocates late or recurrently. It is usually the result of component malposition and/or abductor weakness, the latter, if present, usually being associated with an ununited trochanteric osteotomy and gross trochanteric elevation. The exception (now seldom seen) is the hip with very long-term perfect function, but one inserted by the original Charnley technique in which the aim was zero anteversion of the socket and the stem (the former in order to maximize the HDP area in the walking position in relation to wear). In such hips, the surprising fact is simply the low original incidence of dislocation. Well-inserted hips, done through a posterior approach, can also recurrently dislocate as a function of the inevitable damage to the short external rotators and often to the posterior fibres of gluteus medius; recurrent posterior dislocation is very seldom seen in anterolateral approaches. If it is, it is certainly accompanied by obvious component malposition. The results of surgical treatment for recurrent dislocation are not encouraging and it is essential to have the clearest possible idea from detailed assessment of the case and detailed planning of the reason why the hip recurrently dislocates.

Acetabular augmentation is temptingly easy, but has a high failure rate and should very seldom be done. Although posterior (the usual case) dislocation can usually be prevented, impingement of the neck on the augmentation in extension happens frequently, resulting in fatigue fracture of the screws, movement of the augmentation, and failure. The only circumstances in which it may, perhaps, be considered are where the hip seems to have little amiss, with good component orientation, marginal instability only, such that dislocation occurs infrequently (i.e. the augmentation and screws will be loaded only occasionally), and where the patient's medical state makes a larger operation inadvisable.

Occasionally, malorientation of one component is so obvious that only that needs to be changed, but it is much better to err on the side of changing both.

Head size

This has in fact only a very poor statistical correlation with dislocation, but, nevertheless, a head of at least 28 mm diameter should be used if the head is changed.

The abductors

Assuming that a trochanteric osteotomy is done for the revision, the trochanter should be advanced if possible; this procedure alone has been reported as being successful in certain cases in the treatment of recurrent dislocation. If a trochanteric non-union with elevation is present, a determined attempt should be made to achieve union. This can (in the author's experience) be reasonably hoped for only if the femoral component is changed so as to allow improvement of the trochanteric bed and insertion of wires solidly in new cement. The trochanter needs to be extensively mobilized and a special tool (Fig. 12.18) may be beneficial. To improve the trochanteric bed, it is very helpful if the femoral component is distalized slightly in the femur (Figs 12.19, 12.20). If non-union is present but the trochanter is fragmented, the muscles need to be mobilized, but only a soft tissue reattachment can be done. Under these circumstances, it will be best to use a 32-mm head.

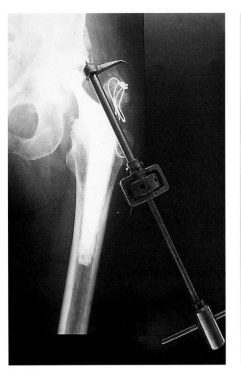

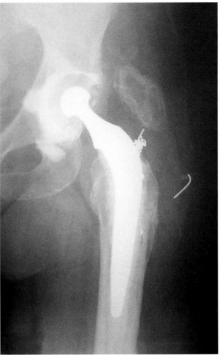

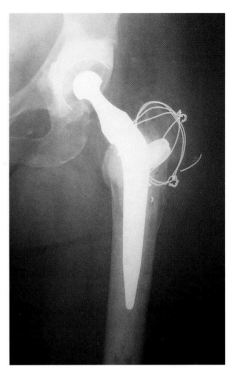

Figure 12.18 – *A hip with recurrent dislocation resulting partly from severe abductor weakness from trochanteric non-union, and the trochanteric distraction jack used to assist in distalizing it before reattachment.*

Figure 12.19 – *A similar case to Figure 12.18.*

Figure 12.20 – *Trochanteric union has been achieved here partly by a complete revision distalizing the femoral component, allowing for a much better trochanteric bed, and sound, cemented, femoral wire fixation. A hip with a 28-mm head would probably have been safer.*

After the operation

Postoperatively, the patient should be kept in bed until removal of the sutures and then put in a solid hip spica, which should be retained for 6 weeks. This is particularly important if an un-united trochanter has been reattached. It may be omitted if severe malorientation of one component has been adequately corrected. The inconvenience, however, of a hip spica to the nursing staff and the patient is amply compensated for by the successful treatment of recurrent dislocation; this is a very worrying and disabling complication for the patient requiring, as it does, repeated hospital admissions.

Femoral fractures

If the fracture was frankly traumatic and the hip previously functioning very well and not loose, then, regardless of the level, the fracture should be accurately reduced and fixed. Fixation, which needs to be solid, can sometimes be achieved by an ASIF plate because, if the femur is sufficiently large, it may be possible to put screws alongside the stem; screws hold well in cement. Nevertheless, a circlage system for plate fixation around the part of the femur containing the stem is preferable. This was the principle in the Partridge plate and band technique, which has now been superseded because its flexibility is not desirable in this situation. At least two excellent systems are at present available, namely the Dall-Miles (Howmedica) and Zimmer systems. Using this type of equipment, the fracture can be anatomically reduced and a very long, rigid plate applied, held by a combination of circlage cables and screws. In the region of the stem, most of the fixation is by the cables, which can be very firmly tensioned because the femur, with its contained implant and well-fixed cement, is effectively solid. Cortical screws can first be inserted to control the position of the plate and rotation at the fracture.

Distally, screws can be inserted bicortically in the usual fashion, reinforced with cables if felt to be desirable. The difference between the two systems is that with the Zimmer equipment the cables pass through holes in the plate and are held with grub screws, whereas with the Howmedica equipment cables go over the top of the plate, being crimped with a sleeve, as in the original Dall-Miles circlage system. The two devices are, in principle, very similar, and whichever is most readily available is recommended. The fracture should be grafted and the patient's leg braced until union is definite. Where the implant is still fixed, but the bone is extremely porotic – for example, in elderly patients after a hemiarthroplasty, the Mennen clasp plate may have an application because normal plate fixation with screws is unlikely to be possible. This device does not, however, have a removal tool and should probably be considered in this stated circumstance only.

In many cases, the implant is loose, the fracture having been partially caused by weakening of the femur from endosteal lysis. Reconstitution of the upper femur by circlage followed by endosteal grafting may be possible in some cases, but a much simpler and more effective solution is to use upper femoral bypass. The author has found the Waldemar Link Reconstruction stem to be very satisfactory in this circumstance, the distal femur being prophylactically circlaged before component impaction. Very careful planning is also needed if the upper femur is very fragmented, in order to assess component insertion depth. Failure to do this might even exceed the length adjustment provided by the modularity of the implant. Radiographs of the intact opposite femur are very helpful. Upper femoral bypass is of course applicable to all cases of femoral fracture, whether or not the component is loose.

Removal of isolated blocks to motion

Very careful assessment, as described in Chapter 8, is needed to make sure that this (Fig. 12.21) is a sensible procedure. It is only very rarely appropriate (about 1% of the author's revisions). A computed tomography (CT) scan gives an imperfect image because of the presence of the implants, but very careful inspection of these films put up together on a large multi-screen radiograph box, alongside the plain radiograph, should give a clear idea of where the bony bars are. The main consideration is whether they are largely anterior or largely posterior. This then determines the position of the patient and the surgical approach, the central problem being that, until the bars are removed (i.e. the procedure is almost complete), the hip will remain immobile and so no change in the view of the hip can be achieved by moving the leg. Second, unless a very neat and anatomically precise dissection is carried out, so that the bars can be carefully exposed (in theory, extraperiosteally) and divided under direct vision near to their ends, the resulting trauma and soft tissue damage, particularly to glutei, will be such that recurrent ossification is very likely. It may be necessary to see the hip from the front

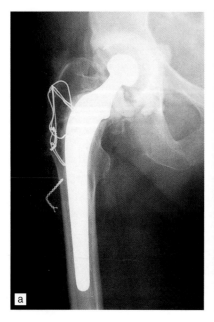
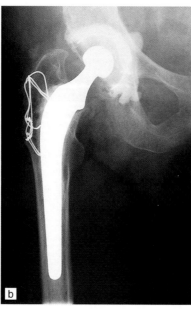

Figure 12.21 – *A patient with pain believed to result from impingement of intra-articular cement and heterotopic (a) bone before and (b) after their removal. Quite severe proximal trochanteric migration (but with healing) is, unfortunately, also present.*

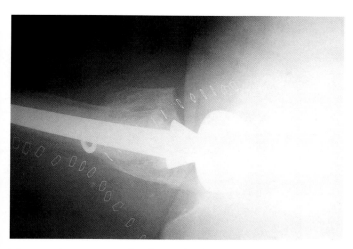

Figure 12.22 – *Lateral radiograph after removal of heterotopic bone. The skin clips show the tri-radiate incision used in this case. The same patient as in Fig. 8.20.*

simultaneously; for this, a tri-radiate skin and fascia lata incision centred on the greater trochanter (Fig. 12.22), akin to an Ollier, is needed, the deep dissection being like that for simultaneous McKee and posterior approaches. The patient may sometimes need to be positioned at a 45° inclination half way between supine and lateral, and a bean bag, of the type that can be moulded and then set in a given position by suction, is best.

The patient needs to have indomethacin in the form of a suppository before the operation and afterwards until he or she is in a position to take it orally (25 mg three times daily), and this should be maintained for at least 10 days. A longer period is sometimes recommended, but is probably not necessary; however, it is essential to have the drug circulating at the time that the bone is removed. If this is not done and indomethacin is started later, early recurrence of the new bone is likely. An alternative is to give radiotherapy. A recent study has shown that one dose may be sufficient. Which of the two is given depends to some degree on the availability of radiotherapy but, nevertheless, there is something a little unattractive about giving this form of treatment for a non-malignant condition. Re-education of the hip muscles by use, for a few days, of a continuous passive motion machine is also sensible, although no data are available about its effectiveness in this situation.

Conversion from Girdlestone pseudarthrosis

The functional results of Girdlestone pseudarthrosis are extremely variable. Pain is not usually a great feature, but patients are often very disabled, requiring two crutches all the time. Although in former days this was accepted as an occasionally inevitable end-stage, it is now increasingly realized that this need not necessarily be the case. Girdlestone conversion is, however, usually far from easy and can be extremely difficult. If the patient is elderly, pain free, and has sufficient stability in the hip to require only one crutch and be able to do a limited active straight leg raise (a situation found only in cases of severe previous sepsis), the hip should almost certainly be left alone. In other cases, however, conversion from pseudarthrosis can produce remarkable results with a very major improvement in the patient's function (Figs 12.23, 12.24). Conversion should be done only in circumstances where there is a good through-put of revision surgery of all grades of complexity. The apparent simplicity caused by the fact that the previous implants have already been removed is extremely misleading. The patient will have had at least two, and often many more, operations. The soft tissue dissection is often very difficult. The soft tissue layers will be confused and the essential planes difficult to establish. This results partly from the fact that the Girdlestone will probably have been done for deep infection, the object of the surgery simply having been to eradicate infection, without regard for the possibility of subsequent insertion of the THR as a

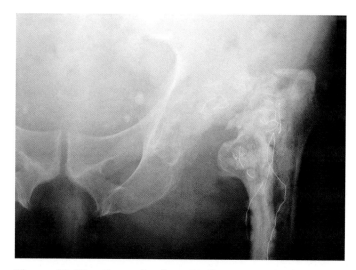

Figure 12.23 – *Conversion from Girdlestone pseudarthrosis. The hip had been infected and chains of beads had been in situ for a very long time. Analysis showed a very long gutter extending down the femur requiring a Waldemar Link reconstruction prosthesis.*

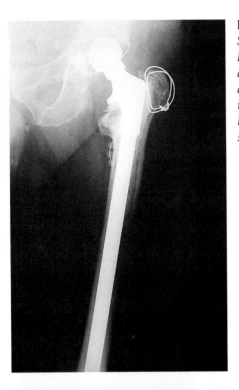

Figure 12.24 – *Same patient as Figure 12.23, after conversion. A short chain of beads was not detected and left behind in the soft tissues.*

corollary, if it is necessary to carry out a Girdlestone, it should be done very carefully, as if for subsequent reconstruction.

To create a functioning THR that is better than the Girdlestone, it is unfortunately necessary to work out the anatomy in detail, however badly it is disorganized (Fig. 12.23). The skeleton will also be deficient in most cases, with erosions, perforations, possibly gutters, and retained cement. The last, unfortunately, is also in less accessible places because otherwise it would already have been removed. The hip is also short. Access to the acetabulum, even when everything has been correctly carried out, can be difficult. The soft tissue has also converted itself into very solid material, much stronger than the underlying osteoporotic bone. Unlike the removal of membrane in a loose THR, soft tissue removal in these circumstances can be taxing, requires sharp dissection or cautery, and takes a long time. The question of one- or two-stage (if infected or previously

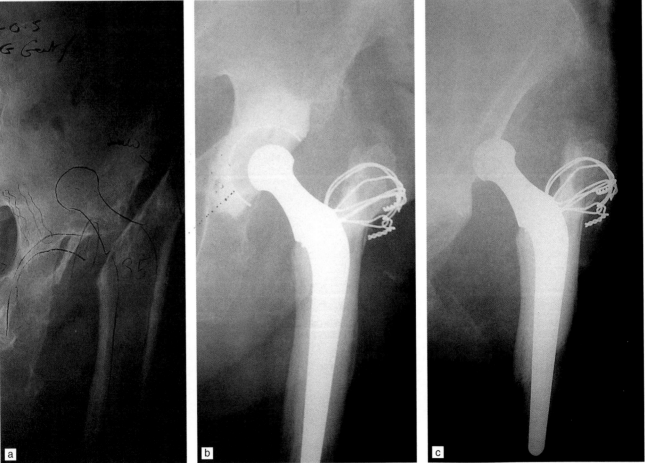

Figure 12.25 – *Conversion (b) from Girdlestone pseudarthrosis (a). There is quite severe acetabular bone loss. It was decided not to use the planned AO reinforcement ring shown on the drawing, and acetabular positioning was probably not ideal. The hip subsequently dislocated, (c) but stabilized after a period in a spica.*

infected), and implant reinsertion techniques, has already been described. Postoperative instability (Fig. 12.25) is likely to be much more of a problem than in other revisions and a 28-mm or larger femoral head should be used if the size of the acetabulum allows this; the patient should be managed postoperatively in a hip spica for 6 weeks, as for revision for recurrent dislocation.

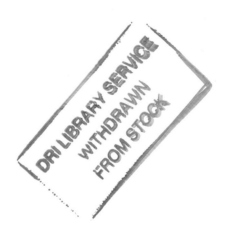

Further reading

Exchange for infection

Steinbrink K. The case for revision arthroplasty using antibiotic-loaded acrylic cement. *Clin Orthop Rel Res* 1990; 261: 19–22.

One-stage exchange

Buchholz HW, Elson RA, Engelbrecht E *et al*. Management of deep infection of total hip replacement. *J Bone Joint Surg* 1981; 63-B: 342–53.

Loty B, Postel M, Evrard J *et al*. One-stage revision of infected total hip replacements with replacement of bone loss by allografts. Study of 90 cases of which 46 used bone allografts. *Int Orthop* 1992; 16: 330–38.

Raut VV, Sine PD, Wroblewski BM. One-stage revision of infected total hip replacements with discharging sinuses. *J Bone Joint Surg (Br)* 1994; 76: 721–24.

Izquierdo RJ and Northmore-Ball MD. Long-term results of revision hip arthroplasty. Survival analysis with special reference to the femoral component. *J Bone Joint Surg (Br)* 1994; 76: 34–9.

Ure KJ, Amstutz C, Nasser S *et al*. Direct-exchange arthroplasty for the treatment of infection after total hip replacement. An average ten-year follow-up. *J Bone Joint Surg (Am)* 1998; 80-A: 961–8.

Two-stage exchange

Antti-Poika I, Joseffson G, Konttinen Y *et al*. Hip arthroplasty infection. Current concepts (review). *Acta Orthop Scand* 1990; 61: 163–9.

Wilde AH. Management of infected knee and hip prostheses (review). *Curr Opin Rheumatol* 1993; 5: 317–21.

Lenoble E, Goutallier D. Replacement of infected total hip prothesis in two stages. *Int Orthop* 1995; 19: 151–6.

Impaction grafting

Gie GA, Lng RS M, Timperley AJ *et al*. Impacted cancellous allografts and cement for revision total hip arthroplasty. *J Bone Joint Surg* 1993; 75-B: 14–21.

Smith EJ, Richardson JB, Learmonth ID *et al*. The initial stability of femoral impaction grafting. *Hip Int* 1996; 6: 166–72.

Heterotopic bone

Ritter MA, Gioe TJ. The effect of indomethacin on para-articular ectopic ossification following total hip arthroplast. *Clin Orthop Rel Res* 1982; 167: 113–17.

Amstutz HC, Fowble VA, Schmalzried TP, Dorey FJ. Short-course Indomethacin prevents heterotopic ossification in a high-risk population following total hip arthroplasty. *J Arthrop* 1997; 12: 126–32.

Healy WL, Lo TC M, DeSimone AA *et al*. Single-Dose irradiation for the prevention of heterotopic ossification after total hip arthroplasty. A comparison of doses of 550 and 700 centigray. *J Bone Joint Surg* 1995; 77-A: 590–95

SECTION IV
Trauma

CHAPTER 13

Trauma: the problem

G. C. Bannister

Proximal femoral fracture is responsible for both the largest number of internal fixations and the greatest proportion of beds occupied in orthopaedic surgery.

Incidence

The incidence of proximal femoral fracture is rising, both as the population ages and per unit population. Dahl [1] noted double the incidence of proximal femoral fracture in Norway between the decades 1948–57 and 1961–70. Lewis [2] recorded a 2.7-fold rise between 1959 and 1977 in England and Wales. Wallace documented an increase of 1.6-fold seven times between 1971 and 1981 in Nottingham, and numbers in the author's unit have risen 1.8-fold between 1981 and 1995.

Projected rise in incidence of proximal femoral fracture

Lord and Sinnett [3], in Australia, recorded a 40-fold difference in the incidence of proximal femoral fractures in patients aged between 35 and 44 years and those over 84, emphasizing that the population over the age of 84 has been estimated to rise by 146% between 1986 and 2011.

Resource implications

Lewis [2] noted that 18% of acute orthopaedic beds in England and Wales were occupied by patients with proximal femoral fracture; Thorngren [4] 33% in Sweden, and Evans [5,6] 50% in Newcastle. More hospital bed days were used in the management of proximal femoral fractures in Sweden than in the treatment of all cancer patients. Lord and Sinnett [3]

estimated that bed usage for proximal femoral fractures, in Australia, would rise by 83% in the decade after the millennium.

Outcome

Anticipation of the outcome after proximal femoral fracture is useful in giving a prognosis to patients and relatives, organizing hospital management and planning discharge. The outcome variables normally measured are mortality, mobility and social independence.

Mortality

Mortality after proximal femoral fracture can be high.

In hospital, mortality rates vary from 2% in Lund [7] to 35.6% in Newcastle [5]. The population sustaining femoral neck fracture is more infirm than age- and sex-matched controls. Mortality rates parallel controls after between 3 months and a year. Gordon [8], in eastern Canada, noted little change after 3 months, Hubble *et al.* [9] in Bristol, England, 4 months, Miller [10] in Charlottesville, USA, 8 months, and White *et al.* [11] in the USA and Jenson *et al.* [12] in Denmark, 1 year.

Cause of death

The cause of death identified *post mortem* assumes importance because it can suggest the potential to reduce mortality. The combined literature comprises a little over 1200 postmortem examinations [13,14]. The cause of death is remarkably constant regardless of geographical location. Thirty seven per cent of patients die of bronchopneumonia, 23% of myocardial infarction or heart failure, and 14% of pulmonary embolism. This suggests that there is a potential for reduction of deaths from bronchopneumonia by early mobilization, and from pulmonary embolism by antithrombotic prophylaxis. Perez *et al.* noted a decline in deaths from bronchopneumonia after the introduction of early mobilization in the early 1980s and, in a series of 581 postmortem examinations, performed over a 40-year period, recorded that 26% of deaths were associated with thromboembolic disorder, compared with 2.4% from haemorrhage. This emphasizes the potential benefits of thromboprophylaxis, but 17% of patients were at risk of haemorrhage if anticoagulated because of concurrent haemorrhagic morbidity. This was predominantly upper gastrointestinal ulceration but included subdural haematoma.

Factors associated with mortality

The differences in mortality in Newcastle and Lund are curious. Both are highly reputable university centres in countries with well-established health services within the same continent. The differences are at least partially explained by population selection. The Lund patients were independent in their own homes before fracture, whereas, in Newcastle [15], there was a disproportionate rate of fracture in residents of institutions and among mentally infirm and house-bound individuals. Current orthopaedic practice is increasingly subject to audit by outside bodies. The author's unit has recently been assessed by a firm of chartered accountants using criteria drawn up the Royal College of Physicians of London [16]. Neither chartered accountants nor physicians normally treat hip fractures; populations vary hugely within cities; published literature from one centre may not be applicable to another. Outside bodies, without experience of managing femoral neck fractures, inevitably rely on published literature. It is thus critical that orthopaedic surgeons are aware of the variables that affect the outcome of proximal femoral neck fracture management, and how they apply in their own geographical and social circumstances.

The appreciation of factors affecting mortality after proximal femoral fracture has changed. Neer [17], in New York, recorded an inpatient mortality rate of 47% in unstable trochanteric and none in stable valgus intracapsular fractures. Reno and Burlington [18] recorded a 47% mortality rate in patients who were non-active, invalid, or semi-invalid before fracture. There was a 43% mortality rate in those with serious medical problems and 29% in those who were considered to be a poor

Table 13.1 *Predetermined factors affecting mortality after total hip fracture*

Factor	Increased risk factor
Impaired social function	6.5
Poor anaesthetic risk	6.3
Dementia	6
Uncontrolled heart failure	6
Medical problems	4
House-bound	3
Male	2

anaesthetic risk. Overall, there was an increase in mortality by a factor of six in uncontrolled heart failure, five in poor anaesthetic risk, and four in those with a serious medical problem. Zuckerman *et al.* [19] and White *et al.* [11] confirmed these findings, whereas Evans *et al.* [15] and Ions and Stevens [20] associated increased mortality with dementia. All authors associate higher death rates with increasing age. Overall (Table 13.1) the risk factors influencing mortality, after hip fracture, appear in descending order to be: impaired social function, poor anaesthetic risk, dementia, uncontrolled heart failure, medical problems, being house-bound, and male sex. Virtually all these factors have been identified by two or more authors.

Although mortality after proximal femoral fracture is largely predetermined by the level of infirmity before injury, hospital practice plays an important role.

Timing of surgery

Returning to postmortem studies, the principal cause of death after proximal femoral fracture is bronchopneumonia. Perez *et al.* [13] note that the mortality rate from bronchopneumonia rose 500% if surgery was delayed by more than 24 hours. Neer [17] suggested that surgery should be carried out as soon as is practicable. Villar *et al.* [21] recorded a trend to higher mortality with delay to surgery, as did Zuckerman *et al.* [19], and Sexson *et al.* [22] in fitter patients. Fox *et al.* [23] prospectively reviewed a population of patients who were frequently cancelled through lack of operating room time and noted an increase of mortality rate from 0% to 17% if surgery was delayed by more than 24 hours. White *et al.* [11] and Rogers *et al.* [24] observed that mortality doubled if surgery was delayed beyond 24 hours. Dolk [25] earlier recorded the same phenomenon, but on subsequent study failed to reproduce the same observations. Zuckerman observed an adjusted hazard ratio of 1.76 if surgery was delayed beyond 3 days. Kenzora [26] recorded increased mortality when surgery was carried out within 24 hours of admission.

The weakness of all these studies is that, apart from the studies of Sexson and Lemner, they failed to identify the infirmity of the population concerned. Patients may have been lying unattended at home and have become dehydrated and hypothermic. In health care systems where there are junior anaesthetists, the more infirm patient may be cancelled because of perceived anaesthetic risk. It would appear that Neer's original observation has stood the test of time, but that more infirm patients should be assessed for correctable medical disorders. Repeated cancellation results in starvation and dehydration, which is poorly tolerated by this infirm group of patients. If surgery is carried out on emergency lists, there should be little prospect of cancellation; if not the fracture should be stabilized on an elective list within 24 hours of admission. Stabilization of the fracture means that the patient is able to walk fully weight-bearing on the injured hip, with walking aids being required only for temporary pain or to assist balance. The practice of leaving patients starved, supine, and waiting for an available operating slot invites bronchopneumonia and can no longer be regarded as acceptable.

Hospital practice

Three studies have compared hospital practice in the management of proximal femoral fracture. Wide differences occur in hospitals in the same city or region (Table 13.2). In Newcastle [15], 53% of patients in one teaching hospital were dead after 6 months compared with 28% in another. Nurse staffing ratios were significantly lower in the hospital with the higher mortality. In East Anglia [27], one hospital, which had a special interest in the management of proximal femoral fracture, had a quarter the mortality of the seven other units measured in the same predominantly rural region. In Bristol, England [28], the 1-year mortality rate at one teaching hospital was 45% compared with 21% at an adjacent affiliated unit. The unit with the higher mortality had rapid turnover of nursing staff whereas

Table 13.2 *Hospital differences in mortality rate*

Author	Year	Location	A	B	Ratio
Evans [15]	1980	Newcastle	53	28	1.9
Bannister *et al.* [28]	1990	Bristol	45	21	2.1
Todd *et al.* [27]	1995	East Anglia	20	5	4

that with the lower rate had two experienced head nurses leading the orthopaedic trauma care team.

Rehabilitation

Rehabilitation units following proximal femoral fracture were developed in the UK in Stoke on Trent and Hastings at a time when patients with proximal femoral fractures occupied acute orthopaedic beds for months. Such units were beacons in the then prevalent atmosphere of nihilism. Kennie *et al.* [29], in a prospective randomized controlled study, lowered mortality, numbers discharged to institutions, and hospital inpatient stay, and returned a higher proportion of patients home. The difference was maintained after a year [30]. These results, however, were not reproduced. Ceder *et al.* [31] in Sweden, and Jensen and Bagger [32] in Denmark, found that rehabilitation units merely protracted hospital admission without long-term benefit.

Sikorski *et al.* [33] took patients with fractures that could be stabilized, with relatives at home, no medical problems, and who lived close to the treating hospital. Fractures were stabilized immediately, patients were discharged home after a mean of 3 days, 72% of the population assessed could be entered into the programme, and the mortality rate was 4% at 1 month and 7% after 3 months. Sikorski *et al.* philosophized 'we are convinced that hospital is not the place for the elderly and that removing these people from their home environment is destructive'. Sikorski is an experienced academic with a particular and long-standing interest in the management of proximal femoral fracture, and his study was motivated purely for improving patient care. Rapid discharge was instituted in the Mid-West of the USA for economic reasons [34]. Hospital remuneration changed from item of service to a total care package, with a consequent reduction of inpatient stay to 12 days. The amount of physiotherapy was slightly reduced; the distance walked before discharge was no more than a mean of 11 metres, and 60% had to be admitted to nursing homes. After a year, 33% of patients were still in such institutions, although the mortality was unchanged.

Fox *et al.* [35] compared two hospitals in the Avon region of Britain. In one, a formidable head nurse discharged patients promptly to available local hospitals and nursing homes, and in the other marginally fit patients were rehabilitated in a well-staffed orthopaedic geriatric unit. After 1 year the mortality rate was 27% in both hospital populations. Patients had returned home from local hospitals and nursing homes, and overall 75% of patients from the hospital with early discharge had retained their preadmission residential status compared with 66% of those from the hospital with the rehabilitation unit. The difference in bed occupancy was sufficient to resource 100 total hip arthroplasties for the population served by the hospital with the early discharge policy.

Pryor and Williams [36] compared home and hospital rehabilitation. Patients were discharged home after about 8 days, or kept in hospital on a general orthopaedic ward for 16 days. No advantage accrued from remaining in hospital for the extra 8 days. Jalovaara *et al.* [37] in Finland, and Stromberg *et al.* [38] in the Stockholm area of Sweden, both found that transfer from orthopaedic to geriatric rehabilitation units protracted inpatient stay, increasing costs without benefits.

What is clear is that patients do at least as well at home as in hospital. Protracted hospital stay is expensive and not advantageous to the patient. Precipitate discharge places patients at risk of long-term institutional care. The correct management is early assessment and home discharge with appropriate support in the community.

Mobility and social function

Death is a categorical variable, and provided that patients can be traced it is relatively easy to measure. Mobility and social dependence are interrelated and very much more difficult to quantify.

Mobility

Miller [10] and Bannister *et al.* [28] found that 51% of patients were as mobile after proximal femoral fracture as they were before. Bannister *et al.* noted that 28% of patients had lost one grade of walking and 65% of

Table 13.3 *Risk of inability to walk on discharge*

Mobility before fracture	Risk of inability to walk (%)	Ratio
Independently shopping	2.4	
Walking outdoors	4	
Walking upstairs	10	
Using walking aids	20	10
Unable to shop	25	11
House bound	46	11

patients aged over 75 were house-bound, whereas 88% of those under 75 were able to manage stairs or better. Keene *et al.* [39] recorded that 40% of those able to walk independently were ultimately able to do so, 34% required a stick, 23% a frame, and 7% were unable to walk at all. Ceder (1980) reported that by 2 weeks there was an excellent indication as to whether or not patients would walk again. Fox *et al.* [35] (Table 13.3) observed that those who shopped independently and were walking outside their own homes, before fracture, were 10–11 times more likely to walk again than those unable to shop or house-bound. Patients who demonstrated a positive will to live in hospital were 10 times more likely to walk again than those who gave up. Of those who were house-bound 46% never walked again, along with 35% of those who gave up, and 25% of those who were unable to shop before injury.

Social function

Jensen and Bagger [32] noted that the social function deteriorated in 47% of patients after proximal femoral fracture. Keene *et al.* [39] recorded that 54% of patients could do their own shopping before injury but that this fell by 39% to 33% after injury. Twenty-eight per cent were house-bound before fracture and 46% after. Bannister *et al.* [28] noted an age-related capacity to retain independence of patients able to manage stairs or better. Ninety-one per cent of those aged between 70 and 79, 77% of those between 80 and 89, and 54% of those over the age of 90 were able to return home. By contrast, 15% or fewer patients who were house-bound and aged over 80 returned home. Social prognosis appears to be established by 6 months and changes very little thereafter [40]. It seems clear that social function, like mobility, is substantially predetermined or declares itself relatively early after fracture.

Given that so much of the outcome of proximal femoral fracture is predetermined, numbers are rising, and protracted hospital stay is not advantageous. It seems sensible to observe hospital practice, reduce bed occupancy, predict outcome from early indicators, and plan rehabilitation early.

Hospital bed usage

Robbins and Donaldson [41] observed the management of proximal femoral fracture in Leicester, England in the early 1980s. Four per cent of all hospital beds and 20% of all orthopaedic beds were occupied by patients suffering from the condition. Of the beds 9.5% were occupied by patients awaiting surgery and 28% by those awaiting discharge.

A decade later Fox *et al.* [35] in Bristol, England observed similar practice in a hospital with low nurse staffing levels and night-time emergency operating in conventional operating rooms, shared with general surgeons; the urgency of whose cases resulted in frequent cancellation of patients with hip fracture. Of hospital bed days, 30% were associated with four factors that could be influenced by surgical practice. Of the excess days, 55% were associated with non-medical delay to surgery, 25% with wound infection, and 20% with broken pressure areas. Cost savings achieved by reducing nursing skill mix and inadequate operating facilities were far outweighed by the complications and protracted bed occupancy associated with such practice. The approach to the management of proximal femoral fracture must be a combination of adequate resource for efficient management and early discharge to make way for new patients. Discharge must not be precipitate but planned according to the individual requirements of the patient, and factors that assist prediction of outcome soon after admission are immensely helpful in organizing the return home or institutional care.

Early prediction of outcome after proximal femoral fracture

Patients who are highly dependent have a mortality rate of between 52% [28] and 60% [42].

Dementia, as measured by a low mental test score, was the single most predictive factor associated with mortality in Newcastle, in two studies [20,43]. However, specificity was poor, with the highest mortality rate being 75% in demented patients over the age of 85 after 6 months. Wallace *et al.* [44] awarded three points each for social circumstances and health, so that those who were dependent and had poor health scored six points. Of patients who scored six points, 87% were dead within a year. Parker and Palmer [45] compared mobility with the mental test score and found it to be slightly more predictive. Of patients with poor mobility, 73% died compared with 71% of those with a low mental test score. Hubble *et al.* [9] associated mortality with increasing immobility: 46% of patients with a frame, 60% of patients mobilizing with a frame plus a helper, 78% of those chair-bound, and 100% of those bed-bound were dead within a year of fracture.

An accurate prediction of early death after hip fracture would spare the patient a painful operative procedure, but the sensitivity and specificity of existing prognostic indicators are insufficiently good to influence treatment. The only patients who can be managed confidently non-operatively are those who are bed-bound with displaced intracapsular fractures. Nothing is to be gained by operating in such cases either in relieving pain or facilitating nursing care.

Capacity to return home

Ceder *et al.* [7] recorded that 81% of those who lived with someone returned home, as did 85% of fit patients, 89% of those who had been sufficiently mobile that they could visit friends before fracture, and 90% of those who could do their shopping. By contrast, 55% of those aged over 80 or in poor health were unable to return home, as were 37% of those who were insufficiently mobile to visit friends, and 43% who were unable to do their own shopping. Of those who could perform acts of daily living within 2 weeks of fracture, 87% returned home, compared with 53% of those who could not. In a subsequent paper [31], a combination of variables, including ability to walk 2 weeks after surgery, living with someone, good general medical condition, and type of fracture, was predictive of return home in 81% of cases. Bannister *et al.* [28] observed that 91% of patients between the ages of 70 and 79 were able to return home compared with 77% of those between 80 and 89, and 54% of those over 90. By contrast, only between 10%

and 15% of those who were house-bound and over 80 before fracture ever returned home. No patient in Wallace's series [46], scoring five or six points, ever returned home. Hubble *et al.* [9] computed tables of variables, which indicated that 76% of male patients returned home, rising to 88% if they walked independently or with a stick before fracture. By contrast, between 61% and 63% of patients over the age of 80 required nursing or residential accommodation within a year of fracture, as did 88–90% of those who had depended on a frame before injury.

It would appear that, regardless of location or era, over 80% of those independent in the community and aged under 80 years, should expect to return to the home from whence they came before fracture. By contrast, those over 80 whose walking was compromised have an under 15% chance of returning home. Such patients almost certainly occupy the 28% of hospital bed days used to care for patients who have completed surgical treatment, identified by Robbins and Donaldson. It is apparent on admission that their chances of successful rehabilitation at home are extremely low and, if they have not begun to walk and perform acts of daily living within 2 weeks, the correct management is to arrange nursing institutional accommodation immediately.

Audit of proximal femoral fracture management

The resource implications of proximal femoral fracture are such that individual orthopaedic surgeons' practices are likely to be examined by health care providers. Information available to such health care providers may well be skewed. Pearse and Woolf [47] assessed the standard of management of proximal femoral fracture throughout the UK, according to the Guidelines of the Royal College of Physicians. Of a maximum of 15 points, three related to routine referral to physicians specializing in geriatric medicine, and two to the grade of surgeon or anaesthetist, regardless of ability. Thus, 20% of the assessment related to orthogeriatric units, of which only one has proved to have superior results to other methods of managing proximal femoral fracture. One point only was allocated for social circumstances, one for medical problems and none for pre-accident mobility at all. Performance throughout the UK varied. The area served by Newcastle as its teaching hospital had clearly

benefited from the lessons learned by Evans in the late 1970s, and scored three times as highly as the two lowest scoring regions.

Table 13.4 *Audit outcome of proximal femoral fracture*

Preoperative state
Social
Living at home
Shopping
Visiting friends
Living with spouse
Doing housework
Requiring home help
Cooking
Requiring meal preparation
Capable of self-care
Reliant on others for care
Residential accommodation (able to walk)
Elderly mentally infirm (able to walk)
Nursing home

Mobility — **Stairs**
Walking unaided
Walking with stick/frame

ASA grading
I   Normal healthy patient
II Mild systemic disease
III Severe systemic disease not incapacitating
IV Incapacitating systemic disease that is a constant threat to life
V   Moribund patient not expected to survive 24 hours with or without surgery

Hospital management
Delay to surgery
Late cancellation of surgery
Reoperation or failed fracture fixation
Postoperative infection
Postoperative pneumonia or heart failure
Time to walking and self-care
Discharge planning
Pressure sores

Community service
Time to assessment of social workers
Time to assessment by nursing home and residential managers
Delay of provision of home care

The weighting of the Guidelines of the Royal College of Physicians is skewed, and the audit correspondingly blunt. Auditors acting on the guidelines failed to distinguish between grades of patient admitted from their own home. No attempt is made to differentiate degrees of independence among patients living at home, and inevitably units serving poorer populations find that such audit instruments fail to take into account the infirmity of the patients they are treating. It is therefore wisest for orthopaedic surgeons to undertake their own audits (Table 13.4). Table 13.4 includes data derived by several authors, and includes the difficulties faced by surgeons in discharging patients from hospital when treatment has been completed. Audit using these variables will give a truer estimate of the standard of management of proximal femoral fractures than criteria produced by outside bodies, ensure that standards of management are maintained and that economically driven changes in hospital resource do not harm the patients in their care.

References

1. Dahl E. Mortality and life expectancy after hip fractures. *Acta Orthop Scand* 1980; S1: 163–70.

2. Lewis AF. Fracture of neck of femur: changing incidence. *Brit Med J* 1981; 283: 1217.

3. Lord SR, Sinnett PF. Femoral neck fractures: admissions, bed use, outcome and projections. *Med J Aust* 1986; 145: 493–6.

4. Thorngren K-G. Optimal treatment of hip fractures. *Acta Orthop Scand* 1991; 62(suppl 241): 31–4.

5. Evans JG. Fractured proximal femur in Newcastle upon Tyne. *Age Ageing* 1979; 8: 16–23.

6. Evans JG, Prudham D, Wandless I. A prospective study of fractured proximal femur: factors predisposing to survival. *Age Ageing* 1979; 8: 246–50.

7. Ceder L, Thorngren K-G, Wallden B. Prognostic indications and early home rehabilitation in elderly patients with hip fractures. *Clin Orthop* 1980; 152: 173–84.

8. Gordon PC. The probability of death following a fracture of the hip. *Can Med Assoc J* 1971; 105: 47–51.

9. Hubble M, Little C, Prothero D, Bannister GC. Predicting the prognosis after proximal femoral fracture. *Ann R Coll Surg Engl* 1995; 77: 355–7.

10. Miller CW. Survival and ambulation following hip fracture. *J Bone Joint Surg* 1978; 60A: 930–4.

11. White BL, Fisher WD, Liquens CD. Rate of mortality for elderly patients after fracture of the hip in the 1980s. *J Bone Joint Surg* 1987; 68A: 1335–40.

12. Jensen JS, Tondevold E, Sorensen P. Social rehabilitation following hip fractures. *Acta Orthop Scand* 1979; 50: 777–85.

13. Perez J, Warwick DJ, Case CP, Bannister GC. Death after femoral neck fracture - an autopsy study. *Injury* 1995; 26: 237–40.

14. Riska EB. Factors influencing primary mortality in the treatment of hip fractures. *Injury* 1970; 2: 107–15.

15. Evans JG, Wandless I, Prudham D. A prospective study of fractured proximal femur. *Public Health London* 1980; 94: 149–54.

16. Royal College of Physicians of London. *Fractured Neck of Femur: Prevention and Management*. London: Royal College of Physicians, 1989.

17. Neer CS II. The surgical treatment of the fractured hip. *Surg Clin North Am* 1951; 31: 499–512.

18. Reno JH, Burlington H. Fractures of the hip – mortality survey. *Am J Surg* 1958; 95: 581–92.

19. Zuckerman JD, Skovron ML, Koval KJ *et al.* Postoperative complications and mortality associated with operative delay in older patients who have a fracture of the hip. *J Bone Joint Surg* 1995; 77A: 1551–6.

20. Ions GK, Stevens J. Prediction of survival in patients with femoral neck fractures. *J Bone Joint Surg* 1987; 69B: 384–7.

21. Villar RN, Allen SM, Barnes SJ. hip fractures in healthy patients: operative delays versus prognosis. *Brit Med J* 1986; 298: 1203–4.

22. Sexson SB, Lemner JT. Factors affecting hip fracture mortality. *J Orthop Trauma* 1988; 1: 298–305.

23. Fox HJ, Pooler J, Prothero D, Bannister GC. Factors affecting the outcome after proximal femoral fractures. *Injury* 1994; 25: 297–300.

24. Rogers FB, Shackford SR, Keller MS. Early fixation reduces morbidity and mortality in elderly patients with hip fractures from low impact falls. *J Trauma* 1995; 39: 261–5.

25. Dolk I. Operation in hip fracture patients – analysis of the time factor. *Injury* 1990; 21: 369–72.

26. Kenzora JE, McCrathy RE, Lowell JD, Sledge CB. Hip fracture mortality. *Clin Orthop* 1984; 186: 45–56.

27. Todd CJ, Freeman CJ, Camillezi-Ferantec *et al.* Differences in mortality after fracture of the hip: the East Anglian audit. *Brit Med J* 1995; 310: 904–8.

28. Bannister GC, Gibson AGF, Ackroyd CE, Newman JH. The fixation and prognosis of trochanteric fractures. *Clin Orthop* 1990; 254: 242–6.

29. Kennie DC, Reid J, Richardson IR *et al.* Effectiveness of geriatric rehabilitative care after fracture of the proximal femur in elderly women: a randomised clinical trial. *Brit Med J* 1988; 297: 1083–6.

30. Reid J, Kennie DC. Geriatric rehabilitative care after fractures of the proximal femur: one year follow up of a randomised clinical trial. *Brit Med J* 1989; 299: 25–6.

31. Ceder L, Svensson K, Thorngren KG. Statistical prediction of rehabilitation in elderly patients with hip fractures. *Clin Orthop* 1980; 152: 185–90.

32. Jensen JS, Bagger J. Long term social prognosis after hip fractures. *Acta Orthop Scand* 1982; 53: 97–101.

33. Sikorski JM, Davis NJ, Senior J. The rapid transit system for patients with fractures of proximal femur. *Brit Med J* 1985; 290: 439–43.

34. Fitzgerald JF, Moore PS, Dittus RS. The care of the elderly with hip fracture. *N Engl J Med* 1988; 319: 1392–7.

35. Fox HJ, Hughes SJ, Pooler J *et al.* Length of hospital stay and outcome after femoral neck fracture – a prospective study comparing the performance of two hospitals. *Injury* 1993; 24: 467–66.

36. Pryor GA, Williams DRR. Rehabilitation after fractures. *J Bone Joint Surg* 1989; 71B: 471–4.

37. Jalovaara S, Berglund-Rodean B, Wingstrand H, Thorngren K-G. Treatment of hip fracture in Finland and Sweden. *Acta Orthop Scand* 1992; 63: 531–5.

38. Stromberg L, Ohlen G, Svensson O. Prospective payment systems and hip fracture treatment costs. *Acta Orthop Scand* 1997; 68: 6–12.

39. Keene GS, Parker MJ, Pryor GA. Mortality and morbidity after hip fractures. *Brit Med J* 1993; 307: 1248–50.

40. Holmberg S, Thorngren K-G. Rehabilitation after femoral neck fracture. *Acta Orthop Scand* 1983; 56: 305–8.

41. Robbins JA, Donaldson LJ. Analysing stages of care in hospital stay for fractured neck of femur. *Lancet* 1984; ii: 1028–9.

42. Jensen JS. Determining factors for the mortality following hip fractures. *Injury* 1984; 15: 411–14.

43. Wood DJ, Ions GH, Quincy JM *et al.* Factors which influence mortality after subcapital hip fracture. *J Bone Joint Surg* 1992; 74B: 199–202.

44. Wallace RGD, Lowry JH, McLeod NW, Mollan RAB. A simple grading system to guide the prognosis after hip fracture in the elderly. *Brit Med J* 1986; 293: 865.

45. Parker MJ, Palmer CR. A new mobility scale for predicting mortality after hip fracture. *J Bone Joint Surg* 1993; 75B: 797–8.

46. Wallace WA. The increasing incidence of fractures of the proximal femur: an orthopaedic epidemic. *Lancet* 1983; 1: 1413–14.

47. Pearse M, Woolf A. Care of elderly patients with a fractured neck of femur. *Health Trends* 1992; 24: 134–6.

CHAPTER 14

Intracapsular fractures

G. C. Bannister

Background

Intracapsular fractures present unique difficulties because fractures disrupt the blood supply to the femoral head and neck, preventing union; if union does occur, it causes subsequent avascular necrosis of the femoral head. The capacity of the hip joint is between 60 and 90 ml so the fracture does not cause shock, although bleeding into the capsule achieves sufficiently high pressures for the residual blood supply to be occluded. Displacement of the fracture usually interrupts the blood supply, increasing the rates of non-union and avascular necrosis.

Undisplaced fractures cause little disturbance of blood supply and, provided they remain stable, they unite in 95% of cases. Conservatively managed displaced intracapsular fractures unite in no more than 25% of cases [1], and it was not until the introduction of the Smith-Petersen trifin nail in 1929 that the union rate for displaced intracapsular fractures became acceptable. Interestingly, Smith-Petersen's figures of 80% union have rarely been achieved in subsequent practice.

Fixation of intracapsular fractures forms a substantial part of the literature, and yet it is one of the most straightforward aspects.

The surgeon needs to obtain stability in all planes; two implants give better rotatory stability than one. The rotatory stability of the three fins of Smith-Petersen's nail is vastly outweighed by the moment of two implants placed within the periphery of the neck. There is evidence from clinical controlled trials that union rates are higher when two implants are used, both with the Smith-Petersen nail [2], and when comparing the dynamic hip screw with cannulated Garden screws. The quest to enhance union by using sliding or compression screws [3,4] has never improved union rates. The MRC

prospective study on the management of displaced intracapsular femoral neck fractures [5] demonstrated slight advantages of cannulated screws over trifin nails and no benefit from the Charnley compression screw. Scandinavian Hip Fracture Registers record equally good results regardless of fixation method.

The unsolved problem in intracapsular femoral neck fracture is identifying whether or not the femoral head is alive. In heads retrieved *post mortem* after fixation of intracapsular fractures, the blood supply to the head is almost universally compromised if not obliterated [6]. Two authors have assessed blood supply to the femoral neck in displaced intracapsular fractures in patients and recorded a 90% union rate in heads with an intact blood supply: Outerbridge [7] using perosseous phlebography and Milligan [8] using vital dye (Kiton green) both demonstrated union rates of 90%. Technetium-labelled phosphate is not reliable for 2–3 weeks which renders its use impractical. At the time of writing, magnetic resonance imaging does not appear to be helpful in the early stages. In practice, perosseous phlebography has not been reproducible outside the hands of the originator and vital dyes are socially unacceptable. The surgeon is thus denied the critical information needed to decide on whether to save, reduce, and internally fix displaced femoral heads or to sacrifice the head opting for prosthetic replacement.

Treatment options

In undisplaced intracapsular fractures, the surgeon may elect to treat either conservatively or by internal fixation. The penalty of using internal fixation is an avascular necrosis rate of 15%, although union is 95% compared with between 80% and 90% [9] for conservatively treated undisplaced fractures. Conservative management of undisplaced intracapsular fractures is now of historical interest because of pressure on hospital beds. Even in patients who have sustained a recent myocardial infarction or have other overwhelming anaesthetic risks, the operation can be carried out under local anaesthesia with infiltration of the skin and periosteum [10].

The displaced intracapsular fracture may be reduced and internally fixed or the head discarded and hemi- or total arthroplasty carried out.

The problem with reduction and fixation is delayed union or non-union. Union may take as long as 10 months and is never complete in under 3 months. Union rates fall with advancing age: 50% of displaced intracapsular fractures in octogenarians, who are predominantly the victim of such injuries, unite. That 50% depends on satisfactory reduction. The acceptable limits of reduction are no more than 5° varus and 10° displacement in any other direction [5]. In general, some 17% of fractures are not reducible closed within these limits or not recognized as being inadequately reduced. Fracture union does not guarantee a pain-free hip so, in general, 30% of patients with displaced intracapsular femoral neck fractures treated by closed reduction and internal fixation, are free of pain. For this reason many centres make no attempt to preserve the head in elderly patients, instead electing for prosthetic replacement. Prosthetic replacement may be hemiarthroplasty, bipolar, or total. Each has its separate complications.

Hemiarthroplasty

Hemiarthroplasty may be uncemented or cemented. The most widely used uncemented hemiarthroplasty is the Austin Moore, initially developed in 1935 as a tumour prosthesis and subsequently published in modern form in 1956. The Moore hemiarthroplasty is a narrow collared prosthesis with a straight stem. As for all uncemented devices, it relies on three-point fixation and achieves this most securely in narrow femoral medullary cavities with good quality bone. This is exactly the type of bone that is not found in patients with intracapsular femoral neck fractures who are universally osteoporotic, and the Moore hemiarthroplasty rarely obtains stable fixation. Some 70% of Moore hemiarthroplasties migrate into a varus position. There is concomitant thigh pain. The Moore, as do all hemiarthroplasties, causes acetabular erosion. The

Austin Moore prosthesis has one major advantage over cemented devices, which is that it can virtually always be removed easily if required. There are three major indications for wishing to remove a Moore hemiarthroplasty: these are dislocation, infection, and acetabular erosion requiring total hip replacement.

Dislocation after hemiarthroplasty is a much feared but relatively rare complication. Most series report between 2% and 4% [11] and dislocation occurs in patients who are intellectually or neurologically impaired. Demented patients, which comprises those with a mental test score of less than three, and those with Parkinson's disease or strokes, all have higher dislocation rates. The surgeon cannot influence the systemic condition from which the patient suffers, and in such cases recurrent dislocation of a hemiarthroplasty is best managed by a Girdlestone excision arthroplasty. A Girdlestone is very much easier to perform if the prosthesis is uncemented than if it is cemented, and the Moore prosthesis is usually easily removed.

Infection rates in displaced intracapsular femoral neck fractures are of the order of 5%. The population is infirm. Operations are generally carried out in conventional, plenum ventilated operating rooms. Although antibiotic prophylaxis is routinely used in modern practice, bacterial resistance and intra-hospital infection is increasing. Infection rates in hip fractures carried out in conventional operating rooms with first- or second-generation cephalosporin antibiotic prophylaxis are of the order of 5%. Infection rates in uncemented prostheses are lower than those in cemented ones. In the first instance, the treatment of an infection is likely to be a Girdlestone prosthesis. An Austin Moore prosthesis is usually more easily removed if such a course has to be taken.

The cemented hemiarthroplasty

The most widely used cemented hemiarthroplasty is the Thompson [12]. This was originally designed with a collar to rest on the trochanters because F.R. Thompson, its originator, had observed resorption of the femoral neck in failed fixation of displaced intracapsular fractures. The Thompson prosthesis has a curved stem and was originally designed to be inserted uncemented. As the stem is curved, it is usually not possible to obtain a uniform cement mantle when polymethylmethacrylate is used to enhance its fixation. When cemented it migrates less than the Moore prosthesis; there is also less thigh pain. Acetabular erosion occurs as in the Moore hemiarthroplasty. If patients survive 5 years, some 20% will have undergone total hip replacement [13], and by inference a very much higher proportion will have eroded their acetabulum and have pain, but be too unfit to consider revision. Some 25% of patients at this time also demonstrate aseptic loosening of the stem.

The cemented Thompson erodes the acetabulum more frequently if the size of the head is too large for the acetabulum or if it is inserted with the neck long [14]. The latter is a common error because both the Moore and stem replacement in total hip arthroplasty preserve the neck and a further 2 cm of the neck at least needs to be resected to seat a Thompson hemiarthroplasty satisfactorily.

If infection ensues, it is of the essence to remove all prosthetic material. The cement in a Thompson hemiarthroplasty grips on thin bone that is easily perforated and cement removal is particularly difficult.

Should the acetabulum erode, conversion of a Thompson hemiarthroplasty to a total hip replacement is a demanding procedure. It is demanding because, if any torsion at all is used in dislocating the hip, the shaft is at risk of fracture at the stress raiser between the thin shaft and the tip of the prosthetic complex. Having dislocated the hip and removed the Thompson prosthesis, the surgeon is then faced with removing cement through a curved track and reimplanting a straight prosthesis in its place. Intraoperative complication rates are high when a cemented Thompson hemiarthroplasty is revised to total hip replacement.

Bipolar prostheses

Bipolar prostheses have a dual joint between a small head, which is attached to the femoral stem and fixed to a large metal-backed mobile head, which articulates with the acetabulum. They were originally designed as treatment for osteoarthritis. Early uncemented polyethylene heads caused acetabular erosion because of high-density polyethylene (HDP) debris and this design is now metal-backed. The Hastings Group [14,15] sought to address acetabular erosion by using a Charnley stem and a metal-backed head of increasing 1-mm increments (the Hastings bipolar hemiarthroplasty). Acetabular erosion

rates were halved, but of the 16 dislocations only three could be reduced closed. Three of the 16 dislocations were late and of these two were intraprosthetic.

Radiological studies show that some bipolar arthroplasties cease to move at both their articulations, functioning as hemiarthroplasties. Their manufacture is more complex, and their cost correspondingly greater. Nevertheless, they are more stable than total hip replacements and pain relief is good. It appears that acetabular erosion rates are rather less with bipolar prostheses than solid metal hemiarthroplasties. If they dislocate, open reduction may be required.

Total hip replacement

Total hip replacement gives excellent relief of pain, a stable hip, and one that is likely to last the duration of an elderly patient's lifetime. The problem with total hip replacement in displaced intracapsular femoral neck fractures in the elderly population has been dislocation [16]. Dislocation rates of the order of 11% are reported, which would appear to represent the inability of the octogenarian to accommodate to the patient requirements of total hip replacement, because a similar rate of dislocation is reported in primary total hip replacement [17]. In an unselected elderly population randomly allocated to closed reduction and screw fixation, hemiarthroplasty, or total hip replacement, the qualitative result was best in those with total hip replacement at the price of a dislocation rate of some 9% [18].

In patients with rheumatoid arthritis, there is no choice but to offer total hip replacement, because union rate after internal fixation is of the order of 10%, and hemiarthroplasty is universally followed by erosion of an already soft acetabulum.

Case selection

Displaced intracapsular fracture is not a condition that lends itself to a unit policy of a single procedure for all cases at all ages. Most patients are around 80 years of age; 12% succumb while in hospital and 30% are dead within a year. Patients usually have multisystem disease. The demands that they place on their hips are restricted by other system failures. Their independence is often parlous and the usual difficulties to follow-up are compounded by changes of address to residential and nursing homes, residence with relatives, and geographical upheaval. There are accordingly very few long-term follow-up studies addressing function.

Four groups seem to emerge that require special consideration.

The young intracapsular fracture

Provided that infection is not introduced in the course of preliminary treatment, the elderly patient has a prospect of excellent pain relief and a stable hip in the vast majority of cases treated by arthroplasty. For that reason, the threshold for discarding the head in elderly people is low, but in the young a completely different approach must be adopted. The results of total hip replacement after trauma in younger patients are the worst in the literature. Injury usually occurs as a result of a highly violent road traffic accident. Patients are often heavily built men who earn their living through manual labour. Life expectancy of a total hip replacement in such a patient is of the order of 5 years, with the prospect of a pseudarthrosis after 10–12 years. In such a situation, the head must be preserved at all costs, its blood supply assessed before it fragments, and the head revascularized if dead.

Intervention must be active and the condition constitutes a surgical emergency. The head should be reduced, open if necessary through an anterior approach, fixed, and the capsule decompressed of haematoma [19]. The patient should be non-weight-bearing. At 3–6 weeks, a technetium scan should be carried out. If this shows that the head is dead, the next approach must be revascularization by either a quadratus femoris transfer or a vascularized free bone flap. If this fails, the only recourse then is a total hip replacement because arthrodesis is now almost never performed, is rarely acceptable to patients in Britain and North America, and is very difficult to achieve with a dead femoral head. If total hip arthroplasty is undertaken, an uncemented acetabular component should be inserted because the results of cemented sockets have been most disappointing in this age range.

Total hip replacement should be undertaken only on the strict proviso that patients retrain for work that is not of a heavy manual nature.

Fit active elderly patients

Fit active elderly people are the population aged over 60

who before fracture are walking unlimited distances in the community, without aids, are independent, coping with stairs, and participating in non-contact sports such as golf or bowls. This population is likely to live more than 5 years, and if a hemiarthroplasty is implanted suffer from acetabular erosion and/or stem loosening. Hemiarthroplasty is absolutely contraindicated in this age range. Case–control studies [20a] confirm grossly inferior results if hemiarthroplasties are inserted into this population. This population comprises no more than 20% of the patients presenting in the author's unit at the time of writing. There are three potential options in the management of this type of patient.

- The fracture can be reduced and internally fixed. If the hip is immediately comfortable this indicates that a stable fixation has been achieved and radiographs of the fracture should be taken regularly. If there is any suggestion that union is not progressing, a technetium bone scan should be carried out to indicate whether the head is viable. If the head is not viable and the hip progressively symptomatic, prompt total hip replacement should be carried out. Patients should not be allowed to degenerate into a state of painful dysfunction. If this is allowed, they lose their capacity to carry out the activities with which they could cope before. The Swedish experience of late total hip replacement after failed internal fixation indicates that only 2% of patients walk without aids.

- Conversely, a primary total hip replacement can be carried out. The technical difficulties encountered are that rather more neck is lost than would normally be resected in a primary joint replacement, but, that apart, results are quite comparable to those after arthritis, and dislocation rates are equivalent in this particular population.

- The final option is bipolar hip replacement. There is evidence [15] that acetabular erosion rates are halved, but this is in unselected population, of whom 80% had been withdrawn from survivorship analysis after 3–4 years. The bipolar hip replacement has advantages and the dislocation rate is lower than in total hip replacement, but it is likely to give slightly higher rates of revision and inferior pain relief.

The aim is to carry out the most definitive procedure possible, because revision 10 years later is inevitably hazardous as the patient is correspondingly older and frailer at that time.

The semi-active elderly person

These patients usually require walking aids, are barely coping with stairs, require assistance about the home, cannot walk more than a quarter of a mile, usually have to be transported to shops, and are 80 years of age or over. They have a limited life expectancy and require a stable hip to allow them to continue to walk the necessary limited distances. A cemented Thompson hemiarthroplasty is the procedure of choice here, because less thigh pain will ensue than with an uncemented Moore hemiarthroplasty.

The barely ambulatory elderly person

These patients are house-bound, able to transfer from bed to chair, and perform their own toilet, but are reliant on others for housework, laundry, and hot meals. A little under 50% of these patients will never walk again or will be room-bound with a frame. A Moore hemiarthroplasty is quite sufficient in this population, because it can be removed easily should chronic dislocation ensue.

The bedridden elderly person

Some 5% of patients are already institutionalized because of inability to walk, and break their hips either falling out of bed or transferring from bed to chair. No useful purpose is served in offering any operative treatment to this population. The hip will cease to be painful after 10–14 days. Pain relief is not improved by surgery. The kindest and most effective treatment is to allow patients to stay in bed until the hip becomes painless, and then to continue with their previous, very limited, mobility.

Clinical management

The outcome of patients with proximal femoral fractures, regardless of site, depends on their state of infirmity before hip fracture and on four aspects of hospital intervention [20b], which in the author's unit have been shown to influence mortality and morbidity:

- Non-medical delay to surgery
- The development of open pressure sores
- Infection
- Failed surgical intervention.

The principal cause of death was bronchopneumonia. If surgery was delayed beyond 24 hours from admission, the death rate from bronchopneumonia rose by 500%

[21]. Pressure sores were associated with prolonged recumbence on hard beds in an accident and emergency department awaiting transfer to a hospital bed. Infection rates in this study were 6% and reoperation rates 2%. Realistically, non-medical delays to surgery can be prevented with bespoke daily operating time allocated for patients with proximal femoral fracture, pressure areas by the use of appropriate mattresses, and infection by the addition of antiseptics to antibiotic prophylaxis at surgery. Patients with proximal femoral fractures tend to be afforded less priority than younger fitter patients with other injuries. Elderly patients have often been lying unattended on a cold floor, after falling and fracturing the hip. They are often dehydrated on arrival at hospital. If they were not already in poor health, they would not have fallen and sustained a hip fracture, and the outcome of their treatment is critically dependent on their state of hydration and surgical nutrition before the additional insult of surgery.

The practice of starving elderly women with proximal femoral fracture for a morning list, and then cancelling, pending an evening emergency list, is reprehensible from every viewpoint. Hospital stay is prolonged and mortality and morbidity increased. Even from a purely financial aspect, there is nothing to commend this practice because the cost of management of patients with proximal femoral fractures is increased as a result of prolonged bed occupancy. Elderly patients with proximal femoral fractures require their surgery to be planned. They should not be starved for more than 6 hours before surgery and should not go without fluids for more than 4 hours.

Operative management

Internal fixation of intracapsular femoral neck fractures

Fractures should be reduced and fixed under image intensification on a fracture table. The non-operated leg is abducted, flexed, and externally rotated to allow maximum access to the image intensifier. If the fracture is undisplaced, the lower limb should be internally rotated so that the patella lies in approximately 15° of internal rotation, because this places the femoral neck in a horizontal position, facilitating fixation in the lateral plane (Fig. 14.1).

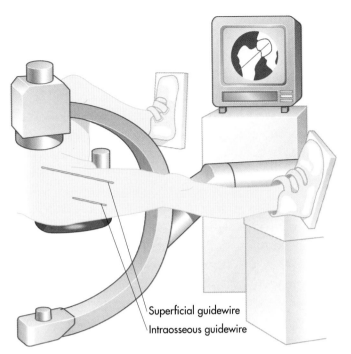

Figure 14.1 – *Placement of limbs for internal fixation of intracapsular femoral neck fractures.*

If the fracture is displaced, it should be gently reduced by traction in extension, external rotation, and abduction, followed by flexion and internal rotation (Fig. 14.2). If the fracture cannot be reduced within 10° of the anatomical on the lateral view or on the anteroposterior (AP) view to within 15° laterally and 5° medially, a further attempt at reduction should be made and, if that fails, depending on the age of the patient, the procedure should be abandoned or open reduction attempted (see below). A guidewire is then placed over the anterior aspect of the femoral neck following a line 2.5 cm distal to the vastus lateralis ridge to the midpoint between the pubic tubercle and the anterosuperior iliac spine, which represents the centre of the hip (Fig. 14.3). This guides the surgeon to the correct site of incision which should be made overlying the middle of the femoral shaft. If two or three cannulated screws are to be inserted, this can be done percutaneously. If the blade or screw plate is to be employed, a limited posterolateral approach should be made (Fig. 14.4). Depending on the available internal fixation device, cannulated screws should be inserted anteriorly and posteriorly, inferiorly, and superiorly (Fig. 14.5), or if a dynamic hip screw is used the head should be stabilized with an additional guidewire during reaming to avoid rotation.

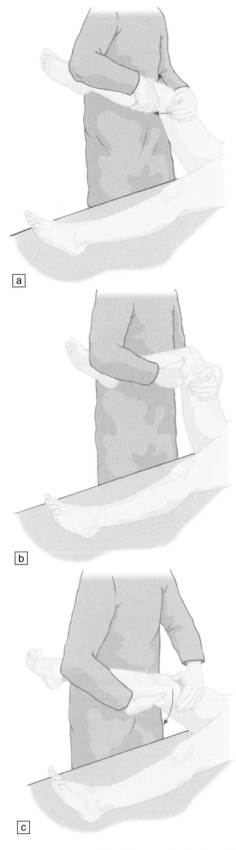

Figure 14.2 – *If the fracture is displaced, it should be gently reduced by traction in extension, external rotation, and abduction, followed by flexion and internal rotation.*

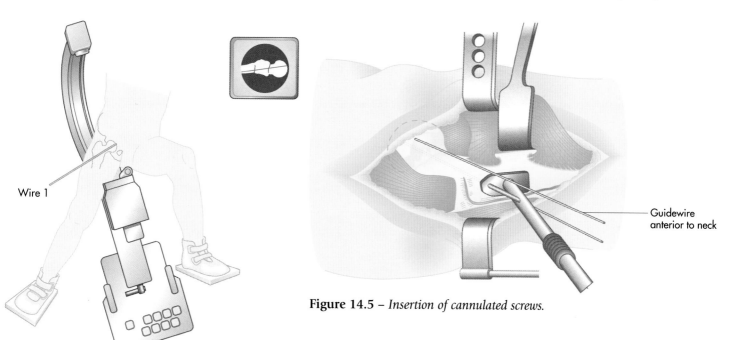

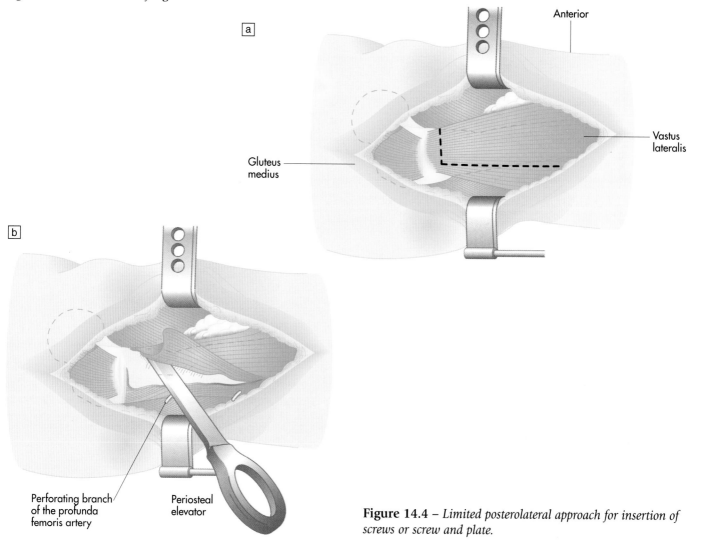

Wire 1

Figure 14.3 – *Placement of a guidewire.*

Guidewire
anterior to neck

Figure 14.5 – *Insertion of cannulated screws.*

[a]

Anterior

Gluteus
medius

Vastus
lateralis

[b]

Perforating branch
of the profunda
femoris artery

Periosteal
elevator

Figure 14.4 – *Limited posterolateral approach for insertion of
screws or screw and plate.*

The dynamic hip screw should be placed absolutely central in the subchondral bone of the head. The patient may sit out of bed the following day or stand if he or she feels so capable. In very young patients, 3 months of eggshell weight-bearing is indicated, because there is a slightly increased union rate with this regimen.

Hemiarthroplasty

The direct lateral approach has a lower incidence of dislocation than the posterior, is widely practised, and is the most sensible option for this procedure. The patient is placed in the lateral position with props holding the sacrum and ischial tuberosities posteriorly and the anterosuperior iliac spines anteriorly. A midline lateral incision is made, beginning l0 cm distal to the greater trochanter, extending 3 cm proximal. The skin is taken in continuity with the fascia lata because this is the fasciocutaneous flap, and the gluteal bursa is dissected off. The proximal 5 cm of vastus lateralis is split with a knife and the incision continued along the anterior third of the greater trochanter, diverting the anterior fibres proximally. The perforating vessel in vastus lateralis is coagulated. Vastus lateralis is elevated from the proximal femoral shaft anteriorly with a periosteal elevator and a bone lever is inserted.

The hip is adducted and externally rotated. Using either a sharp periosteal elevator or a 2-cm osteotome, vastus lateralis is elevated from the anterior aspect of the femoral shaft, taking with it the continuous tendon with the anterior third of gluteus medius and the insertion of gluteus minimus. The fibres of gluteus medius are split anterosuperiorly for no more than 2 cm, leaving a well-formed flap of muscle and fibrous tissue with the capsule of the femoral neck beneath. The plane along the femoral neck is developed anteriorly, medially, and superiorly, a T incision is made in the femoral neck, old blood emerges, and the fractured neck becomes immediately apparent. Sutures are placed in the corner of the T incisions, the superior capsule is resected back further to the piriform fossa, and the neck further exposed by adduction and external rotation. A sharp-ended retractor is placed behind the neck, levering it anteriorly protecting the posterior two-thirds of gluteus. Approximately 1 cm of neck is resected, the fragment being retained. This gives access to the acetabulum and allows the head to be removed. The acetabulum is cleared of bony debris and a swab inserted to protect it from further contamination. The cut fragment of neck

and the fractured head are then placed together on top of the femoral shaft and checked against the collar of the definitive prosthesis, so that the neck resection can be corrected to ensure equal leg length.

The next task is to ensure satisfactory broaching of the femoral medullary canal. Forceful reaming places the femur at great risk of perforation. It is tempting in a heavy patient to settle for inadequate exposure and to commence reaming anteromedially. This temptation should be resisted at all cost because it is extremely unlikely that the canal will ever be satisfactorily reamed and equally likely that the shaft will be perforated. The correct position from which to start reaming and the only position is posterolaterally. The posterior bone lever gives access to the posterolateral aspect of the femoral neck, an opening is made, and a small osteotome and a small blunt curette passed gently down the canal to ensure satisfactory positioning. The canal is then reamed with a larger curette and finally broaches are gently inserted. In an osteoporotic medullary canal, the broaches should pass easily by hand. If the surgeon feels the need to use a hammer forcefully, he should reappraise his alignment immediately.

If an Austin Moore prosthesis is to be inserted, it should be tapped gently down in anatomical anteversion, to appose the neck against the cut calcar femorale. The swab should then be removed from the acetabulum, and the two corners of the capsule pulled aside to allow access for the head to be reduced by a combination of traction and neutral rotation. The capsule is then repaired. The anterior fibres of gluteus medius and vastus lateralis should be repaired through bone. A suitable passage can be made by taking a Kocher bone hook and manipulating it through the greater trochanter from the lateral to the anterior surface. Two or three such holes may be made and the anterior aponeurosis of gluteus medius then overlapped over the posterior to restore the internal rotator mechanism of the hip joint. This should leave spare aponeurosis that will take a further layer of sutures to the aponeurosis of the posterior two-thirds of gluteus medius. The wound is then closed in layers over a drain, which is removed after 24 hours. An abduction wedge should be worn in bed for 3 months, during which time the patient should observe the restrictions imposed on any hip replacement (see below). Patients may begin walking fully weight-bearing, within the limits of comfort, after 48 hours.

Technique for Thompson hemiarthroplasty

The neck should be resected to the level of the lesser trochanter.

When the femoral medullary cavity has been satisfactorily reamed, it should be curetted of loose bone out to the peripheral 3 mm, brushed, restricted 16 cm distal to the cut neck, lavaged with pressure, dried, and bone cement inserted and compressed. The Thompson hemiarthroplasty should be inserted as lateral as possible to ensure that at least 3 mm of cement are interposed between it and the calcar femorale.

Rehabilitation

Just as the management of intracapsular femoral neck fracture must be tailored to the individual patient's need, so must rehabilitation.

The fit active young patient, who has sustained a high violence injury, may reasonably be directed to avoid weight-bearing for 3 months to optimize the chances of fracture union. Such instruction to an elderly woman with parlous memory and multisystem failure, who has already manifestly shown her inability to stand on two feet without falling over, is a counsel of despair. It is the surgeon's duty to provide his physiotherapist with sufficient fracture stability to allow a patient to mobilize.

Fit elderly patients should follow the same regimen as for primary total hip replacement. They should sleep with a pillow between their legs, use a high chair for both sitting and toilet purposes, and avoid driving for 2 months and flexing their hips beyond 90° for ever.

As far as is feasible, slightly impaired elderly patients should follow the same regimen, but when one reaches the more extreme degrees of disability rehabilitation goals change. On average, 50% of patients lose between one and two grades of walking ability after proximal femoral fracture. This means that, if a patient is barely coping in their own home or with relatives with maximum Social Services support, 'meals on wheels', and home help to clean and shop, there is a 50% chance that they will not return to this state. Over 90% of patients who are walking with a frame before they fracture their hips need to be placed in nursing homes within a year of their fracture [22]. It is unkind with this population continually to force patients to walk when they no longer have the energy; the prognosis should be discussed with the patients and relatives as soon as is feasible, and a realistic rehabilitation programme with targets worked out. If patients are not walking within 2–3 weeks, it is most unlikely that they will ever walk again, and it is to everyone's advantage to make arrangements for long-term nursing care outside an acute unit in such circumstances.

Patients who are already bed-bound and in community nursing homes should be returned as soon as possible. An acute hospital unit can do nothing for them and a change of environment merely causes confusional states.

References

1. Phemister DB. Fractures of the neck of the femur. *Surg Gynecol Obstet* 1934; 59: 415.

2. McQuillan WM, Abernethy PJ, Guy JG. Subcapital fractures of the neck of the femur treated by double-divergent fixation. *Br J Surg* 1973; 60: 859–66.

3. Goody-Moreira FE. A special stud-bolt screw for fixation of fractures of the neck of the femur. *J Bone Joint Surg* 1940; 38: 683–97.

4. Charnley J, Blockley NJ, Purser DW. The treatment of displaced fractures of the neck of the femur by compression: a preliminary report. *J Bone Joint Surg* 1957; 39B: 45–65.

5. Barnes R, Brown JT, Garden RS, Nicoll EA. Subcapital fractures of the femur. *J Bone Joint Surg* 1976; 58B: 2–24.

6. Catto M. A histological study of avascular necrosis of the femoral head after transcervical fractures. *J Bone Joint Surg* 1965; 47B: 749–76.

7. Outerbridge RE. Perosseous venography in the diagnosis of viability in subcapital fractures of the femur. *Clin Orthop* 1978; 137: 132–9.

8. Milligan GF. The use of Kiton fast green to measure the viability of the head of the femur after fractures of the neck of the femur. *Injury* 1978; 10: 235–8.

9. Bentley G. Impacted fractures of the neck of the femur. *J Bone Joint Surg* 1968; 50B: 551.

10. Ackroyd CE. The treatment of subcapital femoral fractures with Moore's pins: a study of 34 cases. *Injury* 1973; 5: 100.

11. Sikorski JM, Barrington R. Internal fixation versus hemiarthroplasty for the displaced subcapital fracture of the femur. *J Bone Joint Surg* 1981; 63B: 357–61.

12. Thompson FR. Two and a half years' experience with a vitallium intramedullary hip prosthesis. *J Bone Joint Surg* 1954; 36A: 489–500.

13. Maxted MJ, Denham RA. Failure of the hemiarthroplasty for fractures of the neck of the femur. *Injury* 1984; 15: 224–6.

14. D'Arcy J, Devas M. Treatment of fractures of the femoral neck by replacement with the Thompson prosthesis. *J Bone Joint Surg* 1976; 58B: 279–86.

15. Wetherall RG, Hinves BL. The Hastings bipolar hemiarthroplasty for sub capital fractures of the femoral neck. *J Bone Joint Surg* 1990; 72B:788–93.

16. Sim FH, Stauffer RN. Management of hip fractures by total hip arthroplasty. *Clin Orthop* 1980; 152: 191–7.

17. Newington DP, Bannister GC, Fordyce M. Primary total hip replacement in patients over 80 years of age. *J Bone Joint Surg* 1990; 72B: 450–2.

18. Skinner PW, Riley D, Ellery J *et al.* Displaced subcapital fractures of the femur: a prospective randomised comparison of internal fixation, hemiarthroplasty and total hip replacement. *Injury* 1989; 20: 291–3.

19. Swiontkowski MF, Winquyst RA, Hansen ST Sr. Fractures of the femoral neck in patients between the ages of twelve and forty-nine years. *J Bone Joint Surg* 1984; 66A: 837–46.

20a. Squires B, Bannister G. Displaced intracapsular neck of femur fractures in mobile independent patients: total hip replacement or hemiarthroplasty injury. *Int J Care Injured* 1999; 30: 345–348.

20b. Fox HJ, Pooler J, Prothero D, Bannister GC. Factors affecting the outcome after proximal femoral fractures. *Injury* 1994; 25: 297–300.

21. Perez J, Warwick DJ, Case CP, Bannister GC. Death after femoral neck fracture – an autopsy study. *Injury* 1995; 26: 237–40.

22. Hubble M, Little C, Prothero D, Bannister GC. Predicting the prognosis after proximal femoral fracture. *Ann R Coll Surg Engl* 1995; 77: 355–7.

CHAPTER 15

Trochanteric and subtrochanteric fractures

G. C. Bannister

The blood supply to these fractures is good and non-union in trochanteric fractures is as low as 2%. There is a greater lever arm on the subtrochanteric fractures, which poses significantly greater technical problems in fixation.

Trochanteric fractures

Trochanteric fractures can be managed either conservatively or by internal fixation. Good conservative management is better than poor operative management, but overall results are equally good and rehabilitation after operative treatment is quicker [1].

Conservative management would nowadays be considered only in cases of extreme anaesthetic risk.

The fixation of trochanteric fractures has been revolutionized by the adoption of sliding hip screws. Before that, fixation devices were modifications of the Smith-Petersen trifin nail.

Fixation of trochanteric fractures with fixed length nail plates was fraught with complications, particularly in unstable fracture configurations. There was blood loss that was poorly tolerated by elderly patients, which stimulated a quest for less invasive methods of fixation. In 1981, Hall and Ainscow [2] compared Enders nails with nail-plate fixation, finding reduced operating time, blood loss, mechanical failure, mortality, and hospital stay. However, 12% of patients developed an external rotation deformity of more than 12°.

By this time the sliding hip screw, originally designed to promote compression in intracapsular fractures, was being adopted for trochanteric disruptions. Randomized prospective comparison of Enders nails versus the sliding hip screw confirmed the lower operating time, blood loss, and postoperative medical complications, but was associated with double the rate of reoperation and postoperative pain and knee stiffness in 40% of cases.

The original classification of trochanteric fractures [3] was proposed when management was conservative. The same classification was modified by Jenson et al. [4] for operative treatment using fixed length nail-plate devices.

Before sliding hip screws, it was necessary to obtain good bony apposition to avoid fracture collapse, acetabular penetration, and implant failure. The medial displacement osteotomy [5] was described for four-part fractures and the Sarmiento [6] valgus osteotomy for three-part ones. Sliding hip screws have rendered these procedures obsolete, because, in four-part fractures, the screw allows controlled collapse and, in three-part ones, the strength of the device is sufficient to hold the fracture while union takes place. As the key feature of the sliding screw is the purchase that it obtains on the femoral head, it is axiomatic that the critical part of fixation is to place the screw within 5 mm of the joint surface, absolutely in the centre of the femoral neck or slightly inferiorly [7]. Under no circumstances must the screw be placed superiorly, where the purchase is poor, because it will cut out, and a difficult salvage operation ensues in which it is necessary to implant the screw in the undamaged inferior part of the neck.

Subtrochanteric fractures

Subtrochanteric fractures are sensibly subclassified into true, displaced, transverse, subtrochanteric fractures, or oblique ones, often with comminution extending between the trochanters. The displaced transverse true subtrochanteric fracture is extremely difficult to manage conservatively, because the proximal fragment is displaced into flexion by the psoas and abduction. The abductor mechanism is unopposed by the balancing action of extensors and adductors, which are attached to the distal fragment. Aligning the distal fragment on the proximal means abducting and flexing the distal fragment and applying traction. The patient tends to slide off the bed in the direction of the traction. This can partially be opposed by tucking a sheet around the patient's trunk into the other side of the bed, but problems of managing the fracture in this manner are compounded by the relative inexperience in fracture management by traction in modern orthopaedic practice and limited space on orthopaedic trauma wards.

The overwhelming majority of these injuries are managed by internal fixation. Intramedullary fixation is indicated in transverse, true, subtrochanteric fractures. If intramedullary devices are used in comminuted fractures, the greater trochanter may be sheared off, leaving a highly unstable proximal fixation.

Nailing devices have been employed for both trochanteric and subtrochanteric fracture since Kuntscher and evolved through the Zickel, to the modern variants of which the Gamma nail has been most extensively studied. The problem with K-Y nail-type devices is obtaining accurate purchase in the head of the femur, bursting of the proximal femur in the presence of unsuspected proximal comminution, and fracture of the shaft. The theoretical advantage is that the operation is potentially quicker with less blood loss.

Halder [8] reviewed 123 mixed inter- and subtrochanteric fractures fixed with a Gamma nail, with one non-union, two screw fixations, and three fractures of the greater trochanter. Randomized prospective comparisons of the Gamma nail with the dynamic hip screw revealed no difference in failure of proximal fixation, but increased femoral shaft fractures, in the Gamma nail group [9]. With increasing experience, it appears that complications with the Gamma nail can be reduced, but in general K-Y fixation has a relatively long learning curve and is likely to be associated with complications in the hands of the occasional user.

Technique

Trochanteric fractures using the AO dynamic hip screw

The patient is placed on a fracture table with the uninjured limb abducted, flexed, and externally rotated, to allow an unimpeded anteroposterior (AP) and lateral view of the fracture and the femoral head (Fig. 15.1).

Closed reduction

A little under 50% of trochanteric fractures are stable or minimally displaced and can be reduced easily by closed means. Two- and three-part fractures are best reduced by internal rotation or traction, and four-part fractures in external rotation or neutral (Fig. 15.2).

An incision is made from the distal third of the greater trochanter, 12 cm (Fig. 15.3a) distally, the fascia lata split and vastus lateralis reflected forward from the intermuscular septum (Fig. 15.3b). This technique is a surer one than splitting vastus lateralis, because if splitting takes place the perforating vessels may retract and continue to bleed in the residual posterior muscle, resulting in either excessive intraoperative blood loss or a postoperative haematoma.

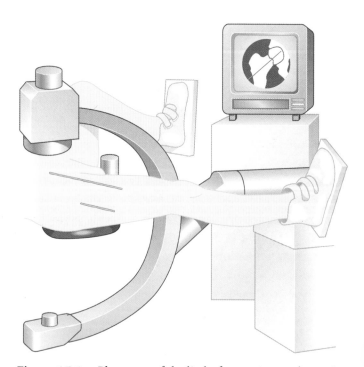

Figure 15.1 – *Placement of the limbs for treating trochanteric fractures with the AO dynamic hip screw.*

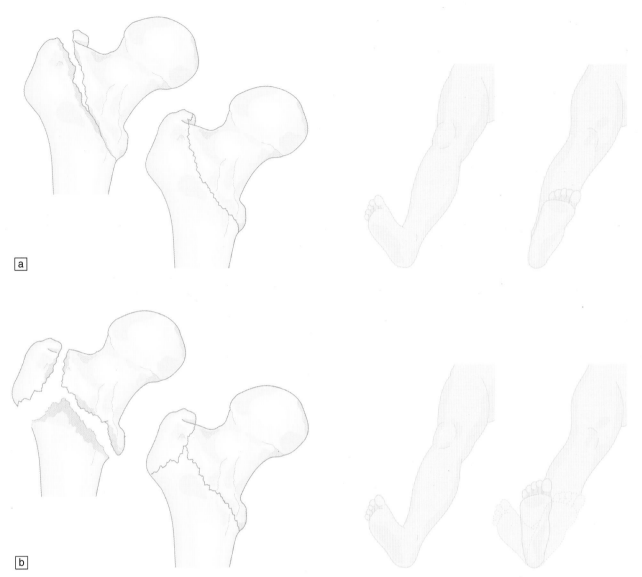

Figure 15.2 – *(a) Two- and (b) three-part fractures are best reduced by internal rotation or traction, and four-part fractures in external rotational or neutral.*

A guidewire is passed through the anterior aspect of the neck, indicating the correct orientation of the guidewire in the sagittal plain (Fig. 15.3c).

The point of entry of the guidewire is generally 2.5 cm distal to the insertion of vastus lateralis, but this is contingent on the standard of reduction that has been obtained. If the femoral neck and head are in varus, despite the best attempts at closed reduction, the 135° guide should be ignored and the guidewire placed centrally in the head-free hand. The plate can then be attached to the screw and the construct used to reduce the femoral shaft on to the plate. The guidewire is placed up to the articular cortex and the femoral neck reamed to within 1 cm of the joint surface. A screw 1 cm shorter than the measured length of the guidewire is selected.

Unless the patient's bone is extremely strong, tapping is not necessary. A firm grip is usually obtained with the dynamic hip screw. The shaft of the dynamic hip screw is hexagonal, and the plate is most easily aligned if the hexagonal opening is aligned with a handle before it is removed from the screw. In three-part fractures, a traction screw is a sensible precaution to oppose the tendency of the fracture to realign in varus. Vastus lateralis naturally falls over the plate and closure over two suction drains, left for 24 hours, concludes the procedure.

Trochanteric fractures in the young

The dynamic hip screw is an excellent device but, by definition, it moves, allows the fracture to settle into a position of maximum stability, and leaves a short leg.

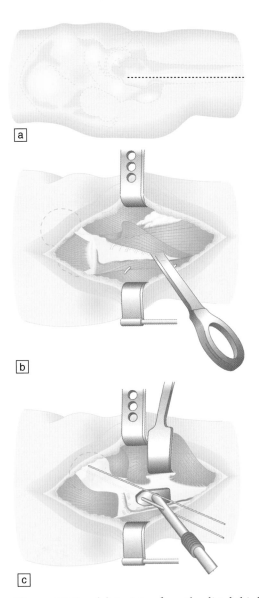

Figure 15.3 – *(a) Incision from the distal third of the greater trochanter. (b) Vastus lateralis is reflected forward from the intermuscular septum. (c) Positioning of the guidewire.*

The average shortening, using the dynamic hip screw, compared with the fixed-length nail plate, is 3.4 cm, compared with 0.4 cm in unstable fractures, and a shoe raise is poorly tolerated in the younger population [10]. Accordingly, in younger patients who can protect weight-bearing for 10 weeks, a fixed-length implant is the treatment of choice. Fixation using the 135° AO blade plate is described. The position on the fracture table is exactly the same as for the dynamic hip screw. A guidewire is placed anteriorly along the neck and 5 mm posterior to this, 2.5 cm distal to the vastus ridge. Three 4.5-mm drill holes are made using an AO guide and joined with a router. A seating chisel is then driven inferiorly on the AP and centrally on the lateral up the femoral neck. The

blade plate is inserted and fixed to the femoral shaft. Closure is as for the dynamic hip screw.

Postoperatively, patients may be fully weight-bearing in stable fractures, but most eggshell weight-bear for 6–10 weeks in unstable fractures.

Fixation of subtrochanteric fractures

True subtrochanteric

There are two technical difficulties about this fixation. The first is to avoid shearing off the greater trochanter leaving the entire fixation unstable, and the second is to ensure good fixation into the femoral neck. The procedure is carried out on a traction table with the patient supine and the non-injured leg externally rotated, flexed, and abducted. A 10-cm incision is made from the midpoint of the greater trochanter, superoposteriorly, splitting gluteus maximus. The tip of the greater trochanter is then located. The correct orientation of the femoral shaft is from posterior to anterior, and an anterior entrance point will result in posterior penetration of the metaphysis. The ideal point of entry is the neck, just anterior to the piriform fossa, but this is round, the gouge tends to slide off it, and the easiest manoeuvre is to remove the tip of the greater trochanter, which lies posterolaterally and, under image intensification, to pass the gouge through the tip of the greater trochanter engaging the neck and metaphysis. The intramedullary canal is further developed with a hand reamer and a fixation device is inserted.

Most fixation devices have a guide through which a screw can be passed into the femoral neck. As in the placement of the dynamic hip screw, it is critical that the screw pass through this guide: it is central to inferior in the neck on the AP view and central laterally. It is very easy for the implant to be inserted not far enough and in retroversion and for the screw to insert posteriorly in the head, from where it will cut out. The orientation of the screw in the sagittal plane can again be assisted by passing a guidewire along the anterior aspect of the neck, which should allow the nail to be positioned in the correct orientation before it is driven home.

If there is any doubt about the degree of proximal comminution, it is wiser to avoid an intramedullary device, because it destroys the cancellous bone of the medullary cavity, leaving a very fragmented fracture that is difficult to reconstruct using other techniques.

Comminuted subtrochanteric fractures

These fractures usually have a butterfly fragment, often

extend into the piriform fossa, and are best treated by open-reduction interfragmentary screw fixation, and a neutralizing dynamic condylar plate or low-angle dynamic hip screw. This is an extremely difficult procedure to carry out on a fracture table because the fracture tends to sag posteriorly, the fragments are difficult to manipulate, the reduction has to be held against gravity, and the only advantage is that a good lateral view of the neck can be obtained to ensure that the screw is in the correct place. This type of fracture is approached very much better with the patient in the lateral position, and the fracture fully exposed through a posterolateral approach.

An image intensifier, with the C arm horizontal, can be brought in to check the position of the fracture. The main fragments are reduced, held with reduction forceps, and fixed with lag screws. A guidewire is placed along the front of the femoral neck to give orientation of the lateral plane and the guidewire to the dynamic condylar plate placed 1.2 cm posteriorly to this. This places the guidewire in the centre of the neck in the sagittal plane. The AP view is checked with the image intensifier and the 95° dynamic condylar plate provides excellent neutralization with multiple proximal screw fixation to prevent shear.

Postoperative regimen

In young patients, eggshell weight-bearing for 6 weeks is indicated. In elderly patients, full weight-bearing within the limits of pain is a compromise that takes into account their poor balance and general debility.

Pathological fractures

Pathological fractures generally involve the metaphyseal region of the bone, because this is the most metabolically active. Patients have a limited life expectancy, the fractures do not unite by conservative measures, and fixation is mandatory. Fixation requirements are exactly the same as for any other fracture of the proximal femur and depend on adequate proximal and distal fixation. In the first instance, a radiograph of the entire femur should be taken to ensure that fixation devices do not create a stress raiser at the level of another metastasis. In general, intermedullary devices are stronger than extramedullary ones. There should be no hesitation in supplementing metal fixation with bone cement, because, unless the tumour is responsive to either radio- or chemotherapy, union will not take place.

It is important to obtain an adequate biopsy for the pathologist and simply sending reamings from the medullary cavity is inadequate. The centre of a large tumour is necrotic and so poorly differentiated that it is impossible for a pathologist to give a precise diagnosis. The best differentiated tumour is in the periphery and multiple biopsies should be taken from this site before the fracture is fixed.

If the head is involved, cemented total hip replacement is the procedure of choice. In all but the most extensive pelvic involvement, it is possible to create an arthroplasty that gives excellent pain relief and good function in the short term.

References

1. Hornby R, Grimley Evans J, Vardon V. Operative or conservative treatment for trochanteric fracture of the femur. *J Bone Joint Surg* 1989; 71B: 619–23.

2. Hall G, Ainscow DAP. Comparison of nail-plate fixation and Enders nailing for intertrochanteric fractures. *J Bone Joint Surg* 1981; 63B: 24–8.

3. Evans EM. Treatment of trochanteric fractures of the femur. *J Bone Joint Surg* 1949; 31B: 190–203.

4. Jenson JJ, Sonne-Holm S, Tondevold E. Unstable trochanteric fractures: a comparative analysis of four methods of internal fixation. *Acta Orthop Scand* 1980; 51: 949–62.

5. Dimon JH, Hughston JC. Unstable intertrochanteric fractures of the hip. *J Bone Joint Surg* 1967; 49A: 440–50.

6. Sarmiento A, Williams EM. The unstable intertrochanteric fracture treatment with a valgus osteotomy and I beam nail-plate. A preliminary report of 100 cases. *J Bone Joint Surg* 1970; 52A: 1309–18.

7. Davis TRC, Sher JL, Horsman A *et al.* Intertrochanteric femoral fractures: mechanical failure after internal fixation. *J Bone Joint Surg* 1990; 72B: 26–31.

8. Halder SC. The Gamma nail for peritrochanteric fractures. *J Bone Joint Surg* 1992; 74B: 340–4.

9. Bridle SH, Patel AD, Bircher M, Calvert PT. Fixation of intertrochanteric fractures of the femur: a randomised prospective comparison of the Gamma nail and the dynamic hip screw. *J Bone Joint Surg* 1991; 73B: 330–4.

10. Bannister GC, Gibson AG, Ackroyd CE, Newman JH. The fixation and prognosis of trochanteric fractures. *Clin Orthop* 1990; 254: 242-6.

CHAPTER 16

Pelvic and acetabular fractures

D. C. Mears

A displaced fracture of the pelvic ring or acetabulum usually represents the aftermath of a motor vehicle accident, an industrial accident, or a fall from a great height. Typically a disruption of the pelvic ring involves the application of an immense force to a patient, who is thereby likely to present with other serious or life-threatening injuries involving the musculoskeletal (85%), respiratory (60%), central nervous (40%), gastrointestinal (30%), urological (12%) and cardiovascular (6%) systems [1,2]. The management of a pelvic ring fracture, therefore, necessitates a concomitant diagnosis and treatment of the other systemic and musculoskeletal injuries. About 50% of acetabular fracture patients have sustained associated injuries, whereas about 30% have experienced injuries to three or more organ systems. Previously Kellam *et al.*, Tile, and others [2–4] have emphasized the need for a meticulous diagnostic protocol that prioritizes the evaluation of diverse organ systems by the degree of urgency. A recent report by Dalal *et al.* [5] provides a correlation of a specific pelvic injury pattern with the statistical likelihood for particular patterns of associated visceral injuries in a way that facilitates the application of diverse diagnostic procedures.

An acetabular fracture is an intra-articular disruption that involves the socket of the hip joint [6]. The injury may be an isolated event or one feature of a more extensive pelvic disruption. Historically, such a fracture was a characteristic sequel to a significant traumatic event. At present, with the favourable impact of public legislation to discourage intoxication while driving [7, 8], the improved safety of automobiles, and the rapid enlargement of the elderly population [9], over half of the fractures arise after minor trauma as the aftermath of a simple fall [10,11]. The latter group is notable for the presence of osteopenic bone and the potential for comminution and impaction. Particularly for patients who are managed with long-term steroids or those who have had radiotherapy around the pelvic ring, an insufficiency fracture of the pelvis or acetabulum or a periprosthetic variant is a formidable management problem [12].

This chapter reviews acute resuscitation after a pelvic ring or acetabular fracture, the radiology, classification and definitive therapeutic management, as well as the principal complications.

Acute evaluation and resuscitation

A pelvic ring disruption is a representative example of a frequent multiple traumatic injury. If an accident is sufficiently forceful to fracture the structurally significant posterior portion of the pelvic ring, there is a strong statistical likelihood that other major organ systems are involved. For a fracture that is open or associated with a major vascular injury, the mortality rates that have been reported in multiple series vary between 5% and 50% [5,13,14]. The wide variability in survival depends on many factors, including the gravity of the injuries, the accessibility to a prompt resuscitation at the scene of the accident, rapid evacuation to the hospital, the degree of sophistication of the accident and emergency department, and the availability of specialized services such as interventional radiology and neurosurgery. The initial assessment and resuscitation of such a polytrauma victim are complex events where evaluation and resuscitation are undertaken in tandem. Multiple organ systems require diagnostic scrutiny and appropriate care in a highly time-dependent way and with an optimal sequence. An elaborate therapeutic protocol for such a polytrauma patient is essential.

The patient requires immediate, accessible, and appropriate treatment from the time of the injury until stabilization in an appropriate accident and emergency room and possibly an intensive care area. The first few hours after the injury are crucial in terms of survival and reduction of late morbidity. If the patient is initially evaluated in an outlying hospital that lacks the appropriate resources, a timely transfer to a major trauma centre is crucial. The resuscitative phase follows established protocols that are subdivided into a primary survey, resuscitation, a secondary survey, and initiation of the definitive care. The systemic priorities and treatment follow the so-called 'ABCs' with management of the airway, bleeding, central nervous system, digestive system, excretory tracts, and fractures. Quantitative assessment of the extent and severity of the traumatic disruptions by the use of an injury severity scale provides the optimal characterization of the life-threatening potential of the accident [4,15,16].

In terms of mortality, the pelvic fractures that constitute the greatest challenge are those accompanied by an associated head injury, intraperitoneal injury, or both. From the orthopaedic perspective, the management of a fractured pelvis associated with secondary bleeding is a recurring problem. The therapeutic alternatives include the use of a pneumatic antishock garment (PASG),

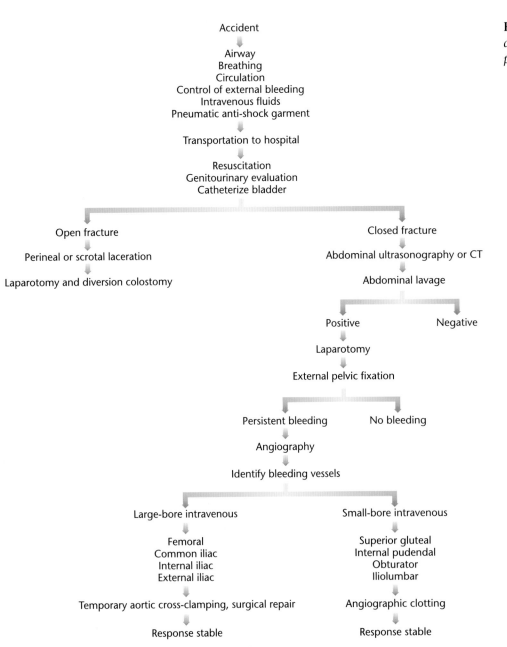

Figure 16.1 – *Algorithm for the control of haemorrhage in the patient with a pelvic fracture.*

external pelvic fixation, diagnostic and therapeutic angiography, and open surgical intervention. Figure 16.1 is an algorithm that outlines a protocol for the control of haemorrhage in a pelvic fracture victim. The role for a PASG is most clearly evident after pelvic trauma where it may afford haemostasis and tamponade, autotransfusion, and increased peripheral vascular resistance [2,4]. Although it is not without risk, its principal shortcomings are decreased visibility and accessibility of the abdomen and lower extremities. Deflation of the PASG is particularly vulnerable for recurrent hypotension in an exsanguinating patient.

The reduction and stabilization of a pelvic fracture can be undertaken by resort to an external wrap such as a sheet, anterior external fixation, internal fixation, a spica cast, and traction. In the acute situation, tying a sheet around the pelvis can provide a readily available and effective temporary method. The alternative spica cast is impractical with its compromise to accessibility. External fixation is meant to facilitate a reduction of the pelvic volume as a site where blood may pool. The volume of a sphere equals $\frac{4}{3} \times \pi r^3$, so that a small reduction of the radius of the pelvis may profoundly decrease the volume [1,17]. Admittedly more recent investigations have confirmed that extravasation of fluid beyond the true pelvis into the thighs or abdomen may occur with or without the presence of an external frame, in view of the traumatic disruption of the ligamentous supports and partitions between neighbouring compartments [18,19]. For the typical unstable pelvic ring with a major posterior injury site, the frame is inadequate to achieve definitive fixation. Nevertheless, its provisional realignment and source of tamponade merit serious consideration. Usually, definitive internal fixation is contraindicated until haemodynamic stability has been achieved.

As an alternative to a classic external fixation device, pelvic clamps have been designed for application in the accident and emergency room [2]. Of the two available designs, the Ganz type with its posterior iliac fixation pins affords the optimal pelvic stability, although the pins jeopardize the neighbouring sciatic nerve, superior gluteal vessels, and intra-abdominal contents. Although the alternative Browner design with its anterior pin placement is mechanically inferior, nevertheless the potential morbidity of the pins is greatly reduced. For most clinical facilities where the role for such a device is highly limited, the use of a classic external frame is

preferred so that the surgical team possesses sufficient experience with the instrumentation. With respect to the relative timing of pelvic reduction and stabilization, and intraperitoneal surgery, the site of greatest blood loss merits the initial application. As a practical guideline a mini-laparotomy that provides a specimen of frank blood prioritizes the intra-abdominal exploration as the initial step. Where the mini-laparotomy is equivocal or negative, external fixation should be applied before the laparotomy. In the latter case, the frame can be designed in such a way that the system of anterior bars can be temporarily manipulated during the laparotomy from a position that is superficial to the abdomen to superficial to the thighs [2,4].

Angiography

Interventional angiography provides a means to identify a specific site of haemorrhage within the retroperitoneal space. Selective internal iliac arteriography can be followed by the insertion of a stent, combined with a gelfoam embolus or autologous clot into a bleeding vessel (Fig. 16.2) [20]. The method is suitable for bleeding vessels of up to 3 or 4 mm in diameter. At present the technique is not consistent with re-cannulation of an essential vessel, such as the common or external iliac artery, for which a direct surgical repair is indicated. Also the method is not suitable for application to a ruptured major vein. Although the relative timing of arteriography versus external pelvic fixation has been debated, the author's personal preference is for external pelvic fixation both to control the retroperitoneal haemorrhage and to immobilize the pelvis, followed by arteriography for cases with persistent bleeding [20].

Open surgical intervention to control haemorrhage possesses three principal indications, one of which pertains to an open pelvic fracture. Either at the site of injury or in the accident and emergency room, the insertion of a sterile pack into the wound may help to restore tamponade as a truly life-saving measure. After the initial resuscitation such an open fracture merits a surgical débridement. In the presence of an open wound that is vulnerable to contamination by faeculent material, notably involving the perineal area and scrotum, a diversion colostomy is indicated [21]. In the presence of a major vascular injury such as the external iliac, common iliac, or internal iliac, a direct surgical repair is

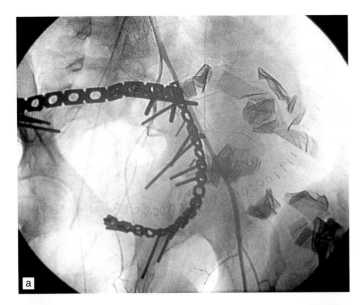

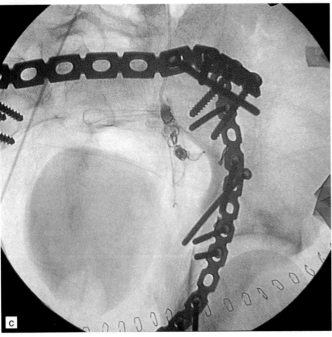

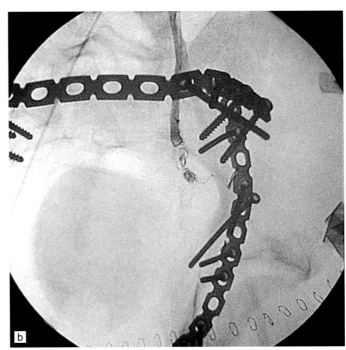

Figure 16.2 – *Multiple anteroposterior (AP) pelvic arteriograms from a 21-year-old man, who had just undergone an open reduction and internal fixation (ORIF) of the sacrum and left acetabulum, displaying bleeding from the left hypogastric artery which is controlled by the insertion of a coiled stent and a gelfoam embolus. (a) Arteriogram with the bleeding vessel; (b) during insertion of the gelfoam embolus; (c) after control of haemorrhage.*

needed. For a patient in extremis from hypovolaemic shock, and provided that a thoracic cause has been eliminated from consideration, an emergency laparotomy is indicated. Temporary proximal control of bleeding can be undertaken if necessary by cross-clamping the aorta for a maximum of 20 min. Supplementary packing of the retroperitoneal space may facilitate haemostasis and identification of a significant vascular injury.

Assessment

At the time of clinical presentation, the pelvic injury is rigorously characterized by its clinical and radiographic features. The direction of the provocative blow and magnitude of the force may be obtained from the history of an alert patient or partly from clinical inspection for sites of contusion or ecchymosis. Such a history may provide insight into the likelihood of the presence of a major unstable pelvic injury, with the potential for concomitant visceral or neurovascular insults or injuries to other organ systems. The pelvic region is examined for evidence of asymmetry, instability, or the presence of an open wound. In the presence of haemodynamic instability, the initial radiographic assessment of the pelvis may be limited to an anteroposterior (AP) view (Fig. 16.3).

Subsequently, a precise characterization of the injury necessitates a minimum radiographic protocol of AP, inlet, and outlet views. For the inlet view of the supine patient, the X-ray beam is directed from the head to the midpelvis at about 45° with respect to the radiographic table. Such a projection is perpendicular to the pelvic brim and illustrates the true pelvic inlet, as well as the

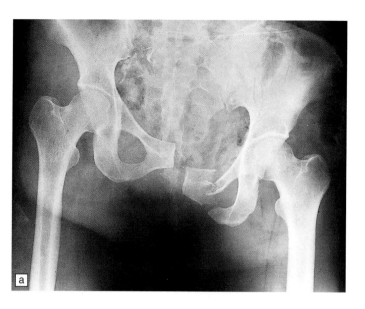

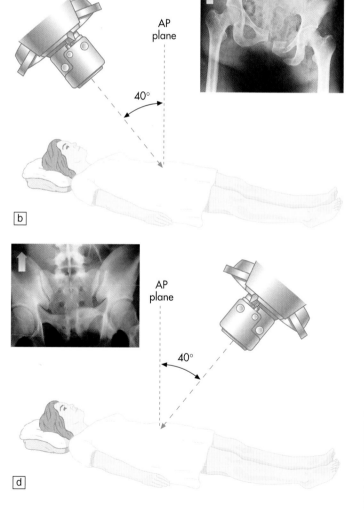

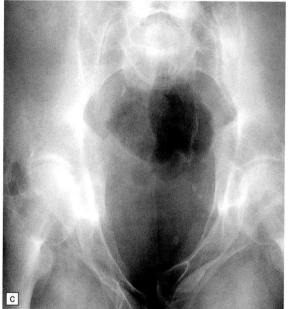

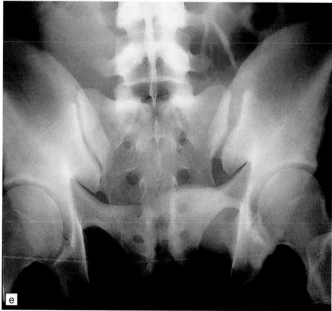

Figure 16.3 – *Standard radiographs for assessment of a pelvic fracture: (a) AP view; (b) schematic inlet view; (c) radiographic inlet view; (d) schematic outlet view; (e) radiographic outlet view.*

AP displacement of the pelvic fracture. For an outlet projection of a supine patient, the beam is directed from the foot to the pubic symphysis at 45° with respect to the radiographic plate. The outlet projection highlights superior displacement of a hemipelvis as well as displacement of the rami. Apparent limb length discrepancy

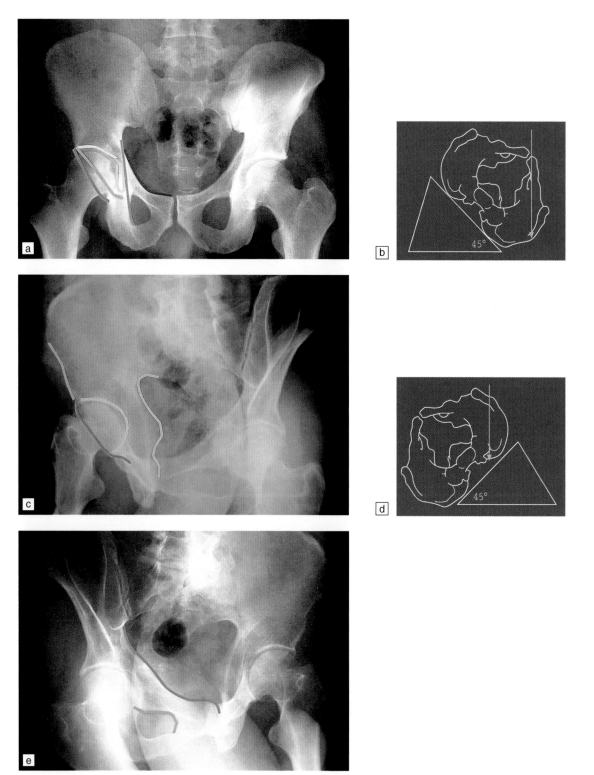

Figure 16.4 – *Standard radiographs for assessment of an acetabular fracture: (a) radiographic AP view; (b) schematic iliac oblique view; (c) radiographic iliac oblique view; (d) schematic obturator oblique view; (e) radiographic obturator oblique view.*

may be secondary to superior displacement of a hemi-pelvis or a sagittal malrotation. Either problem may be accompanied by avulsion fractures of the transverse processes of the lower lumbar vertebra or ramus fractures. For an acetabular disruption, in addition to an AP view, special Judet or obturator and iliac oblique views are obtained by rolling the injured patient carefully from one side to the other to provide a transverse axis of the pelvis of 45° relative to the radiographic table (Fig. 16.4).

Supplementary computed tomography (CT) is indispensable to document sites of pelvic disruption, displacement, and comminution. Whereas a sacral fracture may be undetectable on plain radiographs, it is readily documented by resort to a CT axial scan. Typically five transaxial sections are taken at intervals of about 2 cm to highlight the iliac wings and adjacent sacroiliac joints, the body of the sacrum, the dome of the acetabulum, the midacetabular region, and the rami respectively (Fig. 16.5). For displaced fractures and especially those where surgical reconstruction is anticipated, a three-dimensional CT is valuable (Fig. 16.6) [22]. The optimal three-dimensional CT images are the anterior, posterior, superior, and inferior orthogonal views accompanied by the inlet and outlet 45° oblique projections and the apparent 45° iliac and obturator oblique projections. A

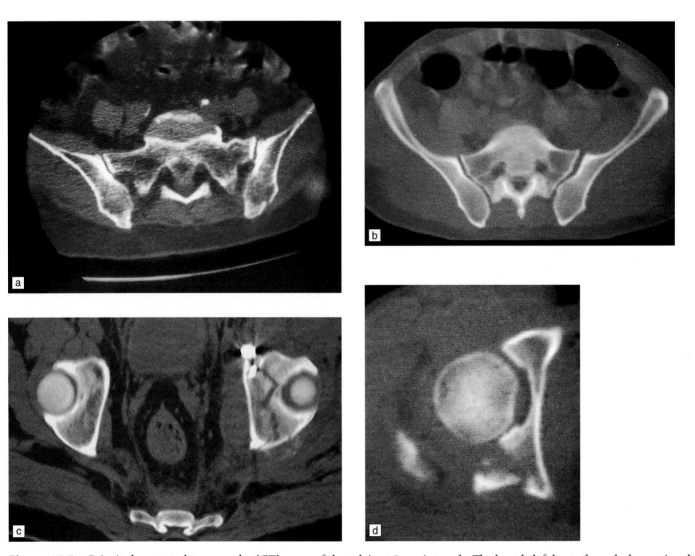

Figure 16.5 – *Principal computed tomography (CT) scans of the pelvis at 2-cm intervals. The least helpful cut, through the rami and symphysis, is not shown. (a) Sacroiliac joints and upper sacrum; (b) first sacral body and sacroiliac joints; (c) acetabular dome; (d) midacetabular level.*

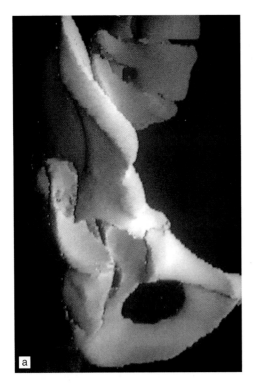

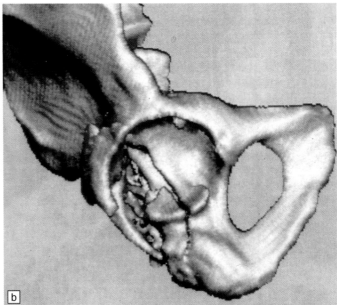

Figure 16.6 – *Examples of three-dimensional CT views: (a) external obturator oblique view of a posterior T fracture; (b) 'dome' view of a posterior wall fracture.*

special 'dome view' is obtained from a projection approximating 20° inferior and 20° anterior to the true lateral view. After a subtraction or so-called disarticulation of the femoral head, the last view presents the acetabulum as a true hemispherical recess.

Classification of injuries

Pelvis

Diverse schemes for classification of pelvic ring disruptions have been based on the anatomical site, the direction of the provocative force, and the degree of resultant instability. The most recent trend has been towards a combination of all these factors. A widely used scheme is that by Pennal, Tile and associates (Fig. 16.7, Table 16.1), wherein the injury is characterized by the vector of the provocative blow corresponding to AP, lateral compressive forces or vertical shearing forces that result from a fall or other unusual injuries [24]. This classification provides insight into the nature of the injury, the morbidity, the potential sites of disruptions, the degrees of pelvic instability, and recommendations for treatment.

The AP compression injury (APC), also known as an external rotation deformity, results from a blow that strikes the posterior ilium or the anterior pelvis to disrupt the symphysis and the anterior sacral ligaments of one or both sacroiliac joints. Usually, the crucial posterior sacroiliac complex is spared so that the injury is vertically stable. Not infrequently, the ipsilateral floor of the hemipelvis, including the sacrospinous and sacrotuberous ligaments, is compromised so that a modest sagittal malrotation of the hemipelvis ensues.

A lateral compression injury (LC) arises from a direct blow to the lateral ilium, typically to provoke an extremely stable impacted fracture of the sacral ala. Most typically, an accompanying anterolateral rotational force provokes an inward rotation of the ipsilateral hemipelvis, so that the ipsilateral pubic rami and occasionally all four rami are disrupted with some overlapping of the fracture fragments. Upon more forceful lateral injuries, the pelvic ring is compromised by an unstable vertical fracture of the lateral ilium, which coincides with the anterior half of the sacroiliac joint.

A vertical shear injury (VS) is a highly unstable disruption with complete posterior ligamentous instability of one or both sacroiliac joints. Usually, the associated anterior injury is a diastasis of the symphysis pubis. Supplementary radiographic findings include avulsion fractures of the sacrospinous and sacrotuberous ligaments from the ischial spine of the adjacent sacrum, as well as avulsion fractures of the transverse processes of the forth and fifth lumbar vertebrae.

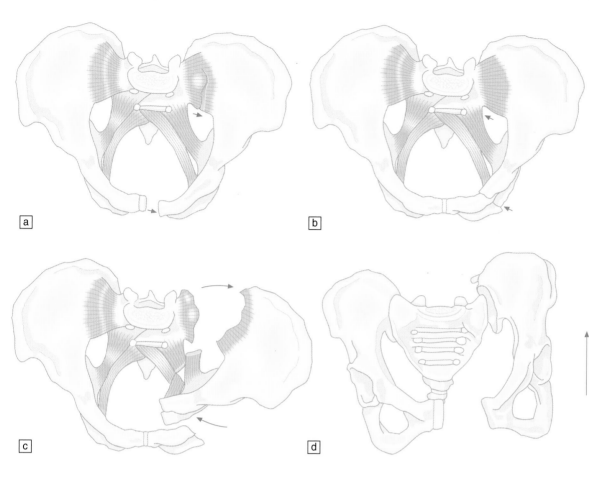

Figure 16.7 – *Schematic illustrations of the Pennal and Tile classification of pelvic fractures: (a) anteroposterior compression (APC) or external rotation injury; (b) stable lateral compression (LC) or internal rotation injury; (c) unstable (LC) or internal rotation injury; (d) unstable vertical shear (VS) disruption.*

Table 16.1 *Tile classification of pelvic disruption [23]*

Type A: stable

A1: fractures of the pelvis not involving the ring
A2: stable, minimally displaced fractures of the ring

Type B: rotationally unstable, vertically stable

B1: open book
B2: lateral compression; ipsilateral
B3: lateral compression; contralateral (bucket handle)

Type C: rotationally and vertically unstable

C1: rotationally and vertically unstable
C2: bilateral
C3: associated with an acetabular fracture

A modified version [2] of the Pennal scheme with input from AO ASIF and SICOT renders it an alphanumeric classification in a way that is highly suitable for meticulous documentation of detailed injury patterns and a correlation with clinical outcome (Fig. 16.8, Table 16.2).

Acetabulum

The widely utilized scheme for characterization of an acetabular fracture by LeTournel and Judet (Fig. 16.9, Table 16.3) identifies two major categories of elementary and associated fractures [6]. In an elementary fracture, all or part of one column is involved to provoke a posterior wall, posterior column, anterior wall, or anterior column fracture. One other elementary pattern is a transverse fracture in which the superior acetabulum is separated from the inferior portion. The associated fracture patterns include combinations of any two of the elementary forms. The five principal examples are a fracture of the posterior column and posterior wall, a transverse and posterior wall fracture, a T-type fracture, a fracture of the anterior column and/or anterior wall associated with a hemitransverse fracture posteriorly, and a complete both column fracture. The last example is where all of the articular surface is disrupted to create at least three major fracture fragments. Characterization of the injuries by these patterns provides insight into the optimal surgical approach and a guideline to prognosis with or without surgical reconstruction. Supplementary

243

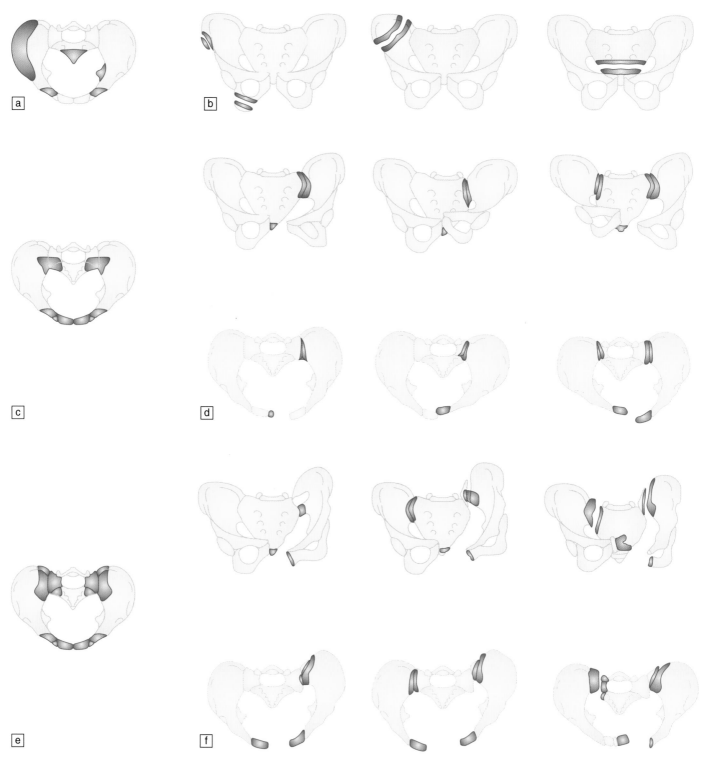

Figure 16.8 – *Schematic illustrations of the Comprehensive Classification System of pelvic fractures. (a) Sites of a type A stable lesion that spares the posterior arch; (b) specific patterns of a type A injury; (c) sites of a type B partially stable lesion with incomplete disruption of the posterior arch; (d) specific patterns of a type B injury; (e) sites of a type C unstable lesion with complete disruption of the posterior arch; (f) specific patterns of a type C injury.*

Table 16.2 *Comprehensive classification of pelvic ring disruptions after AO ASIF, SICOT, and Pennal and Tile [24]*

Type A: stable, posterior arch intact

A1: posterior arch intact, fracture of innominate bone (avulsion)
   A1.1: iliac spine
   A1.2: iliac crest
   A1.3: ischial tuberosity

A2: posterior arch intact, fracture of innominate bone (direct blow)
   A2.1: iliac wing fractures
   A2.2: unilateral fracture of anterior arch
   A2.3: bifocal fracture of anterior arch

A3: posterior arch intact; transverse fracture of sacrum caudal to S2
   A3.1: sacrococcygeal dislocation
   A3.2: sacrum undisplaced
   A3.3: sacrum displaced

Type B: incomplete disruption of posterior arch, partially stable, rotation

B1: external rotation instability, open-book injury, unilateral
   B1.1: sacroiliac joint, anterior disruption
   B1.2: sacral fracture

B2: incomplete disruption of posterior arch, unilateral, internal rotation (lateral compression)
   B2.1: anterior compression fracture, sacrum
   B2.2: partial sacroiliac joint fracture, subluxation
   B2.3: incomplete posterior iliac fracture

B3: incomplete disruption of posterior arch, bilateral
   B3.1: bilateral open-book
   B3.2: open-book, lateral compression
   B3.3: bilateral lateral compression

Type C: complete disruption of posterior arch, unstable

C1: complete disruption of posterior arch, unilateral
   C1.1: fracture through ilium
   C1.2: sacroiliac dislocation and/or fracture dislocation
   C1.3: sacral fracture

C2: bilateral injury, one side rotationally unstable, one side vertically unstable

C3: bilateral injury, both sides completely unstable

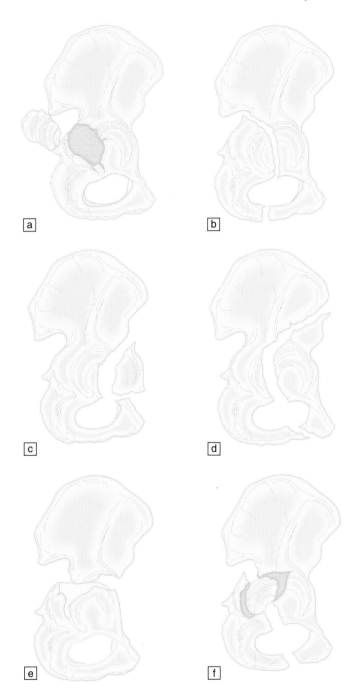

Figure 16.9 – *Schematic illustrations of the LeTournel and Judet classification [6] of acetabular fractures. (a) Posterior wall fracture; (b) posterior column fracture; (c) anterior wall fracture; (d) anterior column fracture; (e) transverse fracture; (f) associated posterior wall and posterior column fracture;*

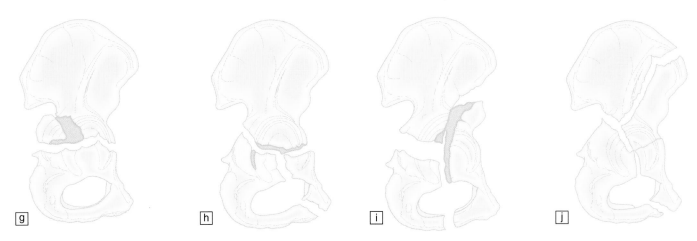

g   h   i   j

Figure 16.9 – *(cont'd) (g) associated posterior wall and transverse fracture; (h) T-shaped fracture; (i) associated anterior column and posterior hemitransverse fracture; (j) both-column fracture.*

Table 16.3 *Classification of acetabular fracture patterns after LeTournel and Judet [6]*

Simple
Posterior wall
Posterior column
Anterior wall
Anterior column
Transverse
Associated
Posterior wall and posterior column
Posterior wall and transverse
T-shaped
Anterior column and posterior hemitransverse
Both column

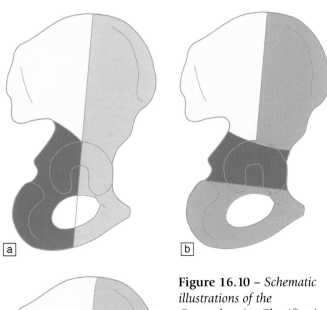

a   b

c

Figure 16.10 – *Schematic illustrations of the Comprehensive Classification System of acetabular fractures. (a) Type A injury: partial articular fracture involving one column; (b) type B injury: partial articular fracture involving both columns; (c) type C injury: complete articular fracture.*

diagnostic features of relevance include the presence of an incarcerated fragment, diffuse comminution and osteopenia, and impaction of the posterior wall or the dome.

More recently, an alpha-numeric identification with input from AO ASIF and SICOT has provided a more detailed characterization of the injury patterns that also attempts to correlate significant features with the prognosis (Fig. 16.10, Table 16.4). Various attempts have been made to quantify the involved segment of the acetabulum and radiographic features that would correspond to an indication for surgery [22,25]. To date none of these has achieved widespread application.

Definitive planning, timing, and decision-making

Once the complete diagnostic survey of the pelvis is

Table 16.4 *Comprehensive classification of acetabular fractures after AO ASIF/SICOT and LeTournel and Judet [6]*

Type A: *Partial articular* fractures, *one column* involved

    A1: posterior wall fracture
    A2: posterior column fracture
    A3: anterior wall or anterior column fracture

Type B: *Partial articular* fracture (transverse or T-type fracture *both columns* involved)

    B1: transverse fracture
    B2: T-shaped fracture
    B3: anterior column plus posterior hemitransverse fracture

Type C: *complete articular* fracture (both-column fracture; floating acetabulum)

    C1: both-column fracture, high variety
    C2: both-column fracture, low variety
    C3: both-column fracture involving the sacroiliac joint

Qualifiers

Additional information can be documented concerning the condition of the articular surfaces, in order to further define the prognosis of the injury. The information should be, as additional qualifiers, identified by Greek letters:

    $\alpha1$: femoral head subluxation, anterior
    $\alpha2$: femoral head subluxation, medial
    $\alpha3$: femoral head subluxation, posterior
    $\beta1$: femoral head dislocation, anterior
    $\beta2$: femoral head dislocation, medial
    $\beta3$: femoral head dislocation, posterior
    $\gamma1$: acetabular surface, chondral lesion
    $\gamma2$: acetabular surface, impacted
    $\delta1$: femoral head, chondral lesion
    $\delta2$: femoral head, impacted
    $\delta3$: femoral head, osteochondral fracture
    $\varepsilon1$: intra-articular fragment requiring surgical removal
    $\phi1$: non-displaced fracture of the acetabulum

From Tile *et al.* [25]

---

completed, an appropriate therapeutic plan is devised where the goals of management include anatomical restoration of the pelvis with sufficient stability so that the patient can be mobilized at least to a bed-to-chair existence, if not a partial weight-bearing gait. For the injuries where preservation of stability and minimal displacement are encountered, a conservative regimen may permit attainment of these goals. With intrinsically unstable injuries, surgical reconstruction should be anticipated as a way of providing substantial alleviation of fracture pain and sufficient mobilization to facilitate pulmonary toilet, and expeditious discharge from the hospital. Acute stabilization of a displaced injury also minimizes the likelihood for a catastrophic late problem such as a painful non-union or malunion of the pelvis.

Timing

Usually, even for a patient with haemodynamic or other forms of acute instability, the general condition is stabilized within a period of 1 or 2 days. Generally, the relevant diagnostic studies can be completed during that course or shortly thereafter. If a surgical reconstruction is indicated, the optimal timing is within a day or two of the time of the injury, which provides sufficient time for the surgical team to marshal the necessary resources and to plan the procedure meticulously. If the surgery is deferred for a more prolonged period, the complications of enforced recumbency, such as thromboembolic problems, urinary tract, or respiratory tract infections, may culminate in a prolonged surgical delay of 1–3 weeks. In such a case, the difficulties in achieving an accurate reduction of the fracture escalate enormously. Particularly for an acetabular fracture where a precise reduction is essential, the quality of the late outcome may be irrevocably compromised. Admittedly, in the exceptional case where a prolonged delay is unavoidable, late surgical reconstruction can be undertaken with an anticipated greater technical difficulty, operative time, and blood loss.

Decision-making

A critical and radiological assessment to define the characteristics of the pelvic injury precisely is essential. For a definition of the optimal clinical management, other factors of relevance include the expertise of the health care team, the desires and expectations of the patient, and aspects of the patient's profile, including age, general health, and haemodynamic status. In some instances, clear alternatives of the potential therapeutic protocol merit review with the patient or the patient's family. If the pelvic or acetabular fracture is combined with other orthopaedic injuries such as a femoral shaft fracture, the therapeutic protocol may necessitate a composite plan that accounts for the diverse injuries.

For a displaced fracture of the acetabulum, in common with other intra-articular fractures, generally an anatomical reduction with stable internal fixation, followed by early motion, is the protocol of choice. Occasionally, the congruity of the hip joint is best restored by conservative means, particularly where the injury is highly comminuted and the bone osteopenic. In contrast, where the weight-bearing roof especially of the posterior aspect of the joint is violated, an open reduction is preferred. After consideration of the precise injury pattern and the prior experience of the surgical team, the risk : benefit ratio of a complex acetabular fracture merits a careful review. On the whole, displaced, posterior fracture dislocations and transverse-based injuries, including T-type fractures, possess such an unusually poor prognosis after conservative treatment that an open method is generally indicated. Perhaps the most difficult type of injury pattern to assess is the true both-column variant which frequently achieves a pattern of so-called secondary congruence (Fig. 16.11). The displaced fragments slide around the femoral head but remain congruent with it [6]. A good functional outcome and long-term prognosis may follow conservative management.

If a surgical reconstruction is undertaken, all the fragments have to be accurately realigned or the surgical

procedure may actually compromise the recovery by the conversion of secondary congruity into an incongruent joint. Non-surgical management merits the greatest consideration for a stable and congruent hip secondary to an undisplaced fracture, a minimally displaced low-anterior column, and rarely a low-transverse fracture or an injury pattern with secondary congruence, notably of a both-column variant.

Definitive treatment of pelvic fractures

The management of a pelvic ring fracture depends on a clear understanding of those injuries that are stable and minimally displaced, in contrast to those that are partly or completely unstable and/or deformed. An example of a stable type A fracture is an avulsion injury, usually as the result of a sporting insult to displace the antero-superior or -inferior spine, the ischial tuberosity, or a segment of the iliac crest. Apart from a case with a markedly displaced and large fragment, conservative treatment is generally indicated. Some of the isolated fractures of the iliac wing or transverse fractures of the inferior sacrum or coccyx and undisplaced fractures of the ilium also respond favourably to conservative treatment.

In the Pennal classification scheme [24], type B injuries are characterized by a rotational deformity and a highly variable degree of instability. By definition, they are stable in the vertical and posterior planes. The most common variant is the lateral compression or internal rotational injury, with ipsi- or bilateral ramus fractures and a highly stable buckle fracture of the sacral ala. This pattern is the most common variant that is seen in an accident and emergency room. The stable sacral component of the injury can be documented on the pelvic inlet view or a CT scan. The vast majority of cases respond favourably to conservative treatment. Nevertheless, an exceptional injury possesses an unacceptable magnitude of internal rotation of the involved hemipelvis, even though it is a stable pattern. Increasingly, it is clear that the initial evaluation merits a documentation of both the degree of pelvic instability and deformity.

From the author's perspective, deformities that exceed 15° of malrotation or 2 cm of linear displacement in any plane merit consideration for an open reduction and internal fixation. For example, an external rotation injury can be characterized by the amount of widening of the symphysis or the degree of malrotation of the hemipelvis. If a diastasis is less than 2.5 cm, typically

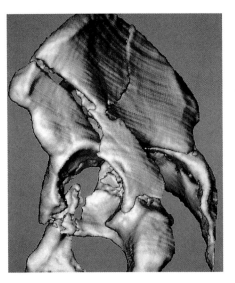

Figure 16.11 –
Three-dimensional CT 'dome' view of a both-column fracture with secondary congruity. For an open reduction, if a partial but incomplete articular reduction ensues, congruity is lost and the prognosis is compromised.

conservative treatment is recommended. When a wider diastasis is encountered, usually an accompanying sagittal malrotation is documented whereby, in an AP view, the involved ramus is apparently higher than the uninvolved side. The sagittal element of the deformity provides a confirmation that the ipsilateral sacrospinous and sacrotuberous ligaments are compromised. If the diastasis is wider than 5 cm, the injury pattern is of either a bilateral nature or, if unilateral, it is a highly unstable disruption in the form of a sacroiliac dislocation or a sacral fracture. If a supplementary deformity is evident in the sagittal or coronal planes, generally the injury pattern is significantly less stable than a variant that displays purely deformity in the transverse plane. Both the injuries that are unstable in a rotational or linear fashion merit serious consideration for internal fixation. Otherwise the likelihood for a late symptomatic non-union and malunion of the pelvic ring is excessive.

As a manifestation of a type C injury, linear deformity is most commonly documented in the AP plane, with a posterior displacement. True vertical displacement of a hemipelvis is highly uncommon. The principal offending injuries are falls from great heights or motor cycle accidents where the driver is in an almost recumbent position. A vertical deformity is readily confused with a much more frequently encountered sagittal malrotation of a hemipelvis (Fig. 16.12). In an AP radiograph, the vertical displacement is consistent with the hemipelvis that is high riding but otherwise a replica of the contralateral side. With sagittal deformity, the ischial tuberosities

are at differing levels although the tops of the iliac crests are fairly symmetrically situated. The involved hemipelvis displays a marked change in the shape of the pelvic brim in an AP view.

Pelvic fixation

Historically, diverse conservative methods such as the application of a pelvic sling or hip spica cast were widely used. The pelvic sling possesses the potential to close the pelvic ring. Nevertheless, with its obligatory enforced recumbency and marked discomfort, it is an outmoded method. The patient is highly vulnerable to decubitus ulcers. Similarly, a hip spica cast possesses very little role for management of an adult. For small children, it can, however, be highly effective to facilitate closure of the pelvic ring. Longitudinal skeletal traction is a useful method to correct vertical displacement, although it does not permit rigorous approximation of the posterior injury. Usually, it is employed as a temporary measure until a definitive internal fixation is performed.

Currently, conservative treatment refers to either a limited period of bedrest or initiation of a partial weight-bearing gait or weight-bearing to tolerance. For the selected patterns of stable injuries and those that do not violate the integrity of the pelvic ring, conservative management is appropriate.

External skeletal fixation
External fixation can be employed as a temporary measure to close the pelvic ring in the presence of haemodynamic instability. In many of these cases, conversion to internal fixation is anticipated once the patient can tolerate such a surgical procedure. Occasionally, external fixation merits consideration as the definitive technique. For example, in the presence of multiple ramus fractures with an unstable posterior hemipelvis and the presence of a diversion colostomy and/or urinary diversion in the lower abdominal wall, external fixation may be the treatment of choice for the anterior stabilization. Overall, external fixation has the greatest role for young adults with dense bone stock. In a child, the disproportionately small pelvis greatly impedes the use of external fixation. In elderly people and others with markedly osteopenic bone, premature loss of fixation of the pins markedly compromises the role of this method. Even in a young adult, typically an

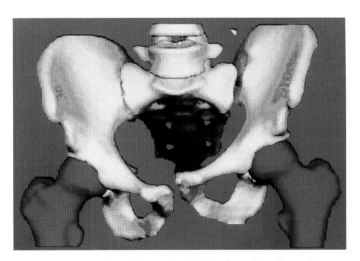

Figure 16.12 – *Three-dimensional CT of a pelvic disruption with sagittal malrotation of the left hemipelvis to distinguish the pattern from the less common vertical shear disruption.*

external fixation merits removal in 4–6 weeks before significant loosening of the pins occurs.

The critical aspect of application of external fixation is the pin–bone interface [1,2]. Unless the pins are solidly anchored in bone, premature loss of fixation is inevitable. Furthermore, such pin sites become infected and thereby eliminate this method of treatment from further consideration. In the emergent situation with the obliquity of the ilium and the presence of a supplementary and ill-defined pelvic deformity, a meticulous technique is needed to ensure that one or two pins are solidly anchored into either hemipelvis. A percutaneous technique is almost guaranteed to provide abysmal alignment and anchorage of the pins in the bone, unless image intensification with iliac and obturator oblique projections are used. In most hospital settings the only way that the procedure can be undertaken in a sterile manner is to perform it in an operating room, with a direct open exposure of the iliac crests. Two of the 5-mm half-pins are inserted into either iliac crest between the anterosuperior spine and the gluteal tubercle under image intensification. A simple radiolucent frame is assembled over the anterior surface of the abdomen, while bearing in mind the larger size of the paunch once the patient is seated. To undertake a closed reduction of the pelvic ring, the patient is turned into a full lateral position so that the influence of gravity is minimized.

Internal fixation

There are numerous techniques of internal fixation of the pelvis available which permit the reconstruction of the wide variety of fracture patterns. With the potential for injury to the adjacent soft tissues, the presence of a colostomy or urinary drainage, and associated musculoskeletal injury, the surgical team needs to be aware of the highly diverse methods that are available and needed for clinical practice. By definition, the typical displaced pelvic disruption possesses crucial posterior instability after a dislocation of the sacroiliac joint or a fracture of the neighbouring portions of the posterior ilium or sacrum. Usually, an anterior accompanying injury involves a diastasis of the symphysis or ramus fractures. In such an example, the pelvic ring can be perceived as having three supporting columns of bone (Fig. 16.13). The anterior column refers to the symphysis and the adjacent superior pubic rami. The middle column refers to the body of the sacrum and the adjacent portions of the sacroiliac joints and the allied posterior ilium. The

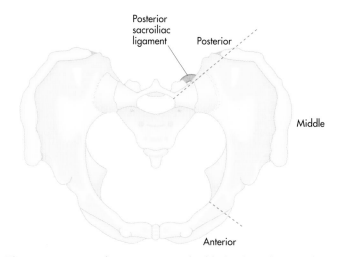

Figure 16.13 – *Schematic view to highlight the columns of the pelvis to aid in the consideration for fixation of unstable injuries.*

posterior column refers to the posterior elements of the sacrum, the posterior sacroiliac ligament and the neighbouring portions of posterior ilium adjacent to the posterosuperior spine.

As a general recommendation two of the three columns are immobilized with internal fixation. Typically, the anterior column injury is surgically exposed, reduced, and plated. This manoeuvre generally provides a satisfactory reduction of the posterior injury. As an alternative, anterior column fixation can be achieved by the use of a simple external frame. Subsequently, either the middle column is stabilized with lag screws or anterior plates or the posterior column is immobilized with a plate or conceivably a traversing bar. One notable exception is in an osteopenic individual such as an elderly person in whom the rami usually afford insufficient structural activity to merit plate fixation. In this case, the middle and posterior columns are immobilized as a preferred strategy of fixation. An understanding of the necessary columns of fixation provides an enhanced flexibility for sites of fixation in which the presence of an open wound or diversion colostomy mandates an alteration to an otherwise anticipated technique of fixation.

Certain complex ring disruptions present with multiple injuries around the pelvic ring. The largest group is a family of bilateral posterior unstable injuries, with a combination of sacroiliac dislocations or unstable fractures involving the sacrum or posterior ilium. Another pattern is where an unstable posterior fracture dislocation is accompanied by an acetabular fracture as well as an anterior injury. Still other cases involve multiple sites of posterior, unstable injuries, and bilateral acetabular fractures. All of these patterns may have various combinations of anterior disruption. Typically, each unstable site merits an open reduction and internal fixation. With ipsilateral superior and inferior ramus fractures, however, generally only the superior ramus is immobilized. By resort to a bilateral ilio-inguinal surgical exposure, the rami as well as the lateral ilium and sacroiliac joint can be exposed for the reduction and fixation. As part of the procedure, percutaneous lag screws can be used to stabilize the sacral body. A supplementary surgical approach may be necessary to expose an accompanying fracture of the posterior acetabular wall or column, or a displaced sacral fracture.

In Figure 16.14, an algorithm outlines the principal strategies that merit consideration for immobilization of diverse pelvic injury patterns.

Surgical approaches to the pelvic ring

A family of specialized surgical approaches is available to address the diverse injury patterns. With the unique surgical hazards around the pelvis, experience gained in the cadaveric laboratory or in a pelvic centre is recommended before embarking on one of the anterior, lateral, and posterior exposures. Although they are fully

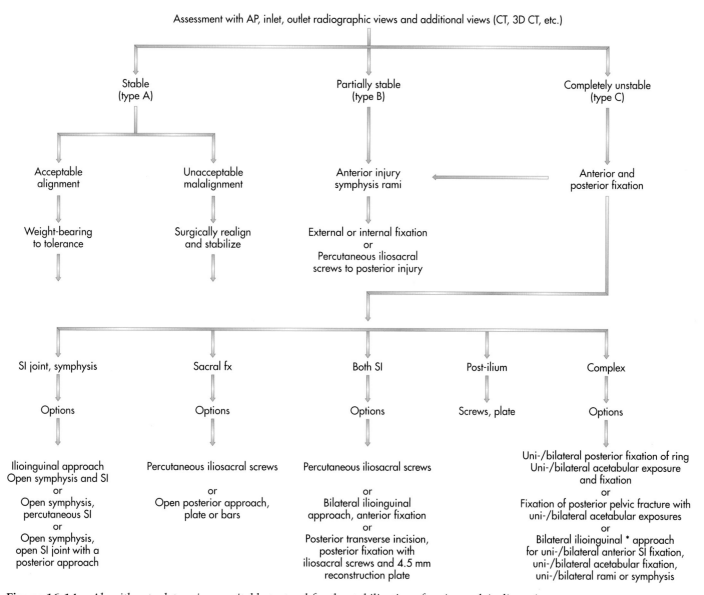

Figure 16.14 – *Algorithm to determine a suitable protocol for the stabilization of various pelvic disruptions.*

described in other available texts [1,2], in brief the anterior approaches include a Pfannenstiel, a uni- or bilateral ilioinguinal, and occasionally a lower midline longitudinal approach. For visualization of the lateral ilium or corresponding internal iliac fossa and adjacent sacroiliac joint, an iliofemoral incision can be used. For a unilateral sacroiliac joint, a posterior exposure is feasible through the use of a longitudinal approach. For bilateral sacroiliac disruptions or a displaced sacral fracture, a transverse posterior incision centred on the posterosuperior spine is preferred.

Of the numerous pelvic fracture patterns, a few more commonly encountered variants merit special description. For a displaced hemipelvis secondary to a diastasis and a dislocated sacroiliac joint, an anterior ilio-inguinal exposure of the symphysis and involved sacroiliac joint permits a simultaneous reduction and stabilization of the injuries (Fig. 16.15). A 3.5- or 3.7-mm reconstruction plate of four or six holes is applied to the pelvic brim. For sacroiliac fixation, generally a two-hole 3.5-mm dynamic compression (DC) plate in combination with 4.5-mm cortical screws provide the optimal rigidity and position of the screws. The 3.5-mm plate is preferred to a 4.5-mm counterpart so that the screws are positioned close to the sacroiliac joint and the corresponding thick column of subchondral bone. With the larger plate, either the medial screw jeopardizes the L5 nerve root as it traverses the sacral ala, or the lateral screw enters the exceedingly thin bone of the lateral ilium. Two of these plates are positioned on the top of the sacral ala and adjacent ilium (Fig. 16.16).

As an alternative fixation technique, percutaneous iliosacral screws can be inserted under biplane image intensification across a disrupted sacroiliac joint or a transforaminal sacral fracture (Fig. 16.17) [27,28]. The method is elegant and minimally invasive, although it raises a potential for significant complications with an errant screw. Undesirable targets include the neural canal, the S1 foramen, the L5 nerve root, and the retroperitoneal space including various neurovascular structures and the rectum. With the common anatomical variants, the distortion that may follow degenerative changes and the potential for supplementary residual displacement of the fracture or dislocation, the anatomy has to be very carefully appreciated. Imaging can be hampered by the presence of an ileus, retained contrast medium, marked obesity, or outdated imaging apparatus. Nevertheless, in enlightened hands, for a broad spectrum of commonly encountered injury patterns, the method permits a relatively benign anterior exposure for anterior fixation and realignment of the pelvic ring, accompanied by a percutaneous posterior fixation. Even in the emergent situation the method may be highly effective.

A significant contraindication is a displaced sacral fracture or one that is comminuted around the foramen. In such a case, a posterior plating (Fig. 16.18) provides appropriate neutralization so that over-compression of the fracture and a potential neurological hazard are avoided [1,28]. For such posterior fixation a 4.5-mm reconstruction plate is positioned across the S1 or S2 sacral bodies. The principal anchorage of fixation screws

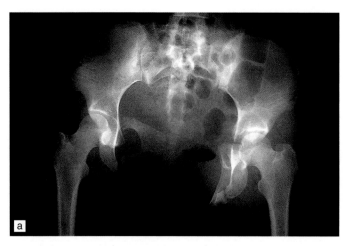

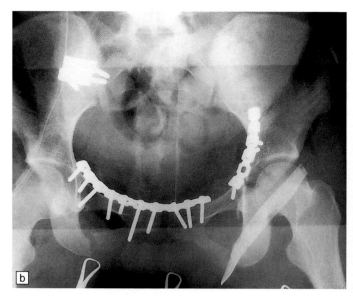

Figure 16.15 – *Plate fixation of a right sacroiliac dislocation, symphyseal fracture-dislocation and a left anterior column fracture in a 28-year-old woman. (a) Preoperative view; (b) intraoperative view.*

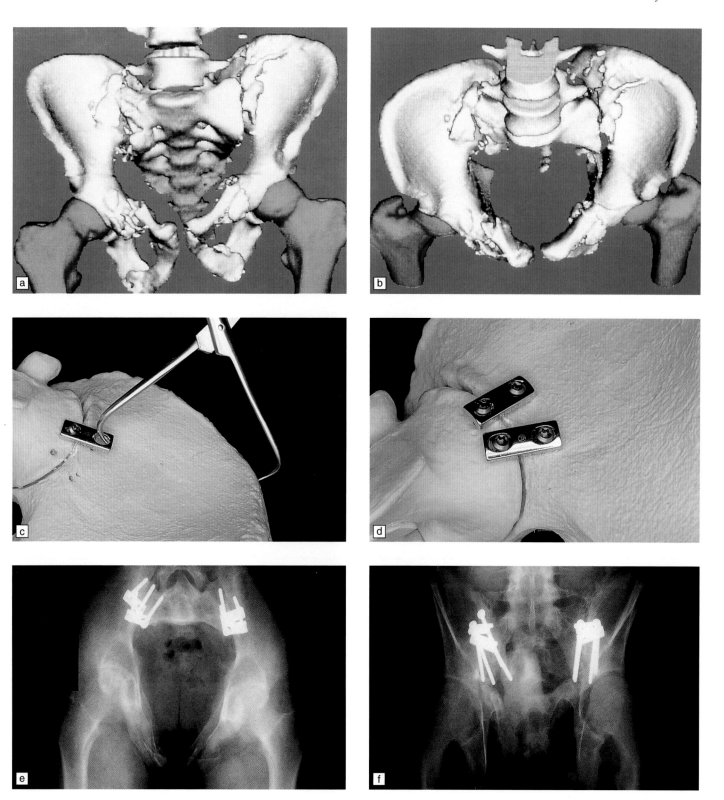

Figure 16.16 – *Plate fixation of a bilateral sacroiliac dislocation in an 18-year-old male. (a) Anterior three-dimensional CT; (b) inlet three-dimensional CT; (c) model of sacroiliac reduction using a two-hole plate; (d) model of sacroiliac fixation with two two-hole plates; (e) postoperative inlet view; (f) postoperative outlet view.*

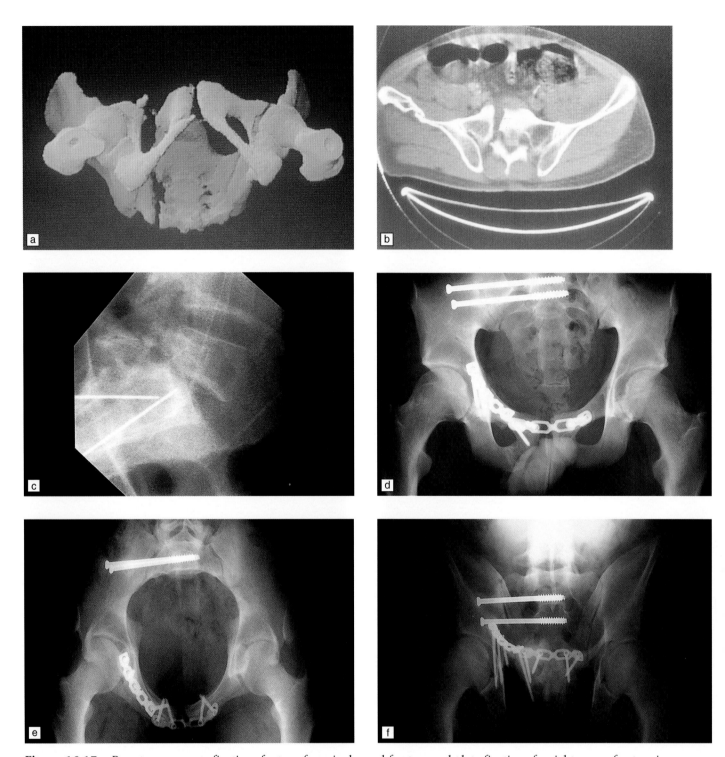

Figure 16.17 – *Percutaneous screw fixation of a transforaminal sacral fracture and plate fixation of a right ramus fracture in a 31-year-old man. (a) Preoperative three-dimensional CT; (b) preoperative CT scan; (c) intraoperative direct lateral sacral view; (d) postoperative AP view; (e) postoperative inlet view; (f) postoperative outlet view.*

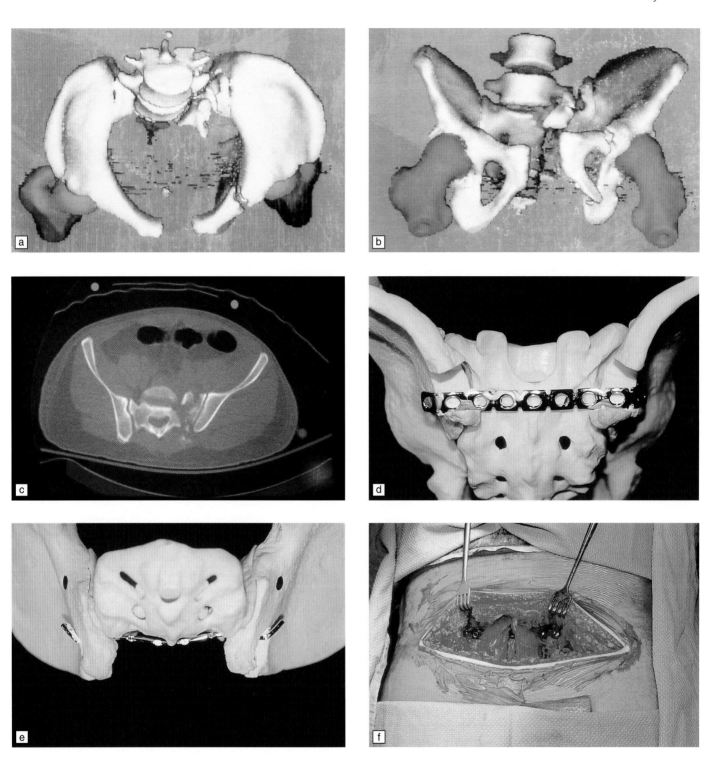

Figure 16.18 – *Transiliac plate fixation of a comminuted vertical sacral fracture and plate fixation of a symphyseal diastasis and left anterior column fracture in a 34-year-old man. (a) Preoperative inlet three-dimensional CT; (b) preoperative outlet three-dimensional CT; (c) preoperative CT scan; (d) model of intraosseous tunnel created for 4.5-mm reconstruction plate; (e) model of contoured plate resting in the intraosseous tunnel; (f) intraoperative view of plate resting beneath the paraspinous muscles; (cont'd)*

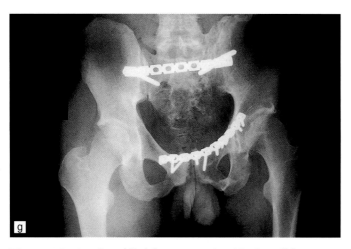

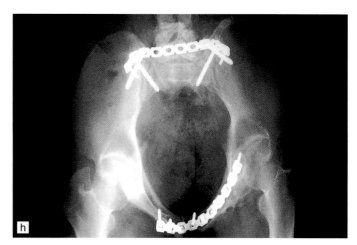

Figure 16.18 – *(cont'd) (g) postoperative AP view; (h) postoperative inlet view.*

is achieved between the inner and outer iliac tables and in the adjacent subchondral bone of the sacral ala.

An alternative method of posterior fixation is a sacral bar that is threaded into the opposing posterosuperior iliac spines [2]. This method possesses several significant shortcomings:

- It does not directly anchor the ilium to the sacrum
- In the presence of bilateral posterior injuries, it does not permit a reattachment of the axial skeleton to the residual pelvic ring
- It is unsuitable for posterior iliac fractures.

As the most common shortcoming, the method is intended for fixation in situ without direct visualization of a posterior disruption such as a sacral fracture. In such a case, a malalignment or 'malfixation' in situ is a

recurring liability. Once a direct posterior exposure is undertaken, posterior plating affords more effective fixation. Also the plate is rarely symptomatic, so that removal is not commonly needed. In contrast the bars require removal in virtually all the cases.

For the complex injury patterns, with any bilateral acetabular fractures accompanying posterior ring disruptions and anterior injuries, a bilateral ilio-inguinal approach is generally preferred [1]. Although the incision necessitates considerable prior experience, nevertheless simultaneous exposure of virtually all the injury patterns provides the highest likelihood of achieving accurate reductions. In most of these cases, the acetabular fractures are anterior column or transverse patterns (Fig. 16.19). The principal fixation is a 3.5- or 3.7-mm

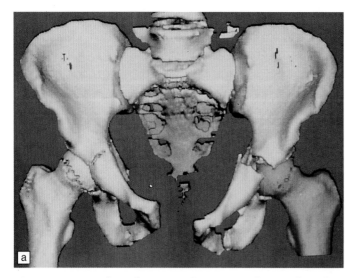

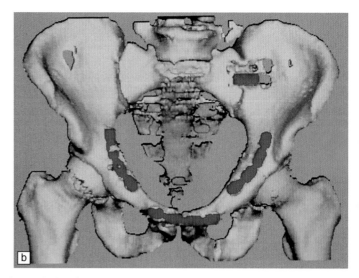

Figure 16.19 – *Three-dimensional CT views of a complex pelvic and acetabular fracture that was managed with a bilateral ilio-inguinal incision. (a) Preoperative view; (b) postoperative view.*

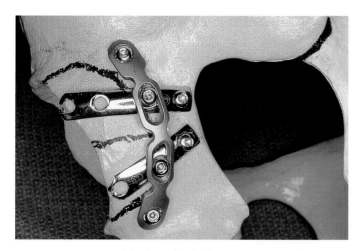

Figure 16.20 – *Model of two-hook plates with an overlying reconstruction plate for posterior wall fixation. The superior hook plate impales the hip joint to illustrate the principal potential complication of the method.*

reconstruction plate with corresponding screws [29]. Bending instrumentation is needed to facilitate three plane contours in an appropriate sequence of a lateral bend, an anteroposterior bend, and a twist. Particularly for application to the undulating pelvic brim, the plate is pre-bent so that it fits perfectly on a life-size pelvic model. Supplementary fixation devices include so-called hook or spring plates, cannulated screws, and cables or large wires. A hook plate [30] is a method to buttress thin segments of bone such as the posterior and anterior acetabular walls (Fig. 16.20). The plate is fashioned

from a 3.5-mm one-third tubular plate by the use of a plate cutter and pliers. Small hooks are fashioned at one end of the plate, which are bent so that they can be embedded into the cortical surface. A mild convexity is added to the plate, so that a screw inserted into the apex of the bend will drive the hooks into the wall fragment. The method is particularly useful for comminuted zones where it is applied in conjunction with an overlying reconstruction plate. It is also useful in proximity to the hip joint where penetration of the joint by an errant screw is a recurring concern [28,31]. Braided cables of 1.6–2.0 mm in diameter provide a method for either the reduction and provisional fixation or definitive fixation of a relatively inaccessible fracture site such as the quadrilateral surface (Fig. 16.21). A Statinski cardiothoracic or vascular clamp provides the optimal passing tool through a hazardous region, such as the greater or lesser sciatic notch or the obturator foramen.

Special problems, such as the presence of an incarcerated fragment or an impacted zone of the acetabulum, are identified. In the presence of impaction, a careful elevation of the fragments or repositioning of an embedded fragment around the reduced femoral head is anticipated. A source of autologous cancellous bone graft such as the greater trochanter is selected for harvesting. The graft is rigorously impacted into the defect before the reduction of the overlying cortical segment.

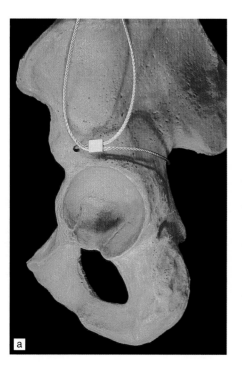
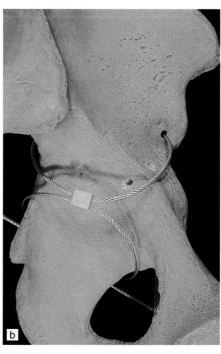

Figure 16.21 – *The use of braided cables to buttress the quadrilateral surface. (a) Direct lateral view; (b) direct medial view.*

Certain authors have recommended the use of two exposures for unusual injury patterns [2]. In the author's experience, the main application is the presence of morbid obesity whereby a very large patient weighs in excess of 135 kg (300 pounds). In this situation, for an injury pattern that presents with displacement of the posterior and anterior columns, a combination of an ilio-inguinal and a Kocher–Langenbeck approach may be preferred. Whichever approach is used, the strategy for minimization of soft tissue stripping needs to be planned so that all of the major bone fragments possess an intact soft tissue pedicle.

To achieve the reduction of an acetabular fracture, a diverse family of specialized bone-holding forceps is available (Fig. 16.22). They are essential for the complex manipulations that represent the most challenging part

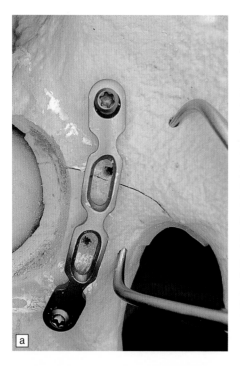

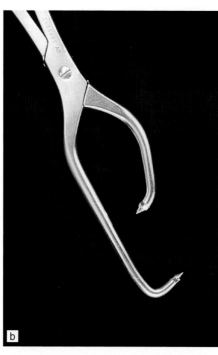

Figure 16.22 – *Tools used in fracture reduction. (a) Tenaculum forceps with jaws inserted into shallow drill holes; (b) eccentric or 'prince-tong' forceps for the quadrilateral surface; (c) screws inserted for use with Lambotte-Farboeuf forceps; (d) reduction with Lambotte-Farboeuf forceps.*

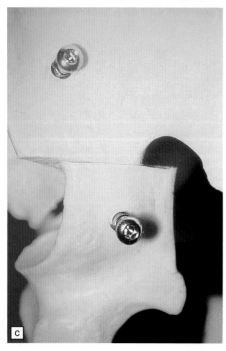

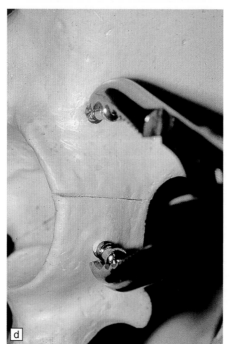

of an acetabular repair. The most valuable collection possesses pointed tips with straight or angled jaws of a highly variable size. Perhaps the most valuable is a large eccentric clamp, the 'prince tong'. Another lion-jawed forceps, the Lambotte-Farboeuf design, can be used to gain rigorous purchase to the iliac crest or another prominent site. Alternatively, a recent design feature is where either jaw of a forceps anchors around a screw head. Opposing screws are inserted into either principal fracture fragment. Once the forceps is applied across the screw heads, it can be used to achieve a reduction.

Still another reduction strategy is to anchor a reconstruction plate to a more remotely situated fracture fragment. A pointed tip or tenaculum-type reduction forceps is applied from the opposing end of the plate around a bony prominence of the other bone fragment. As the jaws are manipulated, a reduction is achieved. Derotation of a fracture fragment such as the posterior column is a recurring technical challenge. Some type of stout pin, such as a Schanz screw or an external fixation pin, can be inserted into the ischial tuberosity. The exposed portion of the pin is manually manipulated, possibly by the addition of a T handle.

Typical patterns of acetabular fixation rely on the unique mechanical environment of the pelvis, with its broad surfaces of cancellous bone and its ring-like structure [1,2, 30,31]. The frictional properties of a reduced fracture afford very considerable intrinsic stability. Bending moments are minimized with the ring-like configuration of the pelvis. Generally, the fracture is significantly united within about 6 weeks, so that the fixation is only needed for a brief period. For the fixation, highly flexible plates made of stainless steel or titanium alloy are preferred. They are readily contoured to the shape of the bone. If the contour is imperfect, the plate may draw down to the bone during tightening of a screw without provoking a secondary deformity of the reduced fracture. When a stiffer plate is used, any imperfection in the contour will translate into a displacement of an anatomically reduced fracture when the corresponding screws are tightened.

Definitive treatment of acetabular fractures

In practice most displaced acetabular fractures merit

consideration for an open reduction and internal fixation. Admittedly, certain elderly and ill patients represent a contraindication. Most contraindications are transient in nature, such as haemodynamic instability or an acute medical problem that merits a deferral for a few days. Once the injury has been rigorously characterized a definitive plan is created. The fracture is drawn on a model plastic pelvis so that its specific site and extent can be appreciated. Two general strategies for acetabular reconstruction have evolved. The author's preference is the use of a radiolucent graphite composite table which facilitates intraoperative image intensification. To achieve a reduction of the fracture, the patient is positioned so that gravity minimizes the displacement that is provoked by the relevant anatomical structures such as the femoral head and upper thigh. For example, for a posterior fracture dislocation, the patient is positioned in an almost prone fashion so that the femoral head rests on the uninvolved anterior acetabulum. In this scenario, the reduction tools are absolutely essential for the correction of deformity by a manipulation of the displaced fragments of bone.

An alternative strategy devised by Judet and LeTournel [6] is the use of a highly specialized fracture table that permits the application of lateral and/or longitudinal traction. Particularly in the presence of central protrusion of the femoral head through an acetabular fracture, the proximal femur can be anatomically reduced. If the capsular attachments across the hip joint are maintained, a corresponding reduction of the acetabulum is achieved. This method minimizes the need for a secondary reduction by resort to bone-holding forceps, although it does not entirely eliminate it. Nevertheless, the instrumentation for traction may hamper a ready manipulation of the lower extremity and the trunk. Also it is vulnerable to excessive secondary forces imposed on the skin with the potential for corresponding cutaneous or neurovascular injury. This problem is particularly notable in the presence of a large patient.

Whichever strategy is used, intraoperative image intensification with a modern high-resolution image intensifier of large field size is essential. The imaging permits an evaluation of the accuracy of the reduction, and the presence of an incarcerated fragment or hardware that violates the hip joint. An iatrogenic injury to the sciatic nerve is a recurring hazard, particularly for the posterior injury patterns. Intraoperative neurological monitoring with somatosensory evoked potentials and continuous electromyographic (EMG) studies is a valuable technique. In many or most of these cases, the sciatic nerve is injured at the time of the accident possibly in an occult manner. In such a case the nerve is unusually susceptible to a second injury with minimal provocation. Neurological monitoring [32–34], particularly with the rapid response of the continuous EMGs, aids the surgeon to identify rapidly the problem and undertake the corrective action. The usual causes of the problem are excessive retraction with a retractor, malpositioning of the extremity with excessive stretching of the sciatic nerve, or occasionally impalement with one of the various sharp tools on the field.

For the acetabular approach specialized surgical exposures are available [1,2]. For the family of posterior injuries a Kocher-Langenbeck approach is preferred. Diverse anterior injury patterns including most both-column fractures are optimally exposed with an ilio-inguinal approach. For displaced transverse and T-type fractures a tri-radiate or extended iliofemoral type of extensile exposure is preferred. The last category affords the optimal exposure to the external and internal surfaces of the hemipelvis. Nevertheless, they provide the greatest risk for devascularization with allied complications of serious postoperative wound infection, avascular necrosis of the acetabulum, heterotopic bone formation, and the provocation of dense scar tissue. Elderly or immunocompromised patients are particularly vulnerable to experience one or both of the first two complications. A markedly obese young adult man who also sustained a closed head injury is particularly vulnerable to experience the last two problems. Recently, both the extended iliofemoral and tri-radiate approaches have been modified in ways that minimize these hazards [35,36]. With both modified formats, the conventional incisions are made. Also, in both modified variants, the gluteal insertions on the greater trochanter and the trochanter itself are preserved. The indication for multiple incisions performed sequentially as a single procedure or as two separate ones is limited. Nevertheless, especially for a morbidly obese individual in whom the fracture involves both columns, such as a T-type or complete both-column variant, this method merits consideration [37,38].

Postoperative care

On the day after surgery, the patient is transferred from a bed to a chair and physiotherapy is initiated. For unilateral injury patterns, a late partial weight-bearing gait is encouraged. Active motion exercises of the hips and the residual joints and lower extremities are undertaken, along with progressive resistance exercises for the hip musculature. Supplementary goals of occupational therapy include assessment for activities of daily living and realization of independent transfers.

In the presence of certain bilateral injury patterns that involve the pelvis and/or residual portions of the lower extremities, an initial 6-week period of bed-to-chair transfers may be indicated. Even in this situation, however, after the 6-week period, weight-bearing to tolerance is usually feasible. Also, at that time, a vigorous programme of progressive resistance exercises with machines is encouraged, which continues for 1 year. Other aerobic exercises, including swimming, the use of a stationary bicycle, and a cross-country skiing machine, are recommended from that time. Radiographs of the pelvis and/or acetabulum are taken at 6- and 12-week intervals, which should document partial and complete healing of the fracture, respectively.

Postoperative anticoagulation is routinely undertaken with low-molecular-weight heparin or warfarin (Coumadin) [39–42]. In the presence of an isolated pelvic fracture with rapid mobilization, anticoagulation is undertaken for 3 weeks. With the greater compromise to activity and in the presence of specific risk factors such as a prior thromboembolic event and morbid obesity, anticoagulation is continued for a correspondingly longer period.

Certain pelvic and acetabular fractures provide a notable risk for postoperative heterotopic bone formation. The specific risk factors include the concomitant presentation of a closed head injury, a young obese man, and prior heterotopic bone formation. The extended lateral acetabular approaches are the primary culprits where the risk for serious heterotopic bone formation is at least 7% [1]. The modified versions of these approaches appear to have substantially decreased this risk. Nevertheless for a high-risk patient, especially a large obese man who has sustained an accompanying closed head injury, an extended lateral surgical approach to the acetabulum is discouraged. From the time of surgery, indomethacin can be given as a prophylactic agent. Alternatively, postoperative irradiation therapy of 700–1000 cGy can be given as a single pulse or in subdivided doses [43,44].

Postoperative drainage from a wound is closely followed. If a wound displays features of a tense haematoma formation with persistent drainage or if early alteration in the appearance of the wound is suggestive of an impending wound infection, the patient is returned to the operating room for an open evacuation of the haematoma, antibiotic irrigation, and débridement as necessary.

Complications of internal fixation of the pelvis and acetabulum

About 70–80% of the surgical reconstructions that are undertaken to manage an acute isolated fracture of the pelvic ring or acetabulum achieve a highly satisfactory functional return with minimal or minor residual pain and resumption of most activities, including a return to gainful employment [6,23,45–50]. Certain cases following multiple trauma are moderately or markedly impaired by residual complications of other injuries, such as trauma to the lower leg or spine, although the pelvic injury realizes an excellent result. Other patients are functionally impaired as a result of a complication of the pelvic trauma or of the ensuing therapeutic regimen. The following subsection addresses this crucial consideration, particularly with respect to iatrogenic complications.

A principal source of complications of internal pelvic fixation is related to the particular surgical exposure. The juxtaposition of major neurovascular structures, as well as the intra-abdominal viscera, combined with the limited familiarity of most orthopaedic surgeons with the pelvic region, provides a special likelihood for allied complications. This problem is aggravated further if the surgery is undertaken after a delayed presentation. The presence of scarified boundaries, heterotopic bone, and abnormalities such as a traumatically induced urinary diverticulum create particularly hazardous conditions. A second family of complications is related to the surgical reduction. A traction injury to the sciatic nerve is particularly likely to follow a posterior fracture dislocation of the hip. Where the sciatic nerve is contused at the time of the traumatic injury, subtle features of nerve deficit, including mild hypaesthesiae of the second and third toes or corresponding mild weakness of the extensor digitorum longus, may hint at the susceptibility of the nerve. With even a limited surgical manipulation or retraction, such a nerve is vulnerable to frank deterioration in its function, to culminate as a complete foot drop with hypaesthesia of the foot and a potential for late dysaesthetic pain in the lower leg and foot. Intraoperative and neurological monitoring may permit an early recognition of such a susceptible nerve and the prompt initiation of a corrective manoeuvre.

A third family of complications is related to the application of the fixation devices. The guidewires or drill bits that are used in conjunction with conventional or cannulated screws are particularly hazardous, especially if the far cortex of the bone is breached. Many columns of pelvic bone, such as the superior pubic ramus, are relatively small so that the target area is limited. Alternatively, in the sacrum the presence of nerve roots and the foramina provides a source of neurological hazard that is in close proximity to the limited available bone stock.

A fourth category of problem pertains to the postsurgical period with problematic wound healing, heterotopic bone around the acetabulum, late post-traumatic arthritis or avascular necrosis of the femoral head or acetabulum, and a late non-union or malunion [2]. Many of these problems represent complications that follow excessive stripping of soft tissue and devascularization of the bone fragments. All of these risks are lessened by the use of either a Kocher-Langenbeck posterior or ilio-inguinal anterior approach for the vast majority of posterior and anterior injury patterns, respectively. With the implementation of modern bone-holding forceps and intraoperative image intensification, usually even the most extensive acute fracture patterns managed by experienced surgeons are amenable to one of these approaches.

Deep venous thrombosis (DVT) is recognized as a common sequel of pelvic and lower extremity trauma. After a pelvic fracture for a patient who does not receive any prophylactic measure, the incidence of DVT proximal to the popliteal trifurcation appears to be about 40–60% [51]. The further complication of a pulmonary embolus (PE) has a reported incidence of 4–22% with a consequential mortality rate of 2–3%. The natural history of DVT is multifactorial and highly variable. The long-term sequelae include postphlebitic syndrome of a variable severity, ranging from a non-specific complaint of heaviness or pain in the leg to objective findings such as oedema, atrophic changes, or ulceration. Once thrombosis is recognized, therapeutic anticoagulation is indicated, typically with initial intravenous heparin followed by a conversion to oral warfarin (Coumadin) and continuing for about 3 months.

A significant number of pelvic fracture victims are not candidates for anticoagulation. Examples include those with ongoing haemorrhage or impending surgery and those with acute or chronic bleeding diathesis. In these situations, the application of vena caval interruption merits careful review. Currently, percutaneous intraluminal methods of caval interruption appear to be highly effective with a very low incidence of confirmed complications [52,53]. A special role for an inferior vena caval (IVC) filter is where surgery is delayed and frequently the patient is transferred to a secondary hospital. Late transport and associated transfers of the patient represent a considerable risk for dislodgement of a deep venous embolus and provocation of a life-threatening pulmonary embolism. If duplex ultrasonography or phlebography confirms the presence of a DVT proximal to the popliteal trifurcation, insertion of an IVC filter is strongly recommended before the transfer.

Conclusions

Detailed therapeutic algorithms are available to guide the acute resuscitation, characterization, and definitive management of pelvic and acetabular fractures. With the time-dependent nature of these problems, the algorithms need to be prepared before the presentation of a patient. Classification schemes permit the recognition of injury patterns that are appropriate for conservative management for those in whom surgical stabilization is indicated. With the broad spectrum of operative approaches, reduction strategies and fixation techniques, most injury patterns, particularly with respect to the pelvic ring, can be effectively managed. Nevertheless, the surgical team requires special training in these complex methods. Certain problems remain at least partly unsolved. For the ever-increasing spectrum of geriatric fractures, the presence of osteopenic bone and comminution hampers an attempt to achieve a structurally sound repair. This problem is amplified by corresponding acetabular fractures where an open reduction and internal fixation may not be practical. For this limited spectrum of cases, an acute total hip arthroplasty with limited internal fixation of the acetabulum may be preferred.

References

1. Mears DC, Rubash HE. *Pelvic and Acetabular Fractures.* Thorofare, NJ: Slack Inc., 1986; 95–161.

2. Tile M. *Fractures of the Pelvis and Acetabulum*, 2nd edn. Baltimore: Williams and Wilkins, 1995; 41–52.

3. Kellam JF, McMurtry RY, Paley D, Tile M. The unstable pelvic fracture: operative treatment. *Orthop Clin N Am* 1987; 18: 25–39.

4. Burgess AR, Eastridge BJ, Young JW *et al.* Pelvic ring disruptions: effective classification and treatment protocols. *J Trauma* 1990; 30: 848–56.

5. Dalal SA, Burgess AR, Siegel JH, Young JW. Pelvic fractures in multiple trauma: classification by mechanism is key to pattern of organ injury, resuscitative requirements and outcome. *J Trauma* 1989; 29: 981–96.

6. LeTournel E, Judet R. *Fractures of the Acetabulum.* New York: Springer, 1993; 25–37.

7. Liu S, Siegel PZ, Brewer RD *et al.* Prevalence of alcohol impaired driving. *JAMA* 1997; 288: 122–5.

8. Reduction in alcohol-related traffic fatalities: United States 1990–1992. *MMWR Morb Mortal Wkly Rep* 1993; 42: 905–909.

9. Lowner JH, Koval KJ. Polytrauma in the elderly. *Clin Orthop Rel Res* 1995; 318: 136–43.

10. Melton LJ, Sampson JM, Morrey BF, Ilstrup DM. Epidemiologic features of pelvic fractures. *Clin Orthop Rel Res* 1981; 155: 43–7.

11. Ragnarrson B, Jacobsson B. Epidemiology of pelvic fractures in a Swedish county. *Acta Orthop Scand* 1992; 63: 277–82.

12. Gotis-Graham I, McGuigan L, Diamond T *et al.* Sacral insufficiency fractures in the elderly. *J Bone Joint Surg* 1994; 76B: 882–7.

13. Bosch U, Pohlemann T, Hoas N, Tscherne H. Klassifikatian und Management des Komplex en Beck en Traumos. *Unfall Chirurg* 1992; 4: 189–94.

14. Hanson PB, Milne JC, Chapman MW. Open fractures of the pelvis. *J Bone Joint Surg* 1991; 73B: 325–34.

15. Champion HR, Sacco WJ, Copes WS *et al.* A revision of the Trauma Score (TS). *J Trauma* 1989; 29: 623–9.

16. Baker SP, O'Neill B, Hadden WJr *et al.* The Injury Severity Score: A method for describing patients with multiple injuries and evaluating emergency care. *J Trauma* 1974; 14: 187–96.

17. Mears DC. Modern concepts of external skeletal fixation of the pelvis. *Clin Orthop Rel Res* 1980; 151: 65–72.

18. Grimm MR, Vrahas MS, Thomas KA. Pressure-volume characteristics of the intact and disrupted pelvic retroperitoneum. *J. Trauma* 1998; 44: 454–59.

19. Moss MC, Bircher MD. Volume changes within the true pelvis, during disruption of the pelvic ring – where does the haemorrhage go? *Injury* 1996; 27 Suppl 1: S-A21-3.

20. Panetta T, Sclafani SJA, Goldstein AS. Percutaneous transcatheter embolization for massive bleeding from pelvic fractures. *J Trauma* 1985; 25: 1021–6.

21. Davidson BS, Simmons GT, Williamson PR, Buerk CA. Pelvic fractures associated with open perineal wounds: a survivable injury. *J Trauma* 1993; 35: 36–9.

22. Mears DC, Ward AJ, Wright MS. The radiological assessment of pelvic and acetabular fractures using three-dimensional computed tomography. *Int J Orthop Trauma* 1992; 2: 196–207.

23. Tile M. Pelvic ring fractures: should they be fixed? *J Bone Joint Surg* 1988; 70B: 1–12.

24. Pennal GF, Tile M, Waddell JP, Garside H. Pelvic disruption: assessment and classification. *Clin Orthop Rel Res* 1980; 151: 12–21.

25. Tile M, Helfet DL, Kellam JF *et al. Comprehensive Classification of Fractures in the Pelvis and Acetabulum.* Berne, Switzerland: Maurice E. Muller Foundation, 1995.

26. Olson SA, Matta JM. The computerized tomography subchondral arc: a new method of assessing acetabular articular continuity after fracture. *J Orthop Trauma* 1993; 7: 402–13.

27. Routt MLC Jr, Kregor PJ, Simonian PT, Mayo KA. Early results of percutaneous iliosacral screws placed with the patient in a supine position. *J Orthop Trauma* 1995; 9: 207–14.

28. Mears DC. The use of cannulated screws for the fixation of pelvic and acetabular fractures. In: Asnis S, Kyle R, eds. *Cannulated Screw Fixation: Mechanics, Operative Techniques, Clinical Implications.* New York: Springer, 1996; 97–145.

29. Matta JM, Saucedo T. Internal fixation of pelvic ring fractures. *Clin Orthop Rel Res* 1989; 242: 83–91.

30. Goulet JA, Mason DL, Roubeau JP, Goldstein SA. Comminuted posterior wall acetabular fractures. A bio-mechanical evaluation of fixation methods *J Bone Joint Surg* 1994; 76A:1457–63.

31. Simonean PT, Roult ML JR, Harrington RM, Tencer AF. Internal fixation of the unstable anterior pelvic ring: a biomechanical comparison of standard plating techniques and retrograde medullary superior pubic ramus screw. *J Orthop Trauma* 1994; 8: 476–82.

32. Vrahas M, Gordon RG, Mears DC *et al.* Intraoperative somatosensory evoked potential monitoring of pelvic and acetabular fractures. *J Orthop Trauma* 1992; 6: 50–8.

33. Helfet DL, Kovalck J, Hosa D *et al.* Intra-operative somatosensory potential monitoring during acute pelvic fractures. *J Orthop Trauma* 1995; 9: 28–34.

34. Helfet DL, Amand N, Malkani ALL, Heige C. Intra-operative monitoring of motor pathway during operative fixation of acute acetabular fractures. *J Orthop Trauma* 1997; 11: 2–6.

35. Mears DC. Acetabular fractures: surgical management. *Curr Orthop* 1996; 10: 81–95.

36. Mears DC, Macleod MD. Fractures – surgical approaches: triradiate and modified triradiate. In: Wiss D, ed. *Masters Techniques in Orthopaedic Surgery.* Philadelphia: Lippincott-Raven, 1998; 697–724.

37. Moroni A, Caja VL, Sabato C, Zinghi G. Surgical treatment of both-column fractures by staged combined ilioinguinal and Kocher-Langenbeck approaches. *Injury* 1995; 26: 219–24.

38. Routt ML, Sivionkowski MF. Operative treatment of complex acetabular fractures: combined anterior and posterior exposures during the same procedure. *J Bone Joint Surg* 1990; 72A: 897–904.

39. Knudson MM, Lewis FR, Clinton A *et al.* Prevention of venous thromboembolism in trauma patients. *J Trauma* 1994; 37: 480–7.

40. Kock HJ, Schmit-Neuerburg KP, Manke J *et al.* Thromboprophylaxis with low-molecular weight heparin in out-patients with plaster-cast immobilization of the leg. *Lancet* 1995; 346: 459–61.

41. Montgomery KD, Potter HG, Helfet DL. The detection and management of proximal deep venous thrombosis in patients with acute acetabular fractures. *J Orthop Trauma* 1997; 11: 330–6.

42. Fishmann AJ, Greeno RA, Brooks LR, Matta JM. Prevention of deep venous thrombosis and pulmonary embolism in acetabular and pelvic fracture surgery. *Clin Orthop Rel Res* 1994; 305: 133–7.

43. Moed BR, Maxey JW. The effect of indomethacin on heterotopic ossification following acetabular fracture surgery. *J Orthop Trauma* 1993; 7: 33–8.

44. Johnson EE, Kay RM, Dorey FJ. Heterotopic ossification prophylaxis following operative treatment of acetabular fractures. *Clin Orthop Rel Res* 1994; 305: 88–95.

45. Henderson RC. The long–term results of non-operatively treated major pelvic disruptions. *J Orthop Trauma* 1989; 3: 41–7.

46. Miranda MA, Riemer BL, Butterfield SL, Burke CL. Pelvic ring injuries: a long term functional outcome study. *Clin Orthop Rel Res* 1996; 329: 152–8.

47. Matta JM. Operative treatment of acetabular fractures through the ilioinguinal approach. *Clin Orthop Rel Res* 1994; 305: 10–19.

48. Matta JM. Fractures of the acetabulum: accuracy of reduction and clinical results in patients managed operatively within three weeks after the injury. *J Bone Joint Surg* 1996; 78A: 1632–45.

49. Mayo KA. Open reduction and internal fixation of the acetabulum: results in 163 fractures. *Clin Orthop Rel Res* 1994; 305: 31–7.

50. Helfet DL, Borrelli J, DiPasquale T, Sanders R. Stabilization of acetabular fractures in elderly patients. *J Bone Joint Surg* 1992; 74A: 753–65.

51. White RH, Goulet JA, Bray TJ *et al.* Deep-vein thrombosis after fracture of the pelvis: assessment with serial duplex-ultrasound screening. *J Bone Joint Surg* 1990; 72A: 495–500.

52. Rosenthal D, McKinsey JF, Levy AM *et al.* Use of the Greenfield filter in patients with major trauma. *Cardiovasc Surg* 1994; 2: 52–5.

53. Webb LX, Rush PT, Fuller SB, Meredith JW. Greenfield filter prophylaxis of pulmonary embolism in patients undergoing surgery for acetabular fracture. *J Orthop Trauma* 1992; 6:139–45.

Index